Language Disorders From a Developmental Perspective

Essays in Honor of Robin S. Chapman

New Directions in Communication Disorders Research: Integrative Approaches
Rhea Paul, Series Editor

Rhea Paul (Ed.) • Language Disorders From a Developmental Perspective: Essays in Honor of Robin S. Chapman

---

For a complete list of titles in LEA's Communication Series, please contact Lawrence Erlbaum Associates, Publishers at www.erlbaum.com

Language Disorders From a Developmental Perspective

Essays in Honor of Robin S. Chapman

Edited by

Rhea Paul

Southern Connecticut University
Yale Child Study Center

LEA
LAWRENCE ERLBAUM ASSOCIATES, PUBLISHERS
2007 Mahwah, New Jersey London

Lawrence Erlbaum Associates, Inc., Publishers
10 Industrial Avenue
Mahwah, New Jersey 07430
www.erlbaum.com

Cover design by Kathryn Houghtaling

Library of Congress Cataloging-in-Publication Data

Language disorders from a developmental perspective : essays in honor of Robin S. Chapman / edited by Rhea Paul.

p. cm. (New directions in communication disorders research)

Includes bibliographical references and index.

ISBN 0-8058-5037-6 (cloth : alk. paper)
1. Language disorders in children. 2. Language acquisition. [DNLM: 1. Chapman, Robin S. 2. Language Development Disorders—Festschrift. 3. Child. WL 340.2 L2856 2006] I. Paul, Rhea. II. Chapman, Robin S. III. Series.

RJ496.L35L344 2006
618.92'855—dc22 2006001841
CIP

Books published by Lawrence Erlbaum Associates are printed on acid-free paper, and their bindings are chosen for strength and durability.

Printed in the United States of America
10 9 8 7 6 5 4 3 2 1

Contents

Preface

With this volume, we are pleased to inaugurate Erlbaum's latest series, New Directions in Communication Disorders Research: Integrative Approaches. In this series, we will attempt to bring a range of perspectives to bear on the issues that confront clinicians and researchers who deal with children's language and its disorders. Our hope is to stretch the boundaries of the field, to include the points of view—not only of those who identify themselves with this endeavor, but also of those whose research can inform the discussion of how and why some children struggle with this most fundamental of human capacities. By creating a *big tent* under which data from a myriad of resources can be considered, we hope to make some small contribution to the ability to support children for whom basic communication does not come naturally.

It is a special pleasure to begin our new series with a book of essays in honor of Robin Chapman. This volume is a testament to the effect that Robin has had on the lives of its contributors, and on the careers of the many other clinicians and researchers whom she has touched over the years. Robin came into the field of communication disorders from a background in developmental psychology. In many ways, this background was more an advantage than a handicap, in that she, more than most in our field, tended to encourage her students to see the child's language development in the broader context. When she came to communication disorders, psycholinguistics tended to view the development of communication in light of the *black box* language acquisition device, or in view of cognitive prerequisite theories that saw the development of language as just an instance of the more general problem of the acquisition of concepts. Robin, though, was insistent in reminding us that children learn language in a world with other people in it who bring things to their attention, give names for their actions and perceptions, insist on politeness, and provide other minds for the child to explore. Many of us came away from the experience of working with Robin with our minds expanded, the envelopes of our narrow notions pushed. For this we were all grateful.

This book reflects Robin's wide-ranging curiosity. Her ability to weave new developments from a variety of fields into cohesive stories, as she called them, has supplied us with continual examples of the ways in which cross-fertilization and collaboration advance knowledge. She encouraged all of us to ask new questions, find new approaches, challenge existing notions. There was never a topic she failed to find interesting, nor was there ever a student she was unable to find some way to appreciate and praise. When discussing potential topics for research or dissertation projects, Robin's most fundamental question was "Yes, but which one seems like more fun?" For many of us, it was her nurturing presence that made graduate school bearable.

Robin's influence on the field of communication disorders cannot be underestimated. She trained or collaborated with a great many of the current faculty of core programs around the country and the world; she continues to collaborate with a wide range of individuals around a broad spectrum of topics. Among those who know her, Robin has a reputation as the possessor of something beyond mere knowledge. I recall at a conference some years ago one of her colleagues opened his remarks by explaining that when he had difficulty figuring out how best the frame the complex set of ideas he wanted to present, he went to Robin because he considered her "wise in many things." This view pervades the perception of all who have worked closely with Robin and had the privilege of experiencing her unique ways of thinking and asking questions.

More than that, though, Robin also served as a model to us of the potential shape of the life of the intellect. Robin enjoys life fully. She never made us feel that to be a successful scientist you had to spend 18 hours a day in the lab or the library, and the other six sleeping. She square danced; she wrote poetry; she delighted in her two sons. She used every minute to the fullest; jogging during her lunch hour to the day care center at the far end of campus to spend some time with her boys when they were little, then jogging back in time for class. For many of us who were part of the first generation of women entering the academic work force in significant numbers, few models of what this life could be like were available to tell us. The obvious relish with which Robin plunged into each new activity inspired us to seek ways of balancing all the things we loved in our own lives, finding pleasure and passion in our work, without sacrificing all other aspects of our existence to it. And Robin made these contributions to our development not only by example. She actively mentored and nurtured students, inviting them into her home, serving as a sounding board as they proceeded through complicated phases of their lives and careers. She was never too busy, though she was sometimes quite bemused, to listen.

Robin has recently begun to cut back on her time as an active researcher, and increase her commitment to poetry, painting, and kayaking. But she continues to serve us and our profession as a presence, a benchmark, and a listening post. Though one of the tiniest people any of us ever met, Robin has had a disproportionate influence on our profession and our lives. Her bird-like figure and voice loom large in our imagination. It is with the greatest pleasure and gratitude that we dedicate the work of this volume to her, and we all hope to have the benefit of her wisdom for many years to come.

—*Rhea Paul*

ACKNOWLEDGMENTS

I would like to extend my thanks to the authors of these chapters for their efforts in creating a volume to honor our teacher and friend, Robin Chapman. Thanks also go to Carolyn Gosse, Patricia McMahon, and Susan DeWitt who assisted with the preparation of the manuscript. Cathleen Petree at Lawrence Erlbaum Associates has been of invaluable assistance in the realization of this project, and has provided support and friendship to me throughout its long gestation.

1

Children's Language Learning: An Interactionist Perspective[1]

Robin S. Chapman
Waisman Center, University of Wisconsin–Madison

The study of child language development is at an exciting moment, one in which new advances in research methods and multiple theoretical perspectives-psychological, linguistic, social, cognitive, anthropological, neurobiological-are converging on a new understanding of how children learn to talk. The older debates of the importance of nature vs. nurture in explanations of language acquisition are giving way to interactionist perspectives (Budwig, 1995; Elman et al., 1996; HirshPasek & Golinkoff, 1996; MacWhinney, 1999; Nelson, 1996; Slobin, Gerhardt, Kyratzis, & Guo, 1996). In a field that has been highly productive in identifying developmental patterns and individual differences but slow to develop explanations that are more than a relabeling of the patterns observed, new work suggests explanations that cross disciplinary boundaries (e.g. M. H.

---

[1]This paper is reprinted with permission from the 2000 *Journal of Child Psychology and Psychiatry and Allied Disciplines, 41,* pp. 33–55. It is included to give a flavor of the depth and scope of thought brought to bear upon the study of child language development and its disorders by Robin Chapman.

Johnson, 1997; Locke, 1993, 1996; Muller, 1996; Pulvermuller, 1999; Seidenberg, 1997; Slobin, 1997a).

This selective discussion of research will consider (a) the historical accounts of language development and variability, (b) the recent advances in methodology that have provided new evidence on children's language development, (c) the recent substantive research on genetic and environmental input to language development that has contributed to the interactionist perspective, and (d) the generalizations to be drawn from that work that support interactionist, emergent, functional approaches to language development.

HISTORICAL ACCOUNTS OF DEVELOPMENT AND VARIABILITY

Child language research has long been noted for its intensive, longitudinal study of free speech samples from individual children, a method particularly suited to revealing developmental trajectories and individual differences (Bloom, 1970, 1993; Brown, 1973). That work, mainly in English, has yielded the outlines of developmental sequence in children's language production in pragmatics (Appendix, Table A); semantics (Appendix, Table B); syntax and morphosyntax (Appendix, Table C); identified dimensions of individual variability and their potential sources (Appendix, Table D); and identified characteristics associated with specific language impairment (Appendix, Table E). These findings are reviewed in many texts (e.g. Barrett, 1999; Berko-Gleason, 1993; Bloom, 1998; Chapman, 1988; Hoff-Ginsberg, 1993; Owens, 1996; Paul, 1995; and, in particular detail for acquisition sequences, Ingram, 1989; for individual differences, Bates, Dale, & Thal, 1995).

The weight of the last 25 years of work has provided evidence for at least two important generalizations about the nature of children's language learning. First, language acquisition follows a course in which *new meanings and communicative functions are first expressed by old means, or forms, of behavior*—whether gesture, vocalization, word, or sentence structure. Second, *new forms of communicative behavior typically emerge to express meanings and communicative intents already in the child's repertoire.* These two generalizations support the strong advice, to parents, that they respond to children's communicative attempts; appropriate form will follow. They also imply an interactionist view: that new motor, cognitive, and social learning serve as precursors to the emergence of particular linguistic forms; that acquisition of linguistic form, in turn, can lead to subsequent development in other spheres (Hirsh-Pasek & Golinkoff, 1996; Jusczyk,1997; Kent, 1992; Slobin et al.,1996); and that a large range of individual differences will result (Bates et al., 1995).

This fundamental understanding-that the new emerges out of old patterns-has informed much of our understanding of change in cognitive development generally, both in older Piagetian (Piaget, 1954) theory of accommodation and assimilation in schema development and contemporary counterparts such as Karmiloff-Smith's (1996) account of developmental redescription or Nelson's (1986) account of generalized event knowledge. Roger Brown (1973) framed it as an issue of cumulative complexity; that which required both X and Y would be learned later than either X or Y, developmentally. The recognition that new learning builds on old has given rise in more recent theory-making to proposals that children "bootstrap" their way into language learning by using existing learning to make an approximate, if not completely correct, initial mapping of one domain onto another (Morgan & Demuth, 1996). Proposals have included (a) *prosodic bootstrapping,* in which prosodic contours (e.g. the mother's typical intonation patterns) or metrical expectations (e.g. of the strong-weak syllable stress pattern typical of English) drive the form of early communicative vocalization (e.g. Kemler-Nelson, HirshPasek, Jusczyk, & Cassidy, 1989) ; (b) *phonological bootstrapping* (called *phonological selectivity* in the literature), in which produced syllable forms and sounds in the child's repertoire drive the early vocabulary acquired (e.g. J. S. Johnson, Lewis, & Hogan, 1997; Schwartz & Leonard, 1982; Schwartz, Leonard, Loeb, & Swanson, 1987); (c) *pragmatic bootstrapping,* in which communicative intent drives differentiation of vocalizations in communicative contexts, and their shift to more conventional form (Greenfield & Smith, 1976; Messer, 1994); (d) *cognitive bootstrapping,* in which conceptual content of early object categories (e.g. round, graspable things) drive the referential boundaries of words, and prototypic event schemas (e.g. peekaboo; greetings; stacking and knocking down) drive the early content of utterances (Slobin, 1981; Thiabaut, Rondal, & Kaens, 1995); (e) *semantic bootstrapping,* in which meaning (e.g. person acting on object to change its location) drives the initial analysis of grammatical form (Pinker, 1987); (f) *lexical bootstrapping,* in which early word combinations are specific to lexical items (e.g. no+Noun) (e.g. Braine, 1976; Lieven, Pine, & Baldwin, 1997; Tomasello, 1992); and (g) *syntactic bootstrapping, in* which co-occurring function words (e.g. articles *the, a)* and bound morphemes (e.g. past tense inflection, plural -s) provide information about form class (e.g. noun or verb) of a novel word (e.g. Behrend, Harris, & Cartwright, 1995; Mandel, Kemler-Nelson, & Jusczyk, 1996; Naigles & Hoff-Ginsberg, 1995). Factors affecting speed of acquisition of any of these subsystems, then, would slow the acquisition of others systems building on them. These proposals are not mutually exclusive but complementary, naming the ways in which old learning can serve, at a later stage, to assist acquisition of the new. The bootstrapping proposals name facets of an ongoing cycle in which communicative means and goals drive the ability to put intended content into form (production), and the ongoing cycle in which world knowledge, word knowledge, and social knowledge drive the ability to make sense of utterance form (Chapman, 1992). Or rather, that is my interpretation of their relationship.

Classical accounts of children's language learning viewed the child as learning rules of language structure, where the elements combined were syntactic in nature, associating phonological form on the one hand with understood meaning on the other (see Chapman et al., 1992, for discussion). The rules of sentence formation accounted for the generativity, or creativity, of children's language, by being applicable to new vocabulary and by being recursive in form, permitting indefinitely long utterances and novel forms. The process of acquisition was viewed as one of generating and applying hypotheses about rules to the construction of sentences. Because conversational partners seldom explicitly marked children's utterances as ill-formed (the problem of *no negative feedback),* it was argued that these hypotheses must be innately constrained by linguistic universals embodied, in recent accounts, by parameters that could be set by brief samples of local language. Exceptions to rules were treated as acquired through a second, "dual-route" association system; this argument continues today, predicated on the assumption that the main route to acquisition is hypothesis-governed, or based on recognizing paradigmatic patterns.

Associated with this view of children's acquisition of language has been the claim, originating with Chomsky (1965, 1980) and maintained by many researchers working from a linguistic perspective (e.g. Meisel, 1995; Pinker, 1994), that language acquisition occurs too rapidly, universally, and uniquely in the human species, in the face of often ill-formed and degenerate input, to be other than innate in origin. The view that language-and syntax in particular-constitutes a unique, universal, abstract, generative competence whose acquisition requires unique genetic contributions to a "language acquisition device" to explain it has persisted despite the empirical demonstrations that language structure is acquired piecemeal, cumulating over vocabulary instances (Braine, 1994), across a protracted time span of many years (for example, grammatical verb inflections appears to be initially acquired one verb at a time). It has persisted in the face of evidence that there are wide variations in how quickly children acquire language and in the face of the variety of ways (autism, mental retardation, specific language impairment) in which particular aspects of acquisition can be impaired in computational, meaning, or pragmatic aspects (Tager-Flusberg, 1994). It has persisted despite studies showing that language input to young children is well-formed, responsive to the child's communicative attempts, well-adapted to the child's current focus of attention and understanding, and rich in contingent reformulations that model corrections to the child's syntactic errors or omissions (Bohannon,

MacWhinney, & Snow, 1990; Snow, 1995). This persistence has only been possible by separating idealized linguistic competence (unaffected by performance variables or memory limitations) from the data on children's language learning, using single instances or tasks as evidence that competence has been acquired. If the empirical facts of variability and frequency discussed here and outlined in the Appendix are to be explained, however, performance must be modeled in both comprehension and production of language—listening and speaking.

A cognitive version of the innatist hypothesis has also persisted (Slobin, 1981), in the interpretation of children's early semantic categories (e.g. agents act on objects in locations; possessor-possession) as universal primitives, given innately; or in the early Constraint theory work on lexical development that ascribed children's biases for word interpretations to universally given assumptions brought to the language learning task (e.g. Clark, 1993; Golinkoff, Jacquet, Hirsh-Pasek, & Nandakumar, 1996; Golinkoff, Mervis, & Hirsh-Pasek, 1994; Markman, 1994). Proposed constraints included, for example, the assumption that the referents of novel nouns would be whole objects, rather than parts of objects; or the mutual exclusivity constraint that new words could not refer to classes of objects with names and new objects could not be named with words already referring to other categories of objects.

Advances in methodology, however, have allowed us to examine the contributions of genetic variation and environmental input in unprecedented scope, directness, and detail. These advances are reviewed here; they provide evidence for a strong interactionist position, with multiple genetic and environmental factors contributing to variation in language learning; and many of the same investigators who originally proposed universal content for, and constraints on, children's language learning have modified their views with the subsequent evidence (e.g. Markson & Bloom, 1997; Mervis & Bertrand, 1995).

RECENT ADVANCES IN METHODOLOGY

Recent research has benefited from expansions in the methods used for study and analysis of children's language development, including generalization of work to multiple languages, cultures, populations of children, contexts of use, and tasks; advances in archiving, sharing, and analyzing data through computerized support; and adoption of new research designs in the study of genetic and environmental influence.

Crosslinguistic studies

Notable in the recent research is the crosslinguistic research on the acquisition of comprehension and production (Bavin, 1995; MacWhinney & Bates, 1989; Slobin, 1985a, b; 1992; 1997b, c), permitting direct tests of the apparent universals of early language development and the teasing apart of cues to sentence structure; and direct tests of the competing explanations for developmental patterns. Research has been carried out cross-linguistically to test theories of the patterning of specific language impairment (e.g. Leonard & Bortolini, 1998), to test the universality of developmental sequence claims (e.g. Slobin, 1997a), and to evaluate the shifting roles of co-occurring cues to meaning in the differing languages (Bates & MacWhinney, 1989).

Leonard and Bortolini (1998) used crosslinguistic methods to test the claims that children with specific language impairment have specific difficulty with verb agreement, extending the developmental time in which they regard verb markings as optional (the Extended Optional Infinitive hypothesis proposed by Rice and Wexler, 1996a, b). Proposing, alternatively, a Surface Hypothesis that the amount of phonetic substance (e.g. syllables rather than single sounds) influences whether children find grammatical morphemes easy to map or not (Leonard, Eyer, Bedore, & Grela, 1997), Leonard and colleagues have carried out studies in which similar grammatical morphemes vary in their perceptual salience across languages, obtaining evidence in support of the Surface account.

MacWhinney and Bates (1989) have investigated the ways that co-occurring cues of word order, grammatical morpheme marking, and animacy vary across languages in their usefulness as predictors of sentence agent and object, demonstrating that both cue strength and distinctiveness contribute to the probability that children will rely on such cues in sentence interpretation. The Competition Model of language processing derived from these studies (Bates & MacWhinney, 1989) was one of the first models of children's language acquisition to account for variation across languages in comprehension and production.

Slobin (1997a) concludes, in his discussion of the origin of children's grammatical notions, that we must broaden our perspective to take into account not only children's conceptual and social understanding and the ways that native languages incorporate that content systematically in grammatical categories. We must also consider the ways that what is learnable by children, and functional culturally, have shaped the history of languages. Further, evidence on children's learning of early semantic-syntactic categories of space, time, and motion has now come from a sufficient number of languages varying in the way they map meaning to structural form (e.g. Bowerman, 1996; Choi, 1991; Choi & Bowerman, 1991) to persuade him that prior formulations (Slobin, 1981) of conceptual universals in children's representations of prototypic event scenes are wrong. For example, the path followed by an object in motion with respect to some background is expressed by verbs in Korean, and, typically, by prepositions in English. Children learning the two languages are equally adept at mapping the notion of path to these "open class" (verb) or "closed class" (grammatical morpheme) categories (Choi & Bowerman, 1991). Thus, the "basic semantic relations" (e.g. agent acting to change the location of an object) of the English-speaking child arise from an interaction of English language structure, the ways that adults talk to children, and the interesting aspects of events. That is, the specific language and conceptual understanding of events interact to give weight and cue value to particular aspects of meaning and form, as Bowerman (1996) has argued persuasively for the origins of children's spatial semantic categories. The broadening of child language research to languages other than English has been critical in developing these interactionist perspectives.

Cultural Variation in Language Acquisition

Early work on stylistic differences in mother-child interaction has been followed up by linguistically, anthropologically, and culturally based investigations of acquisition patterns in a variety of populations-Papua New Guineans, Inuktitut, and members of African-American, Native American, and Latino language and cultures, to name a few, where the varieties of language performance that are culturally valued are many-and sometimes include learning to be quiet, rather than learning to talk. The cultural and linguistic biases of standardized tests for language assessment have been documented, with some improvement in standardization samples and validity in new test revisions.

Importantly, the work informed by sociocultural variation in the reasons for talk that children encounter has revealed a richly varying repertoire of communicative genres and expectations for children's participation in them (or not) (e.g. Heath, 1983). Noteworthy are the variations in storytelling, argument, patterns of prohibition, and gender language reviewed by the collaborators in Susan Ervin-Tripp's festschrift (Slobin et al., 1996). With the sociological perspective on children's language learning has come an understanding of the many and varying discourse structures that are the task of lifelong learning.

Children with Language Disorders

A large body of work on children with language disorders has provided tests of the ways that language acquisition can come apart, and is beginning to offer insight into possible genetic contributions to language learning, as language disorders are studied in particular populations (e.g., Specific Language Impairment, Down syndrome, Williams syndrome, Fragile X, Prader-Willi, autism; Chapman, 1997; Tager-Flusberg, 1994). These studies also offer an opportunity to assess claims of modular linguistic organization, especially when combined with cross-linguistic methods. The work to be reviewed in the next section makes clear that specific language impairment, broadly defined, has strong genetic components; but that variation in normal language acquisition is strongly linked to environmental variation in input.

Contexts of Use

A substantial body of quantitative data has been gathered on characteristics of children's language in conversation with an adult during free play, or in narrative language attempts, showing that narrative language samples are more sensitive to the emergence of more complex syntactic structures (e.g. Leadholm & Miller, 1992). Elicited language sample techniques have been developed for the study of the use of specific structures, including grammatical morphemes, WHquestions, and negation (e.g. Miller, 1981). Much of this work has been driven by a desire to use language samples in assessing children for language disorders. Additionally, work has focused on the qualitative characteristics of language in situations such as the co-construction of narration, mealtime conversations, procedural descriptions, narration of wordless picture books (Berman & Slobin, 1994) and videotaped events, bedtime monologues, requests for clarification, and referential communication. Those working on communicative intervention for children with social deficits have investigated the scripts associated with many everyday activities—taking the bus, making purchases at McDonald's, joining a peer group, requesting toys. Studies of context effects make clear the importance of these variables in influencing language sample structure and vocabulary.

New Task Paradigms to Assess Performance

Early emphasis on establishing the child's linguistic competence led some to choose whatever task seemed to give evidence of language learning most easily-primarily production tasks in which free speech samples were elicited. Recent research has recognized the need to assess both language comprehension and production, as specific language deficits can arise primarily for language production or appear in both processes. Additionally, a wider variety of assessment paradigms have been developed for comprehension, in particular. These include an intermodal preferential looking paradigm (Hirsh-Pasek & Golinkoff, 1996) that bridges earlier habituated sucking and visually reinforced head-turning procedures for assessing children's ability to recognize novelty in linguistic stimuli. The looking paradigm seats the infant on the blindfolded mother's lap, with an interesting light or toy directly ahead to focus the child on midline, and then presents linguistic stimuli from midline with two visual scenes displayed on video at either side. Preferential, or longer, looking (determined by viewers blind to the stimuli) at the scene consonant with the spoken stimulus is taken as evidence of comprehension, permitting assessment as early as 13 months. The method has the disadvantage, if the infant shows a right- or left-side bias, of excluding that participant from the study; it has the advantage of applicability to lexical and syntactic stimuli. A second new paradigm for studying word learning has been the use of "fast mapping" tasks: Quick, incidental learning tasks that introduce a novel object or action and novel word for one or a few trials, followed by tests of comprehension, production, and memory for the event. Comprehension learning has also been demonstrated in fast mapping tasks from 13 months onward (e.g. Kay-Raining Bird & Chapman, 1998).

The emergence of the MacArthur Communicative Development Inventory (Fenson et al., 1991) and variants for other languages has greatly improved our ability to assess children's emerging vocabulary and sentence structure in the 8-30-month range by providing parents with a detailed checklist of early vocabulary items and sentence examples. The norming sample for the MacArthur CDI has permitted the detailed investigation of the relation between growth of the lexicon and early syntax, showing the high correlation between them (Fenson et al., 1994).

Tasks from cognitive psychology have been adapted for assessment of lexical and syntactic processing, including lexical decision making, in which the child judges whether a stimulus is a word; a gating paradigm, in which an initial brief segment of the word is presented with increasing duration, and the child guesses the word (e.g. Dollaghan, 1998; Montgomery, 1999); competing or dual-processing tasks, for example the Competing Language Processing Test, in which the child must judge whether sentences are true or false and also remember the last word of each sentence (Gaulin & Campbell, 1994); and grammatical judgment tasks, in which the child judges whether an instance is, for example, silly or OK. Systematic exploration of the stimulus continuum in naming and identification studies has allowed study of how children categorize exemplars of sounds or words that increasingly depart from good prototypes, or that shift across category boundaries. Priming studies, in which words, semantic categories, or syntactic structures have been presented on prior trials have been used to investigate the interaction of linguistic domains in the modeling of language production and comprehension.

Computer assessment of comprehension through touchscreen selection or, in older children, self-pacing of reading, have allowed study of temporal aspects of processing, though these responses are not, typically, highly practised and hence show a great deal of variability. Not yet reported are applications of the new cameras that permit tracking of eye gaze during comprehension tasks, a paradigm that has revealed very rapid online interpretation of talk, often before a first syllable of a word is complete, when the referent is clear from the context (Eberhard, Spivey-Knowlton, Sedivy, & Tanenhaus, 1995).

Tasks using designs from the child language intervention literature have been used to verify experimentally the patterns of communicative interaction that lead to faster language acquisition, including increased frequencies of the experimenter's modeling of developmentally appropriate target words, grammatical morphemes, or sentence structures; requests to the child to say the model (elicited production); expansions of the child's utterance that supply missing but obligatory semantic and grammatical content; a pattern of following the child's lead through continuing the child's topics and commenting on the child's actions; and recasting of the child's utterances in varying syntactic form (e.g. questions, negations) in pragmatically appropriate ways.

Neuroimaging. Functional imaging studies (PET, fMRI) are beginning to give a picture of the areas of greatest metabolic activity, in terms of glucose consumption or regional blood flow, during language tasks in adults (Binder, 1997; Kent, 1998; Neville & Bavelier, 1998), confirming the activation associated with production and comprehension, respectively, in classical language areas (Broca's and Wernicke's) and extending the areas of cortex implicated in semantic processing, suggesting spatial localization of lexical items by semantic category (Grabowski, Damasio, & Damasio, 1998). Additionally, premotor activation of naming has been shown to occur in picture viewing tasks (Bookheimer et al., 1998), and word listening tasks presented at slow, but not fast, rates (Price et al., 1996). These tasks made no requirement for naming or rehearsing, indicating that language production is automatically tied to both object recognition and word comprehension, when language experience and time permit.

In adults with dyslexia carrying out phonological awareness tasks, fMRI has demonstrated underactivation in posterior regions (Wernicke's area, the angular gyrus, and striate cortex), and relative overactivation in the inferior frontal gyrus, compared to controls, supporting the view that dyslexia is a disorder of phonological processing (Shaywitz et al., 1998). Additional evidence implicating phonological awareness in reading comes from work by these investigators on young adults (Pugh et al., 1997), showing that individual differences in the magnitude of phonological effects on word recognition, as indexed by spelling-to-sound regularity effects on lexical decision latencies and by sensitivity to stimulus length effects, are strongly related to differences in the degree of hemispheric lateralization in two cortical regions.

A problem with the cognitive neuropsychology approach to imaging, and other cognitive assessment in adults is its focus on representational (competence) differences in modularly conceptualized domains, modularity that does not characterize the developing child or children with specific language disorders (Bishop, 1997). Rather, variation in information processing (for example, auditory memory) or learning mechanisms may lead to trade-offs in performance as demands for resources increase or decrease; or the appearance of a selective deficit in material currently being learned, whose locus shifts developmentally.

Currently only EEG work gives a look at activity across the brain in successive real-time trials, in both adults and children, for listening and reading tasks, but ability to locate spatial sources of electrical activity is limited (Mills & Neville, 1997). Ethical concerns limit PET studies using radioactive tracers to children who require imaging for medical reasons, such as brain mapping prior to resections for epileptic seizures (Bookheimer & Dapretto, 1996; Muller et al., 1998). Thus developmental accounts of functional neuroimaged activity are limited. PET studies suggest that motor control becomes more focal with development through the increasing deactivation of nonmotor cortex, and that cerebellum and vermis activation is stronger in adults (Muller et al., 1998). The size of the planum temporale and pars triangularis has been found to be larger in the left hemisphere than the right in individuals with normal language skills; MRI work has demonstrated that the plana temporale are of more equal size in adults with reading disorder (Semrud-Clikeman, 1997). Children with specific language impairment show both more rightward asymmetry of structures and a significantly smaller pars triangularis in the left hemisphere (Gauger, Lombardino, & Leonard, 1997). These findings, of course, are correlational: the structural differences may reflect differences in amount of learning, rather than cause those differences.

The imaging techniques involve trade-offs of spatial and temporal resolution, require the participant to stay still for long periods (under noisy conditions, in the case of fMRI), expose the participant to radioactive substances (PET) and require methods for the normalization of brain structure coordinates (Frank, Damasio, & Grabowski, 1997) and the detection of statistically probable increases in normal activity (Constable et al., 1998). Additionally, baseline tasks must be conceptualized meaningfully if a subtractive design is used in which differing tasks are compared to find activity unique to a particular task. The subtractive methodology, characteristic of PET and fMRI work, has two conceptual disadvantages: the assumption that activity shared with other tasks is not a fundamental part of the language process in question; and the assumption that greater activity always accompanies the task. EEG work has shown the dynamic whole-brain activation that can accompany naming or word comprehension tasks; PET studies have also shown that highly practised activities show reductions in oxygen consumption or glucose use.

The imaging data, taken collectively, are converging on a view of language representations as dynamic patterns of distributed activity that reflect the usual activities (auditory, speaking, visual) and names associated with objects, with spatial separation of activity for differing lexical and syntactic categories. Thus, these methodologies are contributing to a shift in our view of linguistic knowledge from static competence models, or linguistic modules separate from sensorimotor activity, to recognition of the distributed temporal course of listening, speaking, and reading.

Computer Archiving

Cumulative archives of transcripts have been shared in CHILDES, the cooperative database of children's language samples funded by the National Science Foundation, with its associated tiers of timing, phonological, morphemic, syntactic, and pragmatic coding. Digitized storage of associated acoustic files and videotapes of archival data is in progress, and the opportunity to associate temporal analysis of ongoing talk with the written transcripts is supported in the archive. Computerization of transcript analysis has permitted individual investigators to search and analyze large databases of transcripts; among the available programs are those associated with CHILDES (CLAN, CHAT; MacWhinney, 1995; Sokolov & Snow, 1994); the Systematic Analysis of Language Transcripts, or SALT (Miller & Chapman, 1982-1999), PEPPER, a program for phonological analysis (Shriberg, 1986); LARSP (Bishop, 1984); and CSpeech, for acoustic analysis (Milenkovic, 1996).

The effect of shared archives, such as CHILDES, has been criticized as well as praised (Edwards, 1992). When investigators draw inferences from the occurrence of single utterances, as happens in some linguistic methodologies, there is need for absolute reliability concerning the observation (Edwards, 1993). This is not a level achieved for most of the archived data (indeed, for any of our data), and such inferences from single instances are drawn at the investigator's peril. Nor does the archive meet the archival principles that Edwards (1992) advocates, of maximum readability, minimum bias, consistent encoding across corpora, systematic contrastiveness, or comparability in elicitation techniques, transcription, and coding.

Edwards' (1992) call for a single universal standard of transcription and coding was debated in the development of CHILDES and SALT programs; the consensus at the time of program development was already divided, in that the CHILDES project developed a recommended set of codes for the different coding tiers and the SALT project left the definition of codes oven to the investigator, as an integral part of the research task. The agreement that data should be shareable led to the creation of translation programs for the two formats.

The CHILDES archive, consisting of contributed data going back to Roger Brown's transcripts of Adam, Eve, and Sarah, includes examples of the evolving changes in transcription practice and CHILDES standards that have contributed to differential formatting of older corpora (MacWhinney & Snow, 1992), and the differing samples, encoding plans, elicitation techniques, and transcription conventions that meet the differing goals of the original investigators. Thus, this and other archives are best used when corpora are selected with care to meet the secondary investigator's question, with the limitations in sampling of individuals and speaking contexts taken into account. Large databases accumulated from contributed studies are not a substitute for appropriate sampling plans, if standardization of linguistic expectations is desired. The archives are very valuable, however, for the opportunity they offer to shape experimental questions, and to explore, in the longitudinal data sets, individual differences in growth trajectories.

Computer Analysis

The availability of rapid computer analysis of large databases has reshaped theories of language development, allowing computer modeling of the statistical structure of language input (Seidenberg, 1997), simulation of learning by "neural net," or connectionist, models (Marchman, 1997; Marchman, Plunkett, & Goodman, 1997; Plunkett & Marchman, 1993), and the creation of self-organizing learning systems (Callan, Kent, Guenther, & Vorperian, 1997). The connectionist work, reviewed by Plunkett, Karmiloff-Smith, Bates, Elman, and Johnson (1997), has been important for its existence proves that types of learning once thought to be associated with separate learning mechanisms—categorical vs. continuous, semantic features vs. prototypes, associations vs. paradigms, rules vs. exceptions—can in fact both arise from the same connectionist simulation given different histories and frequency of input. Computer analysis has also been instrumental to the discovery of the statistical structure inherent in large databases of text.

Summary

The recent advances in research methods have greatly broadened the database from which inferences about children's language production can be made, substantially improved our ability to assess comprehension and production, offered new insight into brain organization and function during linguistic processing, and increased our ability to model language learning. The work carried out cross-linguistically has suggested that language and children's cognitive processing interactively shape the developmental content and trajectory of lexical and syntactic learning.

EVIDENCE FOR GENETIC CONTRIBUTIONS TO LANGUAGE DEVELOPMENT

Research Methods

Studies of genetic contributions to language development have investigated family aggregation of language impairment, examined large family pedigrees for speech and language impairment, contrasted identical and dizygotic same-sex twins reared together, and evaluated language function in adopted children of parents with language impairment (Rice, 1996; Stromswold's, 1998, review). These studies, taken together, provide evidence of substantial genetic influence in developmental language disorders as well as substantial environmental influence on language learning within the normal range.

Many of the studies have defined developmental language disorder quite broadly as any problem in speech or language. Work continues on refining the definition of the heritable phenotype of specific language impairment, which may itself be a heterogeneous category, defined by poor language performance not accounted for by impaired nonverbal cognition, impaired hearing, speechmotor problems, social deficits, or lack of language input. Bishop (1992) reviews evidence for six different hypotheses of the origins of specific language impairment, contrasting deficits in a specialized linguistic mechanism with explanations based on output, auditory perception, conceptual development, learning strategies, and speech and language capacity in the information processing systems. These hypotheses are equally relevant to explanations of individual differences among children learning language normally, and reflect the contributions of the differing streams of information contributing to communicative skill.

The heterogeneity of the group of children designated as specifically language impaired, who may show differing degrees of discrepant performance from nonverbal spatial cognition measures, and who may or may not show discrepancies between comprehension and production skills, argues for multifactor explanations of specific language impairment. Evidence from the more general categories of child language delay and disorders, including semantic-pragmatic disorders, children with autism, and children with syndrome-specific patterns of language use and mental retardation or learning disorders, also points to multiple causal factors in the acquisition of communicative skill.

Family Aggregation Studies. Stromswold (1998) reviews studies of family aggregation that, taken together, indicate a mean incidence of positive family history for speech and language problems across studies as 46% in the families of children with specific language impairment and 18% in the controls. When family history is defined as having received intervention, 30% of the family members of children with specific language impairment, and 3% of controls, report such a history (Bishop, 1999). Using recently developed diagnostic procedures for determining SLI (Tomblin et al., 1997) and a case control method, Tomblin showed that children with SLI had greater rates of near relatives with language learning problems. Stromswold concludes, in her review, that developmental language disorders are heterogeneous, but show evidence of a significant genetic component.

Children with specific language impairments are at high risk for later impairments in reading as well. Adults with third-generation familial dyslexia, when compared with unaffected age-matched family members, also report more early speech and language problems (Feldman et al., 1993).

Pedigree Studies. In a study of children with specific grammatical language impairment and their families, van der Lely and Stollwerck (1996) concluded that the evidence was consistent with an autosomal dominant inheritance pattern. A pedigree study (Lewis, Cox, & Byard, 1993) of 45 individuals with a history of preschool speech and language disorders was carried out for the affected age groups of preschool, grade school, adolescents, and adults. The degree to which 888 of their family members were also affected was examined, yielding strong evidence for familial transmission. Models of a major gene or multifactorial transmission, however, could not be distinguished in this study. Pedigree studies face the challenges of obtaining accurate classification of family members across generations and across incomplete family recollections. Finding families large enough to give evidence of transmission patterns is a particular challenge.

The first identified genetic contribution to speech and language disorders is a region, named SPCH 1, containing a dominant gene and located on chromosome 7q31. This region is linked to severe motor dyspraxia, language delay accompanied by residual tense and grammar errors, problems in written language, and intellectual deficit in a large British family (Fisher, Vargha-Khadem, Watkins, Monaco, & Pembray, 1998). M. Gopnik (1990) (Gopnik & Crago, 1991) had earlier proposed that the family offered evidence of a gene exclusively affecting performance on grammatical features, but the constellation of severe apraxic speech and broadly defined developmental language problems currently described make a purely linguistic interpretation of the observed deficits too narrow. Tomblin, Shriberg, Nishimura, Zhang, and Murray (1999) have preliminary evidence, however, that specific language impairment in children is linkable to the CFTR subregion within the SPCH 1 region identified by Fisher et al. (1998). Using both a case control comparing distributions of alleles in SLI and control children, and an affected family-based control, asking whether SLI children receive one allele type from their parents more often than another, they obtained significant associations for language disorder, reading disorder, and poor performance on the Nonword Repetition Task, but not on articulatory measures.

Twin Studies of Typically Developing Children. Twin studies exploit the expectation that dizygotic same-sex twins share, on average, 50% of their genetic makeup and identical twins 100%, whereas environmental contributions to language learning are expected to be similar for all pairs. Language and cognitive development were compared longitudinally in twins at 14, 20, and 24 months (Reznick, Corley, & Robinson, 1997). The higher concordance of identical twins than same-sex dizygotic twins for nonverbal cognitive ability indicated that these measures reflected primarily genetic influence. In contrast, concordances for measures of receptive and expressive language were about the same in both groups, indicating primarily environmental contributions to language performance. Genetic influence emerged for receptive language only at 14 months, a time when skills in fast mapping of phonological forms to novel objects are emerging in comprehension (Kay-Raining Bird & Chapman, 1998). Genetic influence emerged for expressive language at 20 and 24 months, when a productive vocabulary spurt, word combinations, and language reflecting understanding of event roles emerge. :Thus it appears that the periods of first rapid acquisition of vocabulary in comprehension (14 months) and production (around 20 months) are linked with genetic contributions, but that subsequent progress in each domain is linked to environmental variation.

Cumulative expressive vocabulary has also been studied in twins (Ganger, Pinker, & Wallis, 1997). In an interim report on parents' daily journals of 24 pairs of identical twins and 21 pairs of same-sex dizygotic twins in the second year of life, Ganger et al. report that cumulative vocabulary growth curves for the first 100 words differ more for dizygotic pairs than monozygotic pairs. This finding is consistent with the heritable component in production vocabulary at 20 and 24 months reported by Reznik et al. (1997).

Twin studies offer evidence of environmental influence in another way as well. Language delays have long been reported in twins (Day, 1932). Twins serve as (inexpert) language models for each other and encounter reduced amounts of individually directed speech, compared to singletons (Tomasello, Manle, & Kruger, 1986). For monozygotic and dizygotic twin pairs (Ganger et al., 1997), mean rate of acquisition fell into the 10-25 percentile range according to comparisons with the MacArthur Communicative Development Inventory, suggesting a 2-4-month delay in early vocabulary acquisition associated with twinship. Bishop and Bishop (1998) review the evidence for twinship itself as a risk factor for language impairment in dizygotic twins; it appears related to slower language development, but not frank and persistent specific language impairment.

Significant delays in social, emotional, or cognitive areas should also be associated with delays in language development, and twin studies in these domains are relevant to the causal modeling of influences on language acquisition. The MacArthur Longitudinal Twin study (Etude et al., 1992) has shown heritable influences at 14 months for toddlers' inhibition to the unfamiliar (shyness), tester activity ratings of toddlers, and parent ratings of temperament. Genetic influence has been found for child empathy and parental ratings of expression of negative, but not positive, emotion. Genetic influences were also demonstrated for behaviors indexing spatial memory, categorization, and word comprehension.

Matheny (1997) cautions that the variation in twin study results for different ages and measures may reflect variation in the reliability of the differing measures (which include differing numbers of items), and urges a more continuous view of the developmental shifts. However, fine-grained study of language acquisition suggests that the points of genetic contribution currently identified may be conceptualized, in each case, as times of the onset of rapid learning of a component of the developing language system, in which one part of the system is being mapped onto another. These putative components include first-year milestones as well as the vocabulary bursts in comprehension at 14 months and vocabulary production at 20 months.

Twin Studies of Children With Language Disorders. The earlier reviewed twin studies examined genetic contributions to normal variation in language performance. Twin studies in which at least one child has a language impairment allow the evaluation of a genetic component to the distinct disorder, as opposed to its contribution to normal variation. In the first twin study of late talkers, Dale and colleagues (Dale et al., 1998) assessed expressive vocabulary at age 2 for more than 3000 twin pairs. For the lowest 5% of the participants, modeling of heritability was estimated at 73%, compared to 25% for the sample as a whole. Shared environment was less important for the language delayed sample (18%), compared to the entire sample (69%), indicating a strong role for genetic influence in child language disorders, and a strong role for environmental factors in normal variation.

Twin data on 90 pairs aged 7-25 years (Bishop, North, & Donlan, 1995), each of which included at least 1 twin with developmental speech or language disorder according to DSM-111-R criteria, revealed a near 100% concordance for monozygotic twins when the definition was broadened to include those with histories of developmental speech or language disorder or a less pronounced verbal-nonverbal disagreement in scores. The comparable concordance rate for dizygotic twins, using this broadened definition, was 50 %. This is a striking finding, which suggests that the phenotypic description of specific language impairment might be usefully broadened, rather than narrowed, in phenotype-genotype investigations. Other studies of twins show similar evidence of a genetic component to poor oral language skills (Lewis & Thompson, 1992; Tomblin & Buckwalter, 1998). Tomblin and Buckwalter also found that dizygotic twins, when compared to singleton sibling pairs with at least one affected member, were more similar to one another in language achievement, indicating that twinning itself affects language learning, as noted earlier.

What factors are associated with language impairment, broadly defined? The contribution of phonological memory to language impairment has been investigated in a study of a subset of the twins of the prior study, aged 7-9 years, with persistent or resolved language impairment (Bishop, North, & Donlan, 1996). These twins were assessed on the Children's Nonword Repetition Test (Gathercole & Baddeley, 1993), a test that is believed to assess phonological short-term memory. The language impaired twins showed impaired performance in nonword repetition compared to age-matched controls, and increasingly so on the items of greater syllable length. Those with resolved language impairment performed as poorly as those with persistent language impairment. Comparison of monozygotic and dizygotic co-twins indicated significant heritability of performance on the Nonword Repetition Test, with greater regression toward the mean in dyzygotic co-twins than identical co-twins. Thus, the Nonword Repetition Test appears to tap the heritable component of specific language impairment, rather than environmental contributions to language skill. In contrast, the Auditory Repetition Test, which asks children to report the order of high and low tones presented at fast or slow rates, appeared related to normal and environmentally influenced variation in the same children (Bishop et al., 1999).

Twin study of children concordant or discordant for autism also suggests the heritability of language impairments (LeCouteur et al., 1996). Language impairments in childhood and social deficits persisting into adulthood were commoner in the monozygotic twin without autism than in the dizygotic.

Adoption Studies. Additional evidence of a role for genetic factors that contribute to the transmission of speech and language disorders comes from a study by Felsenfeld and Plomin (1997), who compared adopted children who had a biological parent with a history of a speech disorder to adopted children who had an affected adoptive parent. Other groups compared included nonadopted children with affected or nonaffected parents. Twenty-five per cent of the children with affected biological parents showed questionable speech, language, or fluency skills at age 7, compared to 9% of the children with no parental history.

Summary. Studies of genetic contributions to language development suggest a strong genetic contribution to expressive language impairment, broadly defined, and other developmental disabilities with language impaired outcomes; but a strong role for environmental contributions to language learning in the normal range. In children just learning to talk, genetic contributions also appear in the first vocabulary learning bursts associated with comprehension (14 months) and production (20-24 months) but disappear subsequently.

THE ROLE OF LANGUAGE INPUT

Prelinguistic Input

Recent work has underscored the importance of the language spoken to children from birth onward-or, indeed, while still in utero; the auditory system is functional at 24-28 weeks' gestational age (Juscyzk, 1997). The effects of this experience are, first, to make the mother's voice familiar to the newborn; infants orient longer to its sound than to another female voice (e.g. Hepper, Scott, & Shahidullah, 1993). Within 3 months, infants learn to associate the mother's speaking style and face, expecting both to be animated and expressive, and to associate mouth shape differences with vowel sound differences, expecting co-occurrence. Infants are effective at discriminating speech-sound differences from a variety of languages at first; they come to develop perceptual expectations for the sounds prototypic of their language in the second half of the first year (Oller, Eilers, Urbano, & Cobo-Lewis, 1997). This mapping appears to influence the repertoire of sounds produced in babbling, leading to predominance of the native language sounds in babbled vocalizations at 8 to 12 months (Kent, 1992).

Saffran, Aslin, and Newport (1996) have recently suggested the answer to a fundamental problem in the field, that of how children can segment words from the acoustic stream, by demonstrating that 8-month-olds can develop expectations for words defined only by the statistical relationships between neighboring speech sounds in 2 minutes of exposure. That is, children are tracking the transitional probabilities from one syllable to the next, which are typically high within words and lower between words. Thus, the statistical, temporal structure of speech addressed to children contains within it cues to word boundaries, which Saffran et al. have demonstrated that infants can learn (see also Jusczyk & Aslin, 1995; Myers et al., 1996). Thus, variation in interaction style, amount, and structure of talk addressed to prelinguistic children may have important influence on subsequent linguistic development (e.g. Hampson & Nelson, 1993; Hayes & Ahrens, 1988; Ingram, 1995; Swanson & Leonard, 1994).

Interaction Style

What are the effects of parents' communicative style on subsequent child language and cognitive development? A number of older correlation studies evaluating relative differences in parents' use of language with their infants and toddlers have identified a conversational speech style associated with more rapid language development (see Chapman, 1981b; Gallaway & Richards, 1994; Hoff-Ginsberg, 1991; Kavanaugh & Jirkovsky, 1982; Pine, 1994) and the variations associated with language-impaired children (Conti-Ramsden, 1985; Hodapp, Evans, & Ward, 1989; Snow, 1995). The components of this linguistically responsive style include *expansion* of children's utterances into well-formed equivalents, supplying the missing grammatical and semantic elements; *recasting* of children's utterances into other syntactic forms, often questions; *commenting* on the child's actions and focus of attention rather than questioning; *following the child's lead* in the choice of play materials, activities, and topic rather than directing the child; and the use of a *referential,* rather than formulaic, speech style (Hampson & Nelson, 1993). These behaviors have become tools for effective language intervention with late talkers and children with specific language impairment (Nelson, Welsh, Camarata, Butkovsky, & Camarata, 1995). Experimental studies have indicated their efficacy in these populations (Fey, Cleave, & Long, 1997; Fey, Cleave, Long, & Hughes, 1993; Fey et al., 1994; Girolometto, Pearce, & Weitzman, 1996; Yoder & Warren, 1998), especially in combination with prompts for talking and the creation of situations requiring communication (e.g milieu training, Kaiser & Gray, 1993).

Conversational Partner

Research has indicated that mothers and fathers are similar in their speech styles, aside from intonational pattern differences (Warren-Leubecker & Bohannon, 1984); siblings, however, use fewer of the conversational moves associated with more rapid language development, and younger siblings use fewer than older (Hoff-Ginsberg & Kreuger, 1991). In households where childcare is carried out mainly by siblings, conversational support for language learning may be more limited. In day-care settings where speech is addressed simultaneously to several children, the finetuning of talk to individual children's focus of attention may be more limited (Clarke-Stewart, Gruber, & Fitzgerald, 1994). Mothers' affective state also influences interaction; neglecting and depressed mothers are less effective conversational partners, and less likely to provide language input, than peers (Bettes, 1988; Christopoulous, Bonvillian, & Crittenden, 1988). Children's shift to school settings demands a very different pattern of participation in talk (Heath, 1983; Wells & Wells, 1984).

Amount of Input

The effects of differences in sheer amount of input have been investigated little until recently. Clarke-Stewart's (1973) early longitudinal study of language input to 18-month-olds from low socioeconomic class households is an exception. Through sampling of the language addressed to children across their waking hours, she demonstrated both wide variation in the amount of language addressed to children-4% to 75% of their waking time-and the context-0% to 25% of their waking time spent in play. These differences were associated with large differences in their children's subsequent production vocabularies and rate of syntactic development. Hoff-Ginsberg (1991, 1992) more recently demonstrated large differences in amount of input associated with socioeconomic class differences in mothers.

Hart and Risley's Study

Hart and Risley (1992, 1995) have recently completed an intensive longitudinal study of parent-child interaction in 42 Midwestern families representing the range of socioeconomic status from families on welfare through working class and professional families, for white and African-American families. An hour a month of unstructured, naturally occurring interactions with the child in the home were observed and tape-recorded each month from 10 to 36 months; Stanford-Binet assessments of IQ (a measure, mainly, of verbal IQ) were carried out at 36 months.

Most striking, among the families, were stable differences in the amount of talk addressed to the children, which ranged from 56 to 793 utterances per hour in the I1-18-month period and 34 to 783 parent utterances when children were 29-36 months old, associated with differences in the amount of time that parents spent in interaction with their children. Similar variation has been reported in Wells' (1985) study of language development and Clarke-Stewart's (1973) study of 18-month-olds in lower-class families. These differences are associated with socioeconomic indices but not sex of child or parent race.

Extrapolating from the observed hour to a 14-hour day, Hart and Risley (1995) estimate that a child spoken to 50 times an hour will hear 700 utterances in a day; a child spoken to 800 times an hour will hear more than 11,000 utterances. In a year, the difference in exposures would cumulatively result in 250,000 utterances versus 4,000,000 utterances; in the 3 years of the study, 1,000,000 versus 12,000,000 utterances. In terms of the estimated cumulative words encountered by children in the study over the first 4 years of life, those in families on welfare encountered an estimated 12,000,000; those in working class families an estimated 28,000,000; and those in professional families an estimated 48,000,000. These constitute overwhelming differences in the amount of language experienced by children in the early language-learning years in different families; and not surprisingly, measures based on amount of talk and its subcategories predict child language outcomes at 3 years and 9 years of age. These data are, of course, correlational rather than causal; it could be argued that these differences arise from genetic differences in the families' predisposition for low-language skills and, concomitantly, amount of talk. However, the studies in which genetic influence has been compared for adopted children with either biological or adopted parents affected by speech and language problems would suggest otherwise (Felsenfeld & Plomin, 1997), as would the effects of experimental interventions altering the language learning environment. The Hart and Risley estimates underscore the importance of public policies providing very early educational experience and the considerations facing families choosing day-care providers.

To investigate the range of parent behaviors that might predict IQ outcomes on the Stanford-Binet, 10 variables reflecting parent communication skills from the HOME Inventory (Bradley & Caldwell, 1984) were selected and the stability of their individual differences demonstrated across the 2-year span (Hart & Risley, 1992). These measures were averaged across the 2-year span, converted to z-scores, and submitted to a principal components analysis that revealed 3 clusters of variables explaining a total of 63% of the variance in verbal IQ. The 3 factors were (1) the amount of parent participation in the child's activity; (2) the parents' performance as a social partner; and (3) the qualitative content of parents' utterances.

Loading strongly on the first factor, amount of parent activity, were the measures of parent presence during the child's activity, parent participation even when carrying out other work, and the total words and different words addressed to the child. These measures were strongly associated with the existing SES level of the family and accounted for 22% of the explained variance in verbal IQ.

Loading strongly on the second factor, the parent's performance as a social partner, were measures of parent responsiveness to children's initiation of communication the percentage of children's initiations that were responded to; the number of parent turns taken within an interactive episode; and the difference between child mean length of utterance (MLU) and parent MLU, the latter typically being about 2.6 to 2.0 morphemes longer than children's utterances. These measures were not associated with existing SES level but accounted for 16% of the explained variance in verbal IQ.

Loading strongly on the third factor, the qualitative content of parents' utterances, were measures of parent repeats (repetitions, expansions, and extensions of the child's utterance), questions, and prohibitions. Prohibitions, in particular, were strongly and negatively related to subsequent child IQ, though they averaged only 4% overall. These measures were strongly related to family SES level and accounted, collectively, for 57% of the explained variance in verbal IQ.

In subsequent analysis, Hart and Risley (1995) examined two additional child outcome variables at age 3: the rate of vocabulary growth (a parameter for trajectory of expressive vocabulary change at age 3, based on the log of acquired vocabulary); and the number of different words used per hour, averaged over months 34-36. Features of parent talk addressed to children were coded for amount per hour and richness, or proportion of total utterances showing the feature.

Features included total utterances; numbers of different words, nouns, verbs, modifiers, and function words; total numbers of words, nouns, verbs, modifiers, and function words; numbers of sentences containing two or more clauses, past verb tense, or future tense; numbers of declaratives, imperatives, or questions; numbers of questions containing WH-words (e.g. what, why, how), yes/no questions, and yes/no questions with the auxiliary element (e.g. do, can) at the front of the sentence; and utterances that initiated topics, responded to child topics, or held the floor. Finally, utterances expressing affirmative or prohibitory tone were counted; included in affirmations were positive comments and repetitions and expansions of the children's talk.

Because most features occurred at proportionately similar rates across families, the frequency with which they occurred typically predicted more variability in child outcomes than the richness, or proportionate, measures. Those features more strongly related to child outcomes were grouped into five derived variables of significant family experience: (1) *language diversity* (number of different nouns and different modifiers per hour); (2) *feedback tone* (affirmatives divided by affirmatives plus prohibitions, per hour); (3) *symbolic emphasis* (sum of nouns, modifiers, and past-tense verbs per hour divided by total utterances); (4) *guidance style* (auxiliary-fronted yes/no questions divided by imperatives plus auxiliary-fronted yes/no questions); and (5) *responsiveness* (proportion of parent responses not preceded by parent initiations).

Amount of language input (language diversity) was more strongly related to vocabulary use; feedback tone to rate of vocabulary growth and IQ. Symbolic emphasis was more strongly related to vocabulary use; guidance style to vocabulary growth and IQ score. Responsiveness was independently related to all three child outcomes. The 5 measures together accounted for 61% of the variance in vocabulary growth and use, and 59% of the variance in Stanford-Binet IQ. In the 29 children followed up in third grade, these same 5 measures accounted for 61% of the variance in children's scores on both the PPVT-R, a measure of vocabulary comprehension, and the TOLD, a test of both expressive and receptive language.

Similar evidence of the importance of variation in mother's sociodemographic characteristics, personality characteristics (including tendency to respond in a socially desirable fashion), and vocabulary use has been reported by Bornstein (Bornstein, Haynes, & Painter, 1998) in predicting a single latent variable vocabulary competence (derived from spontaneous language samples, examiner-assessed comprehension, and maternal report, Bornstein & Haynes, 1998) in 126 children aged 20 months. Structural equation modeling supported several direct and unique predictive relationships: child gender (girls better) and social competence, and maternal attitudes toward parenting, predicted vocabulary competence. Mothers' vocabulary predicted child vocabulary comprehension and maternal report of expressive vocabulary. Mothers' vocabulary itself was positively influenced by SES, maternal verbal intelligence, and mothers' knowledge about parenting. Children's verbal IQ, and to a lesser degree performance IQ, were predicted at 48 months by the vocabulary competence latent variable at 20 months, and by receptive vocabulary specifically.

Situation-Specific Learning

Real variation exists in language addressed to the child during differing situations; Hoff-Ginsberg (1991), for example, has studied mealtime, dressing, book reading, and toy play contexts, showing the exceptional richness of language during the latter two event contexts. Young children learn, and later use, the language addressed to them in specific contexts, for example book reading (Ninio, 1980; Snow & Goldfield, 1983) or familiar scripts (e.g. Short-Myerson & Abbeduto, 1997).

Early Object Names

The early learning of object names by children has been ascribed to the prevalence and salience of nouns in the input. However, crosslinguistic study of the early vocabularies of English and Korean children (Au, Dapretto, & Song, 1994) has shown that far more verbs than nouns appear in salient position in the speech of the Korean adults to 12-17-month-olds, with the reverse true of English adults speaking to English children. Nevertheless, children of both cultures acquired nouns, mostly object names, much faster than verbs. Au interprets this as evidence that constraints on word meanings are important for explaining basic patterns of semantic development across languages. However, Choi and Gopnik (1995) report evidence for an early verb spurt in Korean children, around 18 months, that was not present in previously collected English data, calling into question the universality of early noun vocabularies. (Similarly, Nelson [1973] drew attention to children's first 50-word vocabularies that were not primarily nominal in her expressive-referential distinction.)

Constraint Theories

The constraints on children's learning of word meaning invoked by language researchers take somewhat different form, but a number have in common the view that the novel word is the starting point that drives the search for meaning (Gunnar & Maratsos, 1992). The principles of constraint proposed include (a) a *whole object* assumption that a novel word is referring to an object, rather than its properties, parts, or activities; (b) a *mutual exclusivity* assumption that different words distinguish different object classes, and hence cannot overlap in their denotation (Markman, 1989); (c) a *principle of contrast* (Clark, 1993) that no two words have the same meaning, when "meaning" is taken broadly to include pragmatic aspects of the word's use; and (d) the N3C, *novel name-nameless category principle* (Golinkoff, Mervis, & Hirsh-Pasek, 1994) that links are to be made between novel words and referents for which no names exist. Constraint theories, in their original formulations, were helpful in drawing attention to the many commonalities in how children treated new words. They had the unfortunate property, however, of being framed as all-or-none rules, rather than as response biases or tendencies. Subsequent research has demonstrated many exceptions; for example, the variable and late acquisition of the mutual exclusivity bias (Davidson, Jergovic, Imami, & Theodos, 1997; Merriman & Bowman, 1989); the children's willingness to apply two different novel verbs to the same novel action (Hesketh & Ellis Weismer, 1997); and the importance of conceptual perspective on word choice (Clark, 1997). Although words for dissimilar objects are treated as mutually exclusive, words for related and similar objects are interpreted hierarchically by children at 2 years, indicating that conceptualization of the object relations mediates word interpretation (Waxman & Senghas, 1992). These studies suggest the importance of locating the sources of "constraints" on children's word learning—or their biases of referent interpretation—in the history of children's interactions with objects (e.g. Masur, 1997) and the interlocutor (Clark, 1997).

Cognitive Views

Piagetian-based views take the child's conceptualization of the world, independent of language, as the driving force leading the child to seek out language and the determinant of the resulting extension of terms to referents. The bias toward whole objects as referents could be treated probabilistically, as an outcome of the child's prior sensorimotor experience with objects (their "affordances " for action, in Gibsonian terms). The failure to map verbs as frequently and as early as nouns, then, may thus be related to the earlier gap in comprehension of nouns vs. verbs (10 months vs. 18 months, roughly; Miller, Chapman, Branston, & Reichle, 1980) or to relative frequency of mapping (Tomasello, Akhtar, Dodson, & Rekau, 1997). The comprehension gap between nouns and verbs may then in turn be viewed as reflecting the earlier developmental gap in schemes associated with objects: looking, as opposed to later emerging schemes of grasping, releasing, exploring, and functional use, a developmental progression that associates remembering object-specific actions with objects beginning at about 10 months, after a long history of less differentiated schemes. This argument, of course, is a version of the classical Piagetian view that conceptual development precedes, and drives, semantic development. It is only one of several ways in which the appearance (but not the innateness) of constraints might come about. Recent work on infants' conceptual generalization of properties across classes of basic level objects reveals the importance of the larger conceptual domains of animals and vehicles in children's imitative play-properties, for example, of eating and drinking are generalized to animals, and those of opening with a key or giving a ride are generalized to vehicles (Mandler & McDonough, 1998) and the importance of language-specific mappings of meaning (e.g., Bowerman, 1996).

Interactionist Views

A. Gopnik and Meltzoff (1984) offer a more interactionist version of cognitive constraint theory based on Vygotsky's (1962) views, called the *specificity hypothesis:* Very specific cognitive achievements related to the child's goals are mapped to words consistently modeled in input (e.g., *more, all gone, all done, again).* Recent cross-linguistic work emphasizes the importance of language variation (Choi & Bowerman, 1991; Slobin, 1997a; Weist, Lyytinen, Wysocka, & Atanassova, 1997).

Speaker's Intended Meaning

A third source of "constraint" on the child's attribution of a word to a referent might arise from the child's expectations based on past events of interaction with the speaker (Nelson, 1986). Here, the past history and present experience of speaker intent becomes critical, and one can imagine certain interactional contexts-for example, the game of naming body parts-that might, if extended to novel animals, reveal a context in which a part-response was more typical than a whole-object interpretation: an experiment crying to be carried out.

Eighteen-month-olds are more likely to learn a new word on a single occasion *(fast mapping* is the term Carey and Bartlett [1978] have applied to this early phase of learning) when they are focusing on the referent; introduction of the label when the infant is attending to an alternative object was less successful (Dunham, Dunham, & Curwin, 1993), indicating the facilitating effect of following the child's lead. However, typically developing children are better able to follow a speaker's shift of attention than children with autism, who fail to track the speaker's locus of attention and link novel words with the objects to which they are attending (Baron-Cohen, Baldwin, & Crowson, 1997; Charman et al., 1997).

Joint-Attention Contexts of Early Word Learning

Much recent work has focused on children's word learning in contexts in which both parent and child are attending to a common focus of attention (e.g. Moore & Dunham, 1995; Tomasello & Merriman, 1995). Tomasello, in a series of innovative studies of children's word acquisition in contexts where adult and child are jointly attending to play with objects, has shown that 2-year-olds link novel words to objects or actions that the other speaker is intending to find, or carry out, rather than the mistakenly found, or accidentally accomplished, actions that actually happen (Barton & Tomasello, 1991). This is a very important set of findings, if it can be replicated, for it means that children from a very young age are filtering meaning through their model of the other person's mind their beliefs about her intended actions, objects of attention, and intended communicative goals. This view would assign a critical role to social cognition in the development of the language system.

Notes Toward an Interactionist, Functional, Emergent View of Children's Language Learning

The biobehavioral work on genetic contributions to language development indicates a strong role for cognitive, social, and expressive language-related genetic contributions to language disorder. General learning impairments impair language learning as well, including its computational or formal aspects. Social impairment affects pragmatic appropriate uses of language, communicative engagement with the other, and the mapping of meaning and form in the joint-attention context. The currently identified genetic source of specific language impairment appears to be related to phonological memory. The deficits in the acquisition of expressive vocabulary, syntax, morphology, and phonological awareness in reading and spelling implicate a specific deficit in phonological auditory memory and its feed-forward activation of language production regions.

In contrast, the studies of parent-child interaction reveal the importance of frequent, relatively well-tuned, affectively positive verbal interaction in supporting rapid language acquisition, and the strong effects of variations in language environment on variations in language skill (Huttenlocher, 1998). Early gains or interventions are associated with later more rapid development of the later emerging aspects of the language system; increases in comprehension are linked to later increases in production; increases in vocabulary to later, more rapid acquisition of syntax (e.g. Thal, Bates, Zappia, & Oroz, 1996) ; more rapid acquisition of syntax to later, more rapid development of discourse structures in comprehension and production. The research also indicates the disproportionate influence of punitive and negative communicative interaction on language learning. Even positively heightened emotionality reduces the probability of talk in toddlers (Bloom, 1993). The important roles played by affect in children's language learning are only beginning to be understood.

Experimental studies of the factors influencing initial phases of word learning (fast mapping), demonstrate the importance of social focus of attention and referent novelty on children's early word learning, and raise the question of how the child comes to link word and referent or action (Tomasello & Merriman, 1995). Cross-linguistic and cross-cultural investigations have challenged the field's generalizations about universals of developmental sequence and semantic content, leading us to seek their sources in the child's history of experience rather than in innately given conceptual or grammatical primitives (Berko-Gleason & Ely, 1997; Fivush & Hudson, 1990; Harris, 1992; Huttenlocher, 1998; van den Broek, Bauer, & Bourg, 1997).

Modeling of the statistical dependencies in language addressed to children has demonstrated how rich a source of information is contained there (Brent & Cartwright, 1996); we have not yet modeled the corresponding cooccurrences and transitions of language, action, and speakers within the joint-attention context. Nevertheless, we now know that information on word boundaries is inherent in language structure and learnable by 8-month infants in only minutes of exposure (Saffran et al. 1996). As histories of experience in word recognition build up, higher-order statistical dependencies that correspond to grammatical morphology and syntax structure may become accessible, though surely the mapping, in parallel, of meaning will have to play a role in such emergent structure. What we know from early study of acquisition is how gradually such grammatical morpheme use and new structural forms emerge. A number of researchers in the field who have individually pursued functionalist, developmental accounts of language acquisition are now pooling their efforts to account for language as an emergent property of learning, rather than an innate endowment (Elman et al., 1996; Johnson, 1997; MacWhinney, 1999). Thelen's work (1995) on development as a dynamic process goes even further, emphasizing that learning and development are merely two different windows on continuous activity that is not linear, but nonlinear in its trajectories, so that very small differences in initial conditions can lead to large differences in outcomes.

RECONCEPTUALIZING LEARNING AND DEVELOPMENT

Cognitive Development

Reconceptualization of children's language learning must take place against a background of conceptual shift in more general accounts of children's cognitive development (Siegler, 1998). These shifts include (a) an integration of infancy research with later work on toddlers, preschoolers, and older children; (b) new topics of study, including understanding of motor skill development, thinking as a collaborative process, domain-specific constraints on learning, children's theory of mind, and computer simulation of developmental processes; (c) an increased emphasis on the role of learning in both the biology and psychology of development; (d) emphasis on the extent and importance of variability in children's cognition; (e) an increasing role for formal, domain-specific models; and (f) new or more developed metaphors for the child as an agent of actions, a tinkerer, a scientist, an expert, a storyteller, a goal- directed communicator.

The Mind-Body Problem

More generally, current research and thinking about children's language development is occurring against the backdrop of a major conceptual shift in psychology. At the end of the 20th Century, the Cartesian mind-body distinction that has conveniently separated our domains of discourse, and associated explanations, in biology and behavior, body and mind, and brain and cognition, is dissolving in the repeated demonstrations of interactivity at every analytic level, from the environmental contributions to directional orientation in embryos to genes turned on or off by cellular contexts to the observable biological effects in the brain of mind, thinking, or experiencing. Thus, the imaging studies reveal that physical differences in the activation of the brain accompany behavioral differences, and enriched experience in laboratory animals has been shown to enlarge and reshape brain regions. A consequence of the collapse of the Cartesian distinction is the recognition that behavior-feelings, talk to oneself and others, and meaning-making have physical reality and, conversely, alteration of brain states alters behavior.

Selectional Pressures

In analogous fashion, the insights of neo-Darwinian theory of natural selection are being extended to selection of cultural products (memes); and the co-occurrence of pattern as the organism behaves in an environment is recognized as selectively giving rise to mappings of sensory and motor areas onto sensorimotor association domains that effectively organize brain structure and that are responsive to species-specific and acquired valuation. The emergence of patterns of goal-oriented action in the world through reinforcement systems, or addictive processes, are examples. Thus there is a need for a biological-based, as well as a sociocognitive-based, account of children's language learning. One useful framework is that of Edelman (1988, 1992).

Edelman's Theory of Neuronal Group Selection

Edelman's theory of neuronal group selection (1988, 1992) has been applied to the neural processes underlying the development of language by Kent (1992), in which somatosensory, auditory, and motor receptor sheets are mapped to the cortex and the co-occurring interactions mapped at successively more global levels. The mechanisms of brain and behavior development, in this theory, are three: *developmental selection, experiential selection,* and *reentrant mapping.* Developmental selection leads to the diversification and pruning of local neuronal connectivities that become a primary repertoire of large numbers of neuronal groups with brain regions; behavior then causes a dynamic selection of neuronal groups, strengthening or weakening populations of synapses. Reentrant mapping, in Kent's formulation, is a parallel signaling through ordered anatomical areas between separate maps, creating temporal correlations among the neuronal selections. Reentrant mapping can result in auditory, visual, and tactile sensations, all of which occur in a situational context defined by participants, events, and emotions; that is, reentrant mapping can result in an experiential encyclopedia in which various sensory and motor responses are related to a given experience.

Kent (1992) has shown that the vocal tract is continuously remodeled in the first year of life, with continuing change (at different rates) in skeletal, jaw, tongue and laryngeal structures through adolescence; thus the motor patterns required to achieve the same speech target cannot remain fixed, but must alter to accommodate the changing effects of growth (Kent & Vorperian, 1995). They propose that successful speech motor control is a result of a continuous mapping of speech output onto perceptual targets. Perceptual targets themselves arise in the first year of life out of the experienced input; infants show expectations based on affective display, mouth shape, and vowel co-occurrences by 3 months, prosodic contours by 6 months, and categorical perception conditioned by the native language's distribution of speech sounds by 8 months. Similar learning processes yield categorical perception and prototypicality of central instance interactions, or reduced rates of language learning. Kent's application of Edelman's theory could be extended to the other mappings of maps that must attend the full development of language skill: specific objects and goal; goal and action; action and result, where these are communicative goals, and speaking and listening as actions.

Real Complexity

The detailed accounts of specific disciplines have forced a recognition of complexity and of ongoing change in living organisms. Particular examples include the parallel and recurrent networks of analysis in the visual system, which support not only vision but, in reverse direction, visual imaging; the multiple single-cell recordings of environmentally significant sounds in the auditory cortex, showing that learning can lead to neuronal assemblies functioning as "detectors" of significant information; the analysis of synaptic change upon repeated stimulation resulting in long-term potentiation or depression of neural thresholds; or the dynamics of social interaction with the mother, in which meaning is co-constructed in moment-to-moment tracking of the other's focus of attention and intent.

Dynamics in Real Time

The complexity of these systems, and their ongoing dynamic change, have converged to make complex dynamic systems an attractive new framework within which to conceptualize the ongoing processes (Thelen, 1995; Thelen & Smith, 1994). The mathematics of nonlinear complex systems changing through time demonstrate points of extreme sensitivity to initial conditions, attraction of solutions to restricted regions (points, limit cycles, strange attractors), and shifts in patterns as a function of changes in control parameters that allow many observed facts about development—periods of continuous versus discontinuous change, emergent structural schemes, variation that increases at points of transition to new patterns—to be viewed as arising from the same underlying deterministic system.

Language Learning as a Psychobiological Process

Answers to the question of how children learn language are evolving, then, from multiple perspectives and disciplines, making the field an exciting microcosm for the competing explanatory views whose integration is being forced by new technologies of brain imaging, computer simulation, genome description, and the large archival databases of children's talk. Additionally, new work in the biochemistry and neurobiology of learning and development is deepening our understanding of the many events that must participate in the chain of processes underlying these behavioral terms, and research on children's language disorders in a variety of populations is confirming the variety of ways in which genetic, and other, impairments can be linked to language-learning outcomes. Answers are far from in, but the promise of integrating our understanding of events at the level of social interaction with changes at the levels of brain organization and function, synaptic plasticity, and dendritic growth of synaptic connection, where learning is thought to reside, offers important new ways to think about the acquisition of language comprehension and production skills.

Levels of Analysis

At one level, neural activation, neurohomonal regulation, synaptic plasticity, neurotransmitter and receptor availability, blood supply, and long-term changes in connectivity collectively underlie our behavioral constructs of processing, learning, memory, and resource allocation. At another level, social, consumatory, and instrumental goals of approach and avoidance interact with the affordances (remembered associated actions) of objects and people in the environment to bring about communication, affective response, and biochemical alterations in the functioning of the brain, its regulation and learning, and the immune system. Although we are far from the goal of having realistic dynamic system accounts of the general process of language learning, the behavior of connectionist nets (which can be viewed as dynamic systems) and other nonlinear dynamic systems alter substantially the questions that appear interesting to ask, as old theoretical controversies about the nature of the learner turn into questions about the nature of the experienced world.

Learning Mechanisms

If our generalizations about children's language learning are to emerge from our models of learning, we need to take these models much more seriously and in more complex detail than we have before. In particular, we need to base our models in what is known of real brain structure and function, and of the biochemistry of learning. Table F in the Appendix attempts a very partial listing of the topics in learning that might be addressed. It is based on the view that children's expectations provide a continuous prediction of what will happen next on the basis of past experience, which current experience continually updates and corrects. When that experience is emotionally conditioned, attached to primary drives, or moderately novel in terms of past experiences, learning results. For example, novelty increases plasticity of synapses for a few accompanying seconds, increasing the probability of learning at those moments. Some processes mediate short-term learning. Longer-term learning, arising from the association of events with the many valuation systems, primary and secondary, of the human child, link affective and cognitive processes intimately to the social world. Much of what appears given or innate in young children's developing cognition and language may, on closer inspection, be shown to arise from the statistical structure of the encountered world and the correlations arising in action upon it, in a manner shared with other species (e.g. Kluender, Lott, Holt, & Bloedel, 1998). Such an enterprise is initially discomfiting, in a world of narrow and traditional disciplines of study and discourse; it suggests a reality so multilayered and complex that it is dizzying to think about. And yet, a glimpse of what might be real: "interactions, all the way down" (Elman et al., 1996, Ch. 6).

ACKNOWLEDGMENTS

This work was supported by grant ROI-HD23353 from the National Institutes of Health to R. Chapman; and by grant ROI-DC03731 to Susan Ellis-Weismer. A portion of the review was carried out on sabbatical leave at the Applied Psychology Unit of the Medical Research Council in Cambridge, England. Thanks to Maura Jones and Cynthia Renk for assistance in literature searches, and to Donna Boudreau, Stephanie Cawthorne, Julia Evans, Mina Johnson-Glenberg, Mandy Kay-Raining Bird, Elizabeth Leigh, and Sally Miles for discussion.

APPENDIX: DEVELOPMENTAL SEQUENCE AND VARIABILITY IN CHILDREN'S LANGUAGE LEARNING

TABLE A
Pragmatic Development in Children (Adapted From Chapman, 1988)

First year: Discovering communication

- Discovering that vocalizations and gesture have predictable effects
- Mapping prosodic contour to speaker affect and communicative intent

Order of emergence of early communicative intents in the second year

• Earliest (8–15 months):	requesting objects or activity
	refusing
	commenting
	communicative games
• Middle (16–23 months):	requesting information
	answering questions
	acknowledging response
	repeating
• Late (24 months on):	symbolic play
	evoking absent objects and events
	misrepresenting reality

- Frequency of vocalization in the second year
    - 0–12 months: 25 vocalizations/10 minutes of free play
    - 13–18 months: 50 vocalizations/10 minutes of free play
    - 19–21 months: 75 vocalizations/ 10 minutes of free play

Expansion of conversational speech act categories in the preschool years

• Learning to continue topic:	24 months, through repetition
	36 months, through adding new information

- Learning to respond to requests for clarification
- Request forms:

	2-4, variation in form
	4-7, variation in explicitness of content as function of politeness
	7 on, adding justification from listener's point of view

- Functions of language in peer play, 3-7 years
- Directive: language is used to direct or monitor one's own or another's actions (frequency decreases)
- Interpretative: language is used to report on present and past experiences, and to reason (frequency increases)
- Projective: language is used to predict events, to express empathy, and to create imaginary activities and roles (frequency increases)
- Relational: language is used to maintain one's own status and to interact

School years: Sequences in discourse genres

- Narratives: beginning and ending

  protagonist and setting

  problem and attempts at resolution

  obstacles and affective responses

  linking of multiple episodes

  landscape of consciousness: character's thought

- Referential communication:

	neither listener nor informative attributes taken into account
	informative attributes selected from speaker's point of view
	informative attributes selected from listener's point of view
	ambiguities of pronoun use clarified

TABLE B
Semantic Sequences in Language Development (Adapted From Chapman, 1988)

Semantic content of words in one word speech

- Early one-word period (10–16 months)
  - Appearance, disappearance, recurrence
  - People, pets, interesting objects
  - Affective attitudes
  - Communicative games and routines
- Middle one-word period (16–20 months): agent, action, object of action
  (18–20 months): location, possession
  - Semantic development of early negation
    - Rejection
    - Disappearance
    - Nonexistence
    - Denial

Semantic sequences in multiform speech

- Prevalent semantic relations (18–24 months)
  - Agent-action
  - Action-object
  - Agent-object
  - Action-location
  - Entity-location
  - Possessor-possession
  - Demonstrative-entity
  - Attribute-entity
- Semantic aspects of WH questions (2–5 years)
  - Objects and people (what, who)
  - Basic event questions (who what-doing where)
  - Event explanation (why)
  - Event manner (how)
  - Event time (when)
- Semantic relations between adjacent and conjoined sentences
  - Additive
  - Temporal
  - Causal
  - Contrastive

TABLE C
Syntactic Sequences in Children's Language Development (Adapted From Chapman, 1988)

Major syntactic stages and morphosyntax associated with Brown's five stages[a]

- Basic semantic roles and relations (Stage I)
  - Agent, action, object of action, location
  - Possessive, attributive, demonstrative
- Grammatical morphemes (Early mastered, Stage II)
  - In, on, -in, noun plural
- Syntactic modulation of sentences (Stage III)
  - Auxiliary use in negation, yes-no and WH questions
- Emergence of embedded sentence forms (Stage IV) and mastery of mid-difficulty grammatical morphemes
  - Irregular past, articles the and a, be as an uncontracted main verb
- Emergence of conjoined sentences (Stage V)
- Grammatical morphemes (Late mastered, Stage V+)
  - Regular past tense, third person present, irregular third person, contractible copula be, auxiliary be

[a]Brown's stages correspond to mean lengths of utterances, in morphemes, as follows: Early I, 1.1–1.5; Late I, .5-2.0, II, 2.0–2.5; III, 2.5–3.0; Early IV: 3.0–3.5; Late IV–Early V: 3.5–4.0; Late V: 4.0–4.5.

TABLE D
Variability in Language Learning in Typically Developing Children

Dimensions of individual difference in typical language development

- Analytic vs. gestalt style
- Rate of language learning
- Rate of speech sound development
- Willingness to speak (shyness); Fluency of speaking
- Speaking rate

Asynchronies in typical language development

- Communicative intent emerges prior to first word production
- Comprehension-production gap in the emergence of early vocabulary
- Continuing difference in size of comprehension vs. production vocabulary
- Pragmatic constraints on early word use
- Shift to prototypic scene content in middle one-word period
- Single-word production precedes multiform speech
- Early sentence comprehension better for grammatically complete sentences despite the absence of grammatical inflection in production
- Early sentence production lacks grammatical morphemes ("telegraphic" speech)
- Acquisition of grammatical morphemes is gradual
- Sentence imitation may not reveal structures used in spontaneous speech

Factors correlated with rate of typical language development

- Frequency of language input addressed to child
- Dyad's joint attention to referents
- Responsiveness of input language to child's focus of attention
- Prototypicality of referent
- Conversational rather than directive speech style
- Responsiveness of caregiver to child's communicative intent
- Semantic transparency and consistency of words addressed to child
- Phonological form of input within the child's repertoire
- Expansion of child's utterances
- Extension of child's topic
- Recasting of child's utterances
- Positive affect of speaker
- Child's nonverbal cognitive development
- Child's social engagement with the other
- Child's phonological repertoire

TABLE E
Additional Variability in Children With Specific Language Impairments

Added asynchronies in language impairment

- Slower rate of language development than nonverbal cognitive development
- Slower rate of development in production than comprehension (or not)
- Slower rate of syntactic than lexical development in comprehension (or not)
- Slower rate of syntactic than lexical development in production (or not)
- Slower rate of grammatical morphology acquisition than sentence length in production

Typological differences in language impairment

- Receptive-expressive impairment
- Specific expressive language impairment
- Word-finding problems
- Sentence formulation problems
- Perseveration
- Echolalia
- Deficits in language associated with theory of mind
- Semantic-pragmatic deficit

TABLE F
Proposed Mechanisms of Language Learning in Children

- **What is learned is a dynamic, distributed pattern of cortical activation**

  The static constructs of phonological, lexical, syntactic, and pragmatic description have their real counterparts in cortical activity that happens over time and is distributed across cortical locations.

- **Sensitivity to moderate novelty**

  Novelty is automatically tracked in terms of prior learning and, when encountered, engages attentional resources and biochemical alteration in plasticity of cortical synapses ("learning moments").

- **Social engagement**

  Other people engage the infant's attention, interest, and interactive attempts and, with learning, become the locus for the affective meaning of events, a separate focus of attention, and (later still) a separate understanding of the world.

(continued on next page)

TABLE F *(continued)*

- **Competitive activation of prior learning**

  Cortical activity feeds forward in prior patterns, leading to prediction of the incoming activity, comparison with it, and detection of difference (e.g. in the mismatched negativity component of the auditory event-related potential; or the hippocampus's ongoing modeling of the world and activation of the locus coeruleus when expectations are not met). Activation of one pattern may include inhibition of alternative patterns.

- **Biochemical modulation of synaptic plasticity**

  The probability of learning-that is, synaptic alteration—is modulated by neurotransmitters released in the cortex by (a) the locus coeruleus' response to moderate novelty, increasing plasticity over a brief 2-10-second period through norepinephrine release over the cortex; (b) other limbic or brainstem-modulated neurotransmitters connected to affective valuing systems; and (c) neurotransmitters or neurohormones released in the body through affective response to events that affect attention, engagement, and synaptic plasticity in the brain over periods of minutes or hours; or that lead to cell death.

- **Hebbian associations: the importance of context**

  Patterns of synaptic activation too weak to lead to synaptic firing separately may, jointly present, lead to firing; this is a mechanism whereby co-occurring, or correlated, structure can be extracted from experience.

- **Sensorimotor learning**

  Actions performed on objects leave their trace as "affordances" of the objects —including referential actions or namings through the association of action, goal, and stimuli as distributed activation patterns.

- **Fast-mapping of episodic information**

  Rapid ongoing learning of the objects, people, actions, and locations in a interaction, through activation of expectations based on prior learning (thus, developmental sequences are generated by the perceptual and motor histories of experience and their co-occurrences), joined to the affective significance of the events.

- **Networks of networks**

  Early-learned sensory and motor experience may serve as input to other networks to guide or tune their continuing adjustment.

- **Coherence in the world**

  Apparent "primitives" of experience, such as person and object existence and permanence or the existence of a common spatial framework through which people and objects move, are constructed through the experience of the infant reacting to coherent stimulation provided by the world and her actions in it.

- **Dynamic structure in the world**

  Ongoing learning of changes in the world leads not only to the extraction of "units" that statistically cohere in input but their transitional probabilities, as traces of prior paths of activation whose strength reflects current activated context.

REFERENCES

Au, T. K., Dapretto, M., & Song, Y. K. (1994). Input vs. constraints: Early word acquisition in Korean and English. *Journal of Memory and Language, 33,* 567–582.

Baldwin, D. A. (1993). Early referential understanding: Infants' ability to recognize referential acts for what they are. *Developmental Psychology, 29,* 832–843.

Baron-Cohen, S., Baldwin, D. A., & Crowson, M. (1997). Do children with autism use the speaker's direction of gaze strategy to crack the code of language? *Child Development, 68,* 48–57.

Barrett, M. (Ed.). (1999). *The development of language.* Hove, UK: Psychology Press.

Barton, M. E., & Tomasello, M. (1991). Joint attention and conversation in mother-infant-sibling triads. *Child Development, 62,* 517–29.

Bates, E., Dale, P., & Thal, D. (1995). Individual differences and their implications for theories of language development. In P. Fletcher & B. MacWhinney (Eds.), *The handbook of child language* (pp. 96–151). Oxford: Blackwell Publishers.

Bates, E., & MacWhinney, B. (1989). Functionalism and the competition model. In B. MacWhinney & E. Bates (Eds.), *The crosslinguistic study of sentence processing (pp.* 1–73). Cambridge: Cambridge University Press.

Bavin, E. L. (1995). Language acquisition in crosslinguistic perspective. *Annual Review of Anthropology, 24,* 373–396.

Behrend, D. A., Harris, L. L., & Cartwright, K. B. (1995). Morphological cues to verb meaning: Verb inflections and the initial mapping of verb meanings. *Journal of Child Language, 22,* 89–106.

Berko-Gleason, J. (Ed.). (1993). *The development of language* (3rd ed.). New York: Macmillan Publishing.

Berko-Gleason, J., & Ely, R. (1997). Input and the acquisition of vocabulary: Examining the parental lexicon. In C. Mandell & A. McCabe (Eds.), *The problem of meaning: Behavioral and cognitive perspectives* (pp. 221–260). Amsterdam: North-Holland/Elsevier Science Publishers.

Berman, R., & Slobin, D. (Eds.). (1994). *Relating events in narrative: A crosslinguistic developmental study.* Hillsdale, NJ: Lawrence Erlbaum Associates.

Bettes, B. A. (1988). Maternal depression and motherese: Temporal and intonational features. *Child Development, 59,* 1089–1096.

Binder, J. R. (1997). Neuroanatomy of language processing studied with functional MRI. *Clinical Neuroscience, 4,* 87–94.

Bishop, D. V. M. (1984). Automated LARSP: Computer-assisted grammatical analysis. *British Journal of Disorders of Communication, 19,* 78–87.

Bishop, D. V. M. (1992). The underlying nature of specific language impairment. *Journal of Child Psychology and Psychiatry, 33,* 3–66.

Bishop, D. V. M. (1997). Cognitive neuropsychology and developmental disorders: Uncomfortable bedfellows. *The Quarterly Journal of Experimental Psychology, 50A,* 899–923.

Bishop, D. V. M. (1999). *Genetic and environmental causes of language impairment.* Paper presented to the Symposium on Research in Child Language Disorders, Madison, WI, June.

Bishop, D. V. M., & Bishop, S. J. (1998). "Twin language": A risk factor for language impairment? *Journal of Speech, Language, and Hearing Research, 41,* 150–160.

Bishop, D. V. M., Bishop, S. J., Bright, P., James, C., Delaney, T., & Tallal, P. (1999). Different origin of auditory and phonological processing problems in children with language impairment: Evidence from a twin study. *Journal of Speech, Language, and Hearing Research, 42,* 155–168.

Bishop, D. V. M., North, T., & Donlan, C. (1995). Genetic basis of specific language impairment: Evidence from a twin study. *Developmental Medicine and Child Neurology, 37,* 56–71.

Bishop, D. V. M., North, T., & Donlan, C. (1996). Nonword repetition as a behavioral marker for inherited language impairment: Evidence from a twin study. *Journal of Child Psychology and Psychiatry, 37,* 391–403.

Bloom, L. (1970). *Language development: Form and function of emerging grammars.* Cambridge, MA: MIT Press.

Bloom, L. (1993). *The transition from infancy to language: Acquiring the power of expression.* New York: Cambridge University Press.

Bloom, L. (1998). Language acquisition in its developmental context. In W. Damon, D. Kuhn, & R. Siegler (Eds.), *The handbook of child psychology* (5th ed., pp. 309–370). New York: John Wiley & Sons.

Bohannon, J. N., MacWhinney, B., & Snow, C. (1990). No negative evidence revisited: Beyond learnability or who has to prove what to whom. *Developmental Psychology, 26,* 221–226.

Bookheimer, S. Y., & Dapretto, M. (1996). Functional neuroimaging in children: Current directions and future challenges. In R. Thatcher, G. R. Lyon, J. Rumsey, & N. Krasnegor (Eds.), *Developmental neuroimaging: Mapping the development of brain and behavior* (pp. 143–155). San Diego, CA: Academic Press.

Bookheimer, S. Y., Zeffiro, T. A., Blaxton, T. A., Gaillard, W. D., Malow, B., & Theodore, W. H. (1998). Regional cerebral blood flow during auditory responsive naming: evidence for cross-modality neural activation. *Neuroreport, 9,* 2409–2413.

Bornstein, M. H., & Haynes, O. M. (1998). Vocabulary competence in early childhood: Measurement, latent construct, and predictive validity. *Child Development, 69,* 654–671.

Bornstein, M. H., Haynes, O. M., & Painter, K. M. (1998). Sources of child vocabulary competence: A multivariate model. *Journal of Child Language, 25,* 367–393.

Bowerman, M. (1996). The origins of children's spatial semantic categories: Cognitive vs. linguistic determinants. In J. J. Gumpers & S. C. Levinson (Eds.), *Rethinking linguistic relativity* (pp. 145–176). Cambridge: Cambridge University Press.

Bradley, R. H., & Caldwell, B. M. (1984). 174 children: A study of the relationship between home environment and cognitive development during the first 5 years. In A. Gottfried (Ed.), *Home environment and early cognitive development* (pp. 5–56). Orlando, FL: Academic Press.

Braine, M. D. S. (1976). Children's first word combinations. *Monograph of the Society for Research in Child Development,* Serial no. 164.

Braine, M. D. S. (1994). Is nativism sufficient? *Journal of Child Language, 21,* 1–31.

Brent, M. R., & Cartwright, T. A. (1996). Distributional regularity and phonotactic constraints are useful for segmentation. *Cognition, 61*, 93–125.

Brown, R. (1973). *A first language: The early stages.* Cambridge, MA: Harvard University Press.

Budwig, N. (1995). *A developmental functionalist approach to child language.* Mahwah, NJ: Lawrence Erlbaum Associates.

Callan, D. E., Kent, R. D., Guenther, F. H., & Vorperian, H. K. (1997). A dynamic neural network model of speech production in the developing child. Poster presented at the 134th meeting of the Acoustical Society of American, San Diego, CA. *Abstract: The Journal of the Acoustical Society of America, 102*(5), Pt. 2, 3165.

Carey, S., & Bartlett, E. (1978). Acquiring a single new word. *Papers and Reports on Child Language Development, 15*, 17–29.

Chapman, R. S. (1981a). Exploring children's communicative intents. In J. Miller (Ed.), *Assessing language production in children: Experimental procedures* (pp. 111–138). Austin, TX: Pro-Ed.

Chapman, R. S. (1981b). Mother-child interaction in the second year of life: Its role in language development. In R. Schiefelbusch & D. Bricker (Eds.), *Early language: Acquisition and intervention.* Baltimore, MD: University Park Press.

Chapman, R. S. (1988). Language acquisition in the child. In N. Lass, L. McReynolds, J. Northern, & D. Yoder (Eds.), *Handbook of speech-language pathology and audiology* (pp. 309–353). Toronto: B. C. Decker.

Chapman, R. S. (Ed.) (1992). *Processes in language acquisition and disorders.* St Louis, MO: Mosby-Year Book.

Chapman, R. S. (1997). Language development in children and adolescents with Down syndrome. *Mental Retardation and Developmental Disabilities Research Review, 3*, 307–312.

Chapman, R. S., Streim, N., Crais, E., Salmon, D., Strand, E., & Negri, N. (1992). Child talk: Assumptions of a developmental process model for early language learning. In R. Chapman (Ed.), *Processes in language acquisition and disorders* (pp. 3–19), St Louis, MO: Mosby-Year Book.

Charman, T., Swettenham, J., Baron-Cohen, S., Cox, A., Baird, G., & Drew, A. (1997). Infants with autism: An investigation of empathy, pretend play, joint attention, and imitation. *Developmental Psychology, 33*, 781–789.

Choi, S. (1991). Children's answers to yes-no questions: A developmental study in English, French, and Korean. *Developmental Psychology, 27*, 407–420.

Choi, S., & Bowerman, M. (1991). Learning to express motion events in English and Korean: The influence of languagespecific lexicalization patterns. Special Issue: Lexical and conceptual semantics. *Cognition, 41*, 83–121.

Choi, S., & Gopnik, A. (1995). Early acquisition of verbs in Korean: A cross-linguistic study. *Journal of Child Language, 22*, 497–529.

Chomsky, N. (1965). *Aspects of the theory of syntax.* Cambridge, MA: MIT Press.

Chomsky, N. (1980). *Rules and representations.* New York: Columbia University Press.

Christopoulos, C., Bonvillian, J. D., & Crittenden, P. M. (1988). Maternal language input and child maltreatment. *Infant Mental Health Journal, 9*, 272–286.

Clark, E. (1993). *The lexicon in acquisition.* Cambridge: Cambridge University Press.

Clark, E. (1997). Conceptual perspective and lexical choice in acquisition. *Cognition, 64,* 1–37.

Clarke-Stewart, K. A. (1973). Interactions between mothers and their young children: Characteristics and consequences. *Monographs of the Society for Research in Child Development,* Serial no. 187.

Clarke-Stewart, K. A., Gruber, C. P., & Fitzgerald, L. M. (1994). *Children at home and in day care.* Hillsdale, NJ: Lawrence Erlbaum Associates.

Constable, R. T., Skudlarski, P., Mencl, E., Pugh, K. R., Fulbright, R. K., Lacadie, C., Shaywitz, S. E., & Shaywitz, B. A. (1998). Quantifying and comparing region-of-interest activation patterns in functional brain MR imaging: Methodology considerations. *Magnetic Resonance Imaging, 16,* 289–300.

Conti-Ramsden, G. (1985). Mothers in dialogue with languageimpaired children. Topics *in Language Disorders, 5,* 58–68.

Dale, P. S., Simonoff, E., Bishop, D. V., Eley, T. C., Oliver, B., Price, T. S., Purcell, S., Stevenson, J., & Plomin, R. (1998). Genetic influence on language delay in two-year-old children. *Nature Neuroscience, 1,* 324–328.

Davidson, D., Jergovic, D., Imami, Z., & Theodos, V. (1997). Monolingual and bilingual children's use of the mutual exclusivity constraint. *Journal of Child Language, 24,* 3–24.

Day, E. J. (1932). The development of language in twins. I. A comparison of twins and single children. *Child Development, 3,* 179–199.

Dollaghan, C. (1998). Spoken word recognition in children with specific language impairment. *Applied Psycholinguistics, 19,* 193–207.

Dunham, P. J., Dunham, F., & Curwin, A. (1993). Jointattentional states and lexical acquisition at 18 months. *Developmental Psychology, 29,* 827–831.

Eberhard, K. M., Spivey-Knowlton, M. J., Sedivy, J. C., & Tanenhaus, M. K. (1995). Eye movements as a window into real-time spoken language comprehension in natural contexts. *Journal of Psycholinguistic Research, 24,* 409–436.

Edelman, G. M. (1988). *Neural Darwinism: The theory of neuronal group selection.* New York: Basic Books.

Edelman, G. M. (1992). *Bright air, brilliant fire: On the matter of mind.* New York: Basic Books.

Edwards, J. A. (1992). Computer methods in child language research: Four principles for the use of archived data. *Journal of Child Language, 19,* 435–458.

Edwards, J. A. (1993). Perfecting research techniques in an imperfect world: Response to MacWhinney & Snow. *Journal of Child Language, 20,* 209–216.

Elman, J. L., Bates, E. A., Johnson, M. H., Karmiloff-Smith, A., Parisi, D., & Plunkett, K. (1996). *Rethinking innateness: A connectionist perspective on development.* Cambridge, MA: MIT Press.

Feldman, E., Levin, B. E., Lubs, H., Rabin, M., Lubs, M. L., Jallad, B., & Kusch, A. (1993). Adult familial dyslexia: A retrospective developmental and psychosocial profile. *Journal of Neuropsychiatry and Clinical Neurosciences, 5,* 195–199.

Felsenfeld, S., & Plomin, R. (1997). Epidemiological and offspring analyses of developmental speech disorders using data from the Colorado Adoption Project. *Journal of Speech, Language, and Hearing Research, 40,* 778–791.

Fenson, L., Dale, P. S., Reznick, J. S., Bates, E., Thal, D., & Pethick, S. J. (1994). Variability in early communicative development. *Monographs of the Society for Research in Child Development*, Serial no. 242.

Fenson, L., Dale, P. S., Reznick, J. S., Thal, D., Bates, E., Hartung, J. P., Pethick, S., & Reilly, J. S. (1991). *Technical manual for the MacArthur Communicative Development Inventories*. San Diego, CA: San Diego State University.

Fey, M. E., Cleave, P. L., & Long, S. H. (1997). Two models of grammar facilitation in children with language impairments: Phase 2. *Journal of Speech, Language, and Hearing Research, 40*, 5–19.

Fey, M. E., Cleave, P. L., Long, S. H., & Hughes, D. L. (1993). Two approaches to the facilitation of grammar in children with language impairment: An experimental evaluation. *Journal of Speech and Hearing Research, 36*, 141–157.

Fey, M. E., Cleave, P. L., Ravida, A. L., Long, S. H., Dejmal, A. E., & Easton, D. L. (1994). Effects of grammar facilitation on the phonological performance of children with speech and language impairments. *Journal of Speech and Hearing Research, 37*, 594–607.

Fisher, S. E., Vargha-Khadem, F., Watkins, K. E., Monaco, A. P., & Pembray, M. E. (1998). Localisation of a gene implicated in a severe speech and language disorder. *Nature Genetics, 18*, 168–170.

Fivush, R., & Hudson, J. A. (Eds.). (1990). *Knowing and remembering in young children*. Cambridge: Cambridge University Press.

Frank, R. J., Damasio, H., & Grabowski, T. J. (1997). Brain-vox: An interactive, multimodal visualization and analysis system for neuroanatomical imaging. *Neuroimage, 5*, 13–30.

Gallaway, C., & Richards, B. (Eds.). (1994). *Input and interaction in language acquisition*. Cambridge: Cambridge University Press.

Ganger, J., Pinker, S., & Wallis, E. (1997). Genetic contributions to vocabulary development. Poster presented at the biennial meeting of the Society for Research in Child Development. Washington, DC, April.

Gathercole, S. E., & Baddeley, A. D. (1993). Phonological working memory: A critical building block for reading development and vocabulary acquisition? *European Journal of Psychology of Education, 8*, 259–272.

Gauger, L. M., Lombardino, L. J., & Leonard, C. M. (1997). Brain morphology in children with specific language impairment. *Journal of Speech, Language, and Hearing Research, 40*, 1272–1284.

Gaulin, C. A., & Campbell, T. F. (1994). Procedure for assessing verbal working memory in normal school-age children: Some preliminary data. *Perceptual and Motor Skills, 79*, 55–64.

Girolametto, L., Pearce, P. S., & Weitzman, E. (1996). Interactive focused stimulation for toddlers with expressive vocabulary delays. *Journal of Speech and Hearing Research, 39*, 1274–1283.

Golinkoff, R. M., Jacquet, R. C., Hirsh-Pasek, K., & Nandakumar, R. (1996). Lexical principles may underlie the learning of verbs. *Child Development, 67*, 3101–3119.

Golinkoff, R. M., Mervis, C. B., & Hirsh-Pasek, K. (1994). Early object labels: The case for a developmental lexical principles framework. *Journal of Child Language, 21*, 125–155.

Gopnik, A., & Meltzoff, A. (1984). Semantic and cognitive development in 15- to 21-month-old children. *Journal of Child Language, 11*, 495–513.

Gopnik, M. (1990). Feature-blind grammar and dysphasia. *Nature, 344*, 715.

Gopnik, M., & Crago, M. (1991). Familial aggregation of a developmental language disorder. *Cognition, 39*, 1–50.

Grabowski, T. J., Damasio, H., & Damasio, A. R. (1998). Premotor and prefrontal correlates of category-related lexical retrieval. *Neuroimage, 7*, 232–243.

Greenfield, P., & Smith, J. (1976). *The structure of communication in early language development*. New York: Academic Press.

Gunnar, M. R., & Maratsos, M. (Eds.). (1992). Modularity and constraints in language and cognition. *The Minnesota Symposia on Child Psychology*, Vol. 25. Hillsdale, NJ: Lawrence Erlbaum Associates.

Hampson, J., & Nelson, K. (1993). The relation of maternal language to variation in rate and style of language acquisition. *Journal of Child Language, 20*, 313–342.

Harris, M. (1992). *Language experience and early language development: From input to uptake.* Hillsdale, NJ: Lawrence Erlbaum Associates.

Hart, B., & Risley, T. (1992). American parenting of languagelearning children: Persisting differences in family-child interactions observed in natural home environments. *Developmental Psychology, 28*, 1096–1105.

Hart, B., & Risley, T. (1995). *Meaningful differences in the everyday experience of young American children*. Baltimore, MD: Paul H. Brookes.

Hayes, D. P., & Ahrens, M. G. (1988). Vocabulary simplification for children: A special case of "motherese"? *Journal of Child Language, 15*, 395–410.

Heath, S. B. (1983). *Ways with words: Language, life and work in communities and classrooms*. Cambridge: Cambridge University Press.

Hepper, P. G., Scott, D., & Shahidullah, S. (1993). Newborn and fetal response to maternal voice. Special Issue: Prenatal and perinatal behavior. *Journal of Reproductive and Infant Psychology, 11*, 147–153.

Hesketh, L. J., & Ellis Weismer, S. (1997, November). Do preschoolers evidence mutual exclusivity bias in verb-synonym learning? Poster presented at the American Speech-Language Hearing Association annual convention, Boston, MA.

Hirsh-Pasek, K., & Golinkoff, R. M. (1996). *The origins of grammar: Evidence from early language comprehension*. Cambridge, MA: MIT Press.

Hodapp, R. M., Evans, D. W., & Ward, B. A. (1989). Communicative interaction between teachers and children with severe handicaps. *Mental Retardation, 27*, 388–395.

Hoff-Ginsberg, E. (1991). Mother-child conversation in different social classes and communicative settings. *Child Development, 62*, 282–796.

Hoff-Ginsberg, E. (1992). How should frequency in input be measured? *First Language, 12*, 233–244.

Hoff-Ginsberg, E. (1993). Landmarks in children's language development. In G. Blanken, J. Dittmann, H. Grimm, J. C. Marshall, & C.-W. Wallesch (Eds.), *Linguistic disorders and pathologies: An international handbook* (pp. 558–573). Berlin: Walter de Gruyter.

Hoff-Ginsberg, E., & Krueger, W. M. (1991). Older siblings as conversational partners. *Merrill Palmer Quarterly, 37*, 465–481.

Huttenlocher, J. (1998). Language input and language growth. *Preventive Medicine, 27,* 195–199.

Ingram, D. (1989). *First language acquisition: Method, description, and explanation.* Cambridge: Cambridge University Press.

Ingram, D. (1995). The cultural basis of prosodic modifications to infants and children: A response to Fernald's universalist theory. *Journal of Child Language, 22,* 223–234.

Johnson, J. S., Lewis, L. T., & Hogan, J. C. (1997). A production limitation in syllable number: A longitudinal study of one child's early vocabulary. *Journal of Child Language, 24,* 327–350.

Johnson, M. H. (1997). *Developmental cognitive neuroscience.* Oxford: Blackwell Publishers.

Jusczyk, P. W. (1997). *The discovery of spoken language.* Cambridge, MA: MIT Press.

Jusczyk, P. W., & Aslin, R. N. (1995). Infants' detection of the sound patterns of words in fluent speech. *Cognitive Psychology, 29,* 1–23.

Kaiser, A. P., & Gray, D. B. (1993). *Enhancing children's communication: Research foundations for intervention.* Baltimore, MD: Brookes.

Karmilof Smith, A. (1996). *Beyond modularity: A developmental perspective on cognitive science.* Cambridge, MA: MIT Press.

Kavanaugh, R. D., & Jirkovsky, A. M. (1982). Parental speech to young children: A longitudinal analysis. *Merrill Palmer Quarterly, 28,* 297–311.

Kay-Raining Bird, E., & Chapman, R. S. (1998). Partial representations and phonological selectivity in the comprehension of 13- to 16-month-olds. *First Language, 18,* 105–127.

Kemler-Nelson, D. G., Hirsh-Pasek, K., Jusczyk, P. W., & Cassidy, K. W. (1989). How the prosodic cues in motherese might assist language learning. *Journal of Child Language,* 16, 55–68.

Kent, R. D. (1992). Phonological development as biology and behavior. In R. S. Chapman (Ed.), Processes in language acquisition and disorders (pp. 67–85). St Louis, MO: Mosby Year Book.

Kent, R. D. (1998). Neuroimaging studies of brain activation for language, with an emphasis on functional magnetic resonance imaging: a review. *Foliar Phoniatrica et Logopedica, 50,* 291–304.

Kent, R. D., & Vorperian, H. K. (1995). Development of the craniofacial-oral-laryngeal anatomy: A review. *Journal of Medical Speech Language Pathology, 3,* 145–190.

Kluender, K. R., Lott, A. J., Holt, L. L., & Bloedel, S. L. (1998). Role of experience for language-specific functional mappings of vowel sounds. *Journal of the Acoustical Society of America, 104,* 3568–3582.

Leadholm, B., & Miller, J. F. (1992). *Language sample analysis: The Wisconsin guide.* Madison, WI: Wisconsin Department of Public Instruction.

LeCouteur, A., Bailey, A., Goode, S., Pickles, A., Robertson, S., Gottesman, L., & Rutter, M. (1996). A broader phenotype of autism: The clinical spectrum in twins. *Journal of Child Psychology and Psychiatry, 37,* 785–801.

Leonard, L. B., & Bortolini, U. (1998). Grammatical morphology and the role of weak syllables in the speech of Italian-speaking children with specific language impairment. *Journal of Speech, Language, and Hearing Research, 41,* 1363–1374.

Leonard L. B., Eyer J. A., Bedore, L. M., & Grela, B. G. (1997). Three accounts of the grammatical morpheme difficulties of English-speaking children with specific language impairment. *Journal of Speech, Language, and Hearing Research, 40,* 741–753.

Lewis, B. A., Cox, N. J., & Byard, P. J. (1993). Segregation analysis of speech and language disorders. *Behavior Genetics, 23,* 291–297.

Lewis, B. A., & Thompson, L. A. (1992). A study of developmental speech and language disorders in twins. *Journal of Speech and Hearing Research, 35,* 1086–1094.

Lieven, E. V. M., Pine, J. M., & Baldwin, G. (1997). Lexically based learning and early grammatical development. *Journal of Child Language, 24,* 187–220.

Locke, J. L. (1993). *The child's path to spoken language.* Cambridge, MA: Harvard University Press.

Locke, J. L. (1996). Why do infants begin to talk? Language as an unintended consequence. *Journal of Child Language, 23,* 251–268.

MacWhinney, B. (1995). *The CHILDES project: Tools for analyzing talk* (2nd ed.). Hillsdale, NJ: Lawrence Erlbaum Associates.

MacWhinney, B. (Ed.). (1999). *The emergence of language.* Mahwah, NJ: Lawrence Erlbaum Associates.

MacWhinney, B., & Bates, E. (Eds.). (1989). *The crosslinguistic study of sentence processing.* Cambridge: Cambridge University Press.

MacWhinney, B., & Snow, C. (1992). The wheat and the chaff: Or four confusions regarding CHILDES. *Journal of Child Language, 19,* 459–471.

Mandel, D. R., Kemler-Nelson, D. G., & Jusezyk, P. D. (1996). Infants remember the order of words in a spoken sentence. *Cognitive Development, 11,* 181–196.

Mandler, J. M., & McDonough, L. (1998). On developing a knowledge base in infancy. *Developmental Psychology, 34,* 1274–1288.

Marchman, V. A. (1997). Children's productivity in the English past tense: The role of frequency, phonology, and neighborhood structure. *Cognitive Science, 21,* 283–304.

Marchman, V. A., Plunkett, K., & Goodman, J. (1997). Overregularization in English plural and past tense inflectional morphology: a response to Marcus (1995). *Journal of Child Language, 24,* 767–779.

Markman, E. M. (1989). *Categorization and naming in children.* Cambridge, MA: MIT Press.

Markman, E. M. (1994). Constraints on word meaning in early language acquisition. *Lingua, 92,* 199–227.

Markson, L., & Bloom, P. (1997). Evidence against a dedicated system for word learning in children. *Nature, 385,* 813–815.

Masur, E. F. (1997). Maternal labeling of novel and familiar objects: Implications for children's development of lexical constraints. *Journal of Child Language, 24,* 427–440.

Matheny, A. (1997). Infants' cognitive development: Trajectory and segue. *Monographs of the Society for Research in Child Development, 62*(1), 115–160.

Meisel, J. M. (1995). Parameters in acquisition. In P. Fletcher & B. MacWhinney (Eds.), *The handbook of child language* (pp. 10–35). Oxford: Blackwell Publishers.

Merriman, W. E., & Bowman, L. (1989). The mutual exclusivity bias in children's word learning. *Monographs of the Society for Research in Child Development, 54*, Serial no. 220.

Mervis, C. B., & Bertrand, J. (1995). Acquisition of the novel name-nameless category (N3C) principle by young children who have Down syndrome. American *Journal on Mental Retardation, 100*, 231–243.

Messer, D. J. (1994). *The development of communication: From social interaction to language.* Chichester, UK.: John Wiley & Sons.

Milenkovic, P. (1996). *CSpeech [Computer program to analyze acoustics of speech].* Madison, WI: Waisman Center, University of Wisconsin.

Miller, J. F. (1981). *Assessing language production in children: Experimental procedures.* Austin, TX: Pro-Ed.

Miller, J. F., & Chapman, R. S. (1982–1999). Systematic Analysis of Language Transcripts (SALT). [Computer software for IBM, Apple Macintosh, VAX/VMS, and Windows environments]. Madison, WI: Language Analysis Laboratory, University of Wisconsin.

Miller, J. F., Chapman, R. S., Branston, M., & Reichle, J. (1980). Language comprehension in sensorimotor stages V and VI. *Journal of Speech and Hearing Research, 23*, 284–311.

Mills, D. L., & Neville, H. J. (1997). Electrophysiological studies of language and language impairment. *Seminars in Pediatric Neurology, 4*, 125–134.

Montgomery, J. W. (1999). Recognition of gated words by children with specific language impairment: An examination of lexical mapping. *Journal of Speech, Language, and Hearing Research, 42*, 735–743.

Moore, C., & Dunham, P. J. (Eds.). (1995). *Joint attention: Its origins and role in development.* Hillsdale, NJ: Lawrence Erlbaum Associates.

Morgan, J. L., & Demuth, K. (Eds.). (1996). *Signal to syntax: Bootstrapping from speech to grammar in early acquisition.* Mahwah, NJ: Lawrence Erlbaum Associates.

Muller, R. A. (1996). Innateness, autonomy, universality? Neurobiological approaches to language. *Behavioral and Brain Sciences, 19*, 611–631.

Muller, R. A., Rothermel, R. D., Behen, M. E., Muzik, O., Mangner, T. J., & Chugani, H. T. (1998). Developmental changes of cortical and cerebellar motor control: A clinical positron emission tomography study with children and adults. *Journal of Child Neurology, 13*, 550–556.

Myers, J., Jusczyk, P. W., Kemler-Nelson, D. G., Charles Luce, J., Woodward, A. L., & Hirsh-Pasek, K. (1996). Infants' sensitivity to word boundaries in fluent speech. *Journal of Child Language, 23*, 1–30.

Naigles, L. R., & Hoff-Ginsberg, E. (1995). Input to verb learning: Evidence for the plausibility of syntactic bootstrapping. *Developmental Psychology, 31*, 827–837.

Nelson, K. A. (1973). Structure and strategy in learning to talk. Monographs of the Society for Research in Child Development, Serial no. 149.

Nelson, K. A. (Ed.). (1986). *Event knowledge: Structure and function in development.* Hillsdale, NJ: Lawrence Erlbaum Associates.

Nelson, K. A. (1996). *Language in cognitive development: The emergence of the mediated mind*. Cambridge: Cambridge University Press.

Nelson, K. E., Camarata, S. M., Welsh, J., Butkovsky, L., & Camarata, M. (1996). Effects of imitative and conversational recasting treatment on the acquisition of grammar in children with specific language impairment and younger language-normal children. *Journal of Speech and Hearing Research, 39*, 850–859.

Nelson, K. E., Welsh, J., Camarata, S. M., Butkovsky, L., & Camarata, M. (1995). Available input for language-impaired children and younger children of matched language levels. *First Language, 15*, 1–17.

Neville, H., & Bavelier, D. (1998). Neural organization and plasticity of language. *Current Opinion in Neurobiology, 8*, 254–258.

Ninio, A. (1980). Picture-book reading in mother-infant dyads belonging to two subgroups in Israel. *Child Development, 51*, 587–590.

Oller, D. K., Eilers, R. E., Urbano, R., & Cobo-Lewis, A. B. (1997). Development of precursors to speech in infants exposed to two languages. *Journal of Child Language, 24*, 407–126.

Owens, R. E., Jr. (1996). *Language development: An introduction*. Boston, MA: Allyn & Bacon.

Paul, R. (1995). *Language disorders from infancy through adolescence: Assessment and intervention*. St Louis, MO: Mosby-Year Book.

Piaget, J. (1954). *The construction of reality in the child*. New York: Basic Books.

Pine, J. (1994). Environmental correlates of variation in lexical style: Interactional style and the structure of the input. *Applied Psycholinguistics, 15*, 355–370.

Pinker, S. (1987). The bootstrapping problem in language acquisition. In B. MacWhinney (Ed.), *Mechanisms of language acquisition* (pp. 399–441). Hillsdale, NJ: Lawrence Erlbaum Associates.

Pinker, S. (1994). *The language instinct*. New York: William Morrow.

Plunkett, K., Karmilof Smith, A., Bates, E., Elman, J. L., & Johnson, M. H. (1997). Connectionism and developmental psychology. *Journal of Child Psychology and Psychiatry, 38*, 53–80.

Plunkett, K., & Marchman, V. (1993). From rote learning to system building: Acquiring verb morphology in children and connectionist nets. *Cognition, 48*, 21–69.

Price, C. J., Wise, R. J. S., Warburton, E. A., Moore, C. J., Howard, D., Patterson, K., Frackowiak, R. S. J., & Friston, K. J. (1996). Hearing and saying: The functional neuroanatomy of auditory word processing. *Brain, 119*, 919–931.

Pugh, K. R., Shaywitz, B. A., Shaywitz, S. E., Shankweiler, D. P., Katz, L., Fletcher, J. M., Skudlarski, P., Fulbright, R. K., Constable, R. T., Bronen, R. A., Lacadie, C., & Gore, J. C. (1997). Predicting reading performance from neuroimaging profiles: The cerebral basis of phonological effects in printed word identification. *Journal of Experimental Psychology: Human Perception and Performance, 23*, 299–318.

Pulvermuller, F. (1999). Words in the brain's language. *Behavioral and Brain Sciences, 22*, 253–279.

Reznick, J. S., Corley, R., & Robinson, J. (1997). A longitudinal twin study of intelligence in the second year. Monographs of the Society for Research in Child Development, Serial no. 249.

Rice, M. L. (Ed.). (1996). *Toward a genetics of language.* Mahwah, NJ: Lawrence Erlbaum Associates.

Rice, M. L., & Wexler, K. (1996a). Toward tense as a clinical marker of specific language impairment in English-speaking children. *Journal of Speech and Hearing Research, 39,* 1239–1257.

Rice, M. L., & Wexler, K. (1996b). A phenotype of specific language impairment: Extended optional infinitives. In M. L. Rice (Ed.), *Toward a genetics of language* (pp. 215–237). Mahwah, NJ: Lawrence Erlbaum Associates.

Saffran, J. R., Aslin, R. N., & Newport, E. L. (1996). Statistical learning by 8-month-old infants. *Science, 274,* 1926–1928.

Schwartz, R., & Leonard, L. B. (1982). Do children pick and choose? An examination of phonological selection and avoidance in early lexical acquisition. *Journal of Child Language, 9,* 319–336.

Schwartz, R., Leonard, L. B., Loeb, D., & Swanson, L. (1987). Attempted sounds are sometimes not: An expanded view of phonological selection and avoidance. *Journal of Child Language, 14,* 411–418.

Seidenberg, M. S. (1997). Language acquisition and use: Learning and applying probabilistic constraints. *Science, 275,* 1599–1603.

Semrud-Clikeman, M. (1997). Evidence from imaging on the relationship between brain structure and developmental language disorders. *Seminars in Pediatric Neurology, 4,* 117–124.

Shaywitz, S. E., Shaywitz, B. A., Pugh, K. R., Fulbright, R. K., Constable, R. T., Mencl, W. E., Shankweiler, D. P., Liberman, A. M., Skudlarski, P., Fletcher, J. M., Katz, L., Marchione, K. E., Lacadie, C., Gatenby, C., & Gore, J. C. (1998). Functional disruption in the organization of the brain for reading in dyslexia. *Proceedings of the National Academy of Sciences of the United States of America, 95,* 2636–2641.

Short-Meyerson, K. J., & Abbeduto, L. J. (1997). Preschoolers' communication during scripted interactions. *Journal of Child Language, 24,* 469–494.

Shriberg, L. D. (1986). *PEPPER: Programs to examine phonetic and phonologic evaluation records.* Hillsdale, NJ: Lawrence Erlbaum Associates.

Siegler, R. S. (1998). Foreword to Volume 2: Cognition, perception, and language. In W. Damon, D. Kuhn, & R. Siegler (Eds.), *The handbook of child psychology* (5th ed.), Vol. 2 (pp. xxi–xxiv). New York: John Wiley & Sons.

Slobin, D. (1981). The origins of grammatical encoding of events. *Behavioral Development: A Series of Monographs,* 185–199.

Slobin, D. (Ed.). (1985a). *The crosslinguistic study of language acquisition: Vol. 1.* The data. Hillsdale, NJ: Lawrence Erlbaum Associates.

Slobin, D. (Ed.). (1985b). *The crosslinguistic study of language acquisition: Vol. 2.* Theoretical issues. Hillsdale, NJ: Lawrence Erlbaum Associates.

Slobin, D. (Ed.). (1992). *The crosslinguistic study of language acquisition: Vol. 3.* Hillsdale, NJ: Lawrence Erlbaum Associates.

Slobin, D. (1997a). The origins of grammaticizable notions: Beyond the individual mind. In D. I. Slobin (Ed.), *The crosslinguistic study of language acquisition, Vol. 5: Expanding the contexts* (pp. 265–324). Mahwah, NJ: Lawrence Erlbaum Associates.

Slobin, D. (Ed.). (1997b). *The crosslinguistic study of language acquisition: Vol. 4.* Mahwah, NJ: Lawrence Erlbaum Associates.

Slobin, D. (Ed.). (1997c). *The crosslinguistic study of language acquisition, Vol. 5: Expanding the contexts.* Mahwah, NJ: Lawrence Erlbaum Associates.

Slobin, D., Gerhardt, J., Kyratzis, A., & Guo, J. (1996). *Social interaction, social context, and language: Essays in honor of Susan Ervin-Tripp.* Mahwah, NJ: Lawrence Erlbaum Associates.

Snow, C. (1995). Issues in the study of input: Finetuning, universality, individual and developmental differences, and necessary causes. In P. Fletcher & B. MacWhinney (Eds.), *The handbook of child language* (pp. 180–193). Oxford: Blackwell Publishers.

Snow, C., & Goldfield, B. A. (1983). Turn the page please: Situation-specific language acquisition. *Journal of Child Language, 10,* 551–569.

Sokolov, J. I., & Snow, C. E. (Eds.) (1994). *Handbook of research in language development using CHILDES.* Hillsdale, NJ: Lawrence Erlbaum Associates.

Stromswold, K. (1998). Genetics of spoken language disorders. *Human Biology, 70,* 297–324.

Swanson, L. A., & Leonard, L. B. (1994). Duration of functionword vowels in mothers' speech to young children. *Journal of Speech and Hearing Research, 37,* 1294–1405.

Tager-Flusberg, H. (Ed.). (1994). *Constraints on language acquisition: Studies of atypical children.* Hillsdale, NJ: Lawrence Erlbaum Associates.

Thal, D. J., Bates, E., Zappia, M. J., & Oroz, M. (1996). Ties between lexical and grammatical development: Evidence from early talkers. *Journal of Child Language, 23,* 349–368.

Thelen, E. (1995). Motor development: A new synthesis. *American Psychologist, 50,* 79–95.

Thelen, E., & Smith, L. B. (1994). *A dynamic systems approach to the development of cognition and action.* Cambridge, MA: MIT Press.

Thiabaut, J. P., Rondal, J. A., & Kaens, A. M. (1995). Actionality and mental imagery in children's comprehension of declaratives. *Journal of Child Language, 22,* 189–210.

Tomasello, M. (1992). *First verbs: A case study of early grammatical development.* Cambridge: Cambridge University Press.

Tomasello, M., Akhtar, N., Dodson, K., & Rekau, L. (1997). Differential productivity in young children's use of nouns and verbs. *Journal of* Child *Language, 24,* 373–388.

Tomasello, M., Mannle, S., & Kruger, A. (1986). Linguistic environment of 1- to 2-year-old twins. *Developmental Psy*chology, 22, 169–176.

Tomasello, M., & Merriman, W. E. (Eds.). (1995). *Beyond names for things: Young children's acquisition of verbs.* Hillsdale, NJ: Lawrence Erlbaum Associates.

Tomblin, J. B., & Buckwalter, P. R. (1998). Heritability of poor language achievement among twins. *Journal of Speech, Language, and Hearing Research, 41,* 188–199.

Tomblin, J. B., Records, N. L., Buckwalter, P., Zhang, X., Smith, E., & O'Brien, M. (1997). Prevalence of specific language impairment in kindergarten children. *Journal of Speech, Language, and Hearing Research, 40,* 1245–1260.

Tomblin, J. D., Shriberg, L., Nishimura, C., Zhang, X., & Murray, J. (1999). *Association of speck language impairment with loci at* 7q31. Poster presented at the Third International Symposium of Speech and Language Impairments: From Theory to Practice. York, UK, March.

van den Broek, P. W., Bauer, P. J., & Bourg, T. (1997). *Developmental spans in event comprehension and representation.* Mahwah, NJ: Lawrence Erlbaum Associates.

van der Lely, H. K. J., & Stollwerck, L. (1996). A grammatical specific language impairment in children: An autosomal dominant inheritance? *Brain and Language, 52,* 484–504.

Vygotsky, L. S. (1962). *Thought and language.* New York: Wiley.

Warren-Leubecker, A., & Bohannon, J. N. (1984). Intonation patterns in child-directed speech: Mother-father differences. Child *Development, 55,* 1379–1385.

Waxman, S. R., & Senghas, A. (1992). Relations among word meanings in early lexical development. *Developmental Psy*chology, *28,* 862–873.

Weist, R. M., Lyytinen, P., Wysocka, J., & Atanassova, M. (1997). The interaction of language and thought in children's language acquisition: A crosslinguistic study. *Journal of Child Language, 24,* 81–122.

Wells, G. (1985). *Language development in the pre-school years.* Cambridge: Cambridge University Press.

Wells, G., & Wells, J. (1984). Learning to talk and talking to learn. *Theory into Practice, 23,* 190–197.

Yoder, P., & Warren, S. (1998). Maternal responsivity predicts the prelinguistic communication intervention that facilitates generalized intentional communication. *Journal of Speech, Language, and Hearing Research, 41,* 1207–1219.

2

In the Mouths of Babes: Anatomic, Motor, and Sensory Foundations of Speech Development in Children

Ray D. Kent
Houri K. Vorperian
Waisman Center, University of Wisconsin-Madison

A central question in the understanding of speech development in children is: What is the nature of the perception–action linkage underlying speech and how is this linkage adapted to a child's changing abilities in perception, motor control, and language? By *perception–action* linkage we mean the association between auditory and visual perception and the motor patterns that serve the same behavioral goal or target. To some degree, perception and motor action can develop independently, but ultimately they are coordinated in the complex behavior of speech. The goal of this chapter is to present a model of the processes of perception-action linkage in early speech development. This model addresses especially three critical components: the auditory system, motor control of the vocal tract, and language exposure. The visual system is not covered to the same depth, but its contribution should not be neglected because speech can be seen as well as heard. Each of these components has its own intrinsic dynamics, owing to the normal processes of development, but it is the interaction among them that must be understood as a critical foundation for the development of spoken language. We proceed from the assumption that sensory-motor neural maps are established and refined during development, and it is in the mutual adaptation of these maps that the perception–action linkage of speech is found.

SENSORY MAPS

A sensory map is a neural representation of sensory information. Because the sensory map is shaped by cognitive and experiential factors, it is not necessarily a veridical representation of incoming stimuli. As suggested by Guenther, Husain, Cohen, and Shinn-Cunningham (1999), the auditory space will become distorted as it is reorganized during category learning. Sensory maps for speech sounds are built from several sources of information, but especially from the models of speech provided by adults and by a child's self-produced vocalizations. Similarly, Pierrehumbert (2003) proposed that perceptual categories "are initiated bottom-up from statistical modes in use of the phonetic space" (p. 115), and that this bottom-up initiation is effective due to the perception–production loop that operates in the speech community. The child confronts an immediate challenge in reconciling these two acoustically dissimilar sets of stimuli (self-produced and adult-produced) because of differences in length of the vocal tract. Infants and adults cannot produce exactly the same acoustic pattern, even for a sound that is judged to be phonetically similar. In short, the child's auditory map of speech must solve the speaker normalization problem, so that phonetically equivalent signals can be recognized even if they differ in acoustic properties such as formant frequencies for vowels and spectral concentrations for fricatives.

Development of Auditory Function—Behavioral Studies

The ear is functional by 5 months gestational age, but this precocious sensory ability does not necessarily mean that children have a fully mature auditory system. To the contrary, it appears that auditory function has a rather lengthy maturational process extending to at least the age of 12 years. This conclusion is based on developmental improvements in pure-tone thresholds (Maxon & Hochberg, 1982; Siegenthaler, 1969), intensity discrimination (Maxon & Hochberg, 1982), temporal resolution (Wightman, Allen, Dolan, Kistler, & Jamieson, 1989), frequency resolution (Allen, Wightman, Kistler, & Dolan, 1989; Maxon & Hochberg, 1982), backward masking (Hartley, Hill, & Moore, 2003), spectral pattern discrimination (Allen & Wightman, 1992) difference limens for formant frequency (Eguchi, 1976), and an auditory test battery that includes speech stimuli (Stollman, van Velzen, Simkens, Snik, & van den Broek, 2004). However, it has been suggested that developmental improvements in auditory function may reflect attentional or other aspects of processing rather than enhanced auditory resolution per se (Hartley et al., 2003; Wightman et al., 1989), and this is an important issue in interpreting developmental changes in auditory function. Hartley et al. (2003) suggested that differences in processing efficiency alone are sufficient to account for maturational differences. This interpretation is compatible with reports of large variability in children's auditory behavior. It seems that variations in attention are more likely to occur than variations in sensory resolution.

The protracted course of auditory maturation may seem to stand in contrast to the conclusions reached in studies of infant speech perception. These studies generally show that neonates are capable of distinguishing most of the acoustic contrasts used in the world's languages but that infants lose the sensitivity to some nonnative contrasts by the end of the first year of life (Werker & Pegg, 1992; Werker & Tees, 1984). These conclusions indicate that the auditory map for speech sounds is substantially reorganized in early infancy to support the perception of sounds in the ambient language. Following this reorganization, the auditory system undergoes progressive refinement.

Infants' auditory capability is sufficient to recognize phonetic detail in the production of familiar words (Swingley, 2003) and to support fast mapping (Chambers, Onishi, & Fisher, 2003; Saffran & Thiessen, 2003). The development of attentional allocation in infancy is relevant to understanding how certain sounds are preferred over others. Attentional preference for the mother's voice over unfamiliar women's voices is present by 4 months of age (Purhonen, Kilpelainen-Lees, Valkonen-Korhonen, Karhu, & Lehtonen, 2004), and infants at 11months of age are capable of shifting their attention to familiar words within 250 ms of their presentation (Thierry, Vihman, & Roberts, 2003). Data from functional magnetic resonance imaging (fMRI) experiments indicate a functional dichotomy in auditory cortical fields: (a) mesial fields that provide a highly veridical analysis of acoustic events, and (b) lateral fields that analyze sounds in terms of behavioral relevance (Petkov et al., 2004). The latter presumably would serve attentional processes. Conceivably, part of the maturational process in audition would be the effective selection of mesial versus lateral fields depending on experience and task. Consideration of these mechanisms might account for the observation that overhearing a second language in childhood facilitates pronunciation of that language when it is learned in adulthood (Knightley, Jun, Oh, & Au, 2003).

In summary, maturation of the auditory system extends until at least 12 years of age. It appears that an account of this protracted course of auditory development must consider not only refinements in sensory resolution but also the effect of attentional mechanisms. Possibly, the latter are more important than the former in explaining maturational changes in performance. The formation of sensory maps for speech sounds is strongly influenced by statistical patterns in heard speech (Anderson, Morgan, & White, 2003), and these influences account for a major degree of the reorganization of the auditory map that occurs developmentally.

Development of Auditory Function—Neural Correlates

Behavioral maturation in auditory function is related to neural maturation, and the latter is coming to be better understood. Moore (2002) studied the maturation of the human auditory cortex from midgestation to early adulthood by immunostaining axonal filaments. From these data, three developmental periods were identified: (a) A prenatal period characterized by maturation of axons only in the marginal layer; these axons drive the development of cells in deeper cortical layers but do not transmit external stimuli. (b) In early childhood (6 months to 5 years), afferent information from thalamocortical fibers to deeper cortical layers is the first cortical input from lower levels of the auditory system. (c) During later childhood (5 to 12 years), a greater complexity of cortical processing is enabled by the maturation of commissural and association axons in the superficial cortical layers. Language-related areas of the cortex may be the last to mature. Measurements of gray-matter density accomplished with MRI have shown that the posterior temporal cortices have a more protracted maturation than any other cortical region (Sowell et al., 2003).

Auditory–Visual Maps

Auditory–visual maps are neural representations of combined auditory and visual input. Audio–visual interaction is relevant here both because of studies that demonstrate an interaction between audition and vision and because speech information can by conveyed by parallel auditory and visual information. The McGurk effect is a well-known example of auditory–visual integration in speech. It is a phenomenon in which the perception of an auditory stimulus is altered by incongruent visual information on speech articulation (e.g., subjects usually report /da/ when they hear /ba/ but see a speaker's face saying /ga/). Because the McGurk effect has been demonstrated in 5-month-old infants (Rosenblum, Schmuckler, & Johnson, 1997), it seems not to require substantial experience with hearing and seeing speech. In this respect, it is perhaps similar to infant imitations of adult facial gestures, a seemingly precocious sensorimotor accomplishment (Meltzoff & Moore, 1977, 1983). The integration of auditory and visual information appears to involve different regions of the brain depending on which aspect of integration is at hand. Ventral areas are associated with audiovisual synchrony, whereas more dorsal areas are related to spatial multisensory interactions (Macaluso, George, Dolan, Spence, & Driver (2004).

Auditory–visual maps are not the only combined representation of sensory modalities. One can also conceive of auditory–kinesthetic or visual–kinesthetic maps. Because speech is associated with plurimodal afference, several kinds of sensory interaction are possible and may be related to the robustness of speech in the face of various kinds of feedback disruption (e.g., mandibular nerve blockade, superficial anesthesia, auditory masking, hearing loss). Auditory–visual maps are emphasized in this chapter because of their relevance to experimental paradigms such as the McGurk effect. It is likely that children construct speech-relevant auditory–visual maps through their experience in hearing and seeing speech produced by others.

Summary

The auditory system demonstrates a capacity for a relatively early adjustment to the phonetic properties of a child's language environment, so that by the time an infant is only a year old, there is a strong orientation to the ambient language. However, auditory resolution is refined over virtually all of childhood, apparently interacting with attentional systems. Auditory information is highly important to speech development, but it interacts with visual information, even at early stages of development. Maturational changes can be understood in terms of sensory maps that are reorganized with respect to patterns of auditory and visual information. Interaction between auditory and visual maps gives rise to auditory–visual maps that provide for the integration of sensory information. The task that remains is to reconcile these sensory maps with motor representations.

MOTOR MAPS

A motor map is a neural representation of motor control over a given system. Such a map can be adjusted developmentally in accord with the requirements for motor behaviors. The motor map for speech represents the control capabilities over the 100 or so muscles that are involved in speech production and the phonetic requirements of the language in question. These motor maps are constructed from knowledge of muscle activation patterns that generate sound and give shape to the vocal tract. The maps cannot be static because they must be adjusted to the growth and development of the speech production system, and to the possibility of learning another language. This system is complex not only in its variety of muscular components (i.e., the muscles of the respiratory, phonatory, and articulatory systems) but also in the remarkable variety of its muscle fiber types. The latter aspect of variety has only recently been documented in any detail and is reviewed later in this section.

Growth and Development of the Vocal Tract

The term *vocal tract* is an acoustic concept that incorporates all the oral and pharyngeal structures located superiorly to the laryngeal source. Therefore, a description on anatomic development of the vocal tract implies the examination of all the anatomic structures that constitute it. The vocal tract of the infant or child is not merely a miniature version of the adult vocal tract. Not only is there a threefold increase in vocal tract length from infancy to adulthood, but there is an accompanying change in its geometric proportions whereby the infant vocal tract resembles a single tube model that evolves into a the classic two-tube adult model after anatomic restructuring of the vocal tract is complete (Bosma, 1975, 1976, 1985; Crelin, 1973, 1976; Fant, 1960; Fried, Kelly, & Strome, 1982; Helmholtz, 1954; Kent, 1981; Kent & Vorperian, 1995; Laitman & Crelin, 1976; Lieberman, 1977, 1984). Understanding the progression of such anatomic reorganization is challenging because it appears that the different vocal tract structures have different growth rates or growth patterns such that adult sizes are achieved at different ages, ranging from about 7 to 18 years (Fitch & Giedd, 1999; Kent & Vorperian, 1995; Lieberman, McCarthy, Hiiemae, & Palmer, 2001). Of ultimate interest, however, is understanding the relational growth of the different structures for the purpose of understanding the biological foundation of speech, given that speech is produced within the physical constraints of the vocal tract structures (Kent, 1984; Lieberman, Klatt, & Wilson, 1969; Liberman, Laitman, Reidenberg, & Gannon, 1992). Such knowledge should help delineate the structural foundations of the motor control of the vocal tract (Vorperian, 2000; Vorperian et al., 2005). The young child has the task of learning to produce speech using an apparatus that is undergoing change. Two complex levels of anatomic development are addressed in this section on motor maps: macroanatomic and microanatomic, with the latter including molecular biology. The macroanatomic features are reviewed briefly in the following subsection.

Development of Vocal Tract Anatomy

The vocal tract is composed of a number of anatomic structures, both hard and soft tissue structures, in the oral and pharyngeal region. The structures typically included are the lips, anterior oral cavity (composed of the hard palate and the anterior portion of the tongue specifically the tongue tip and the blade), and posterior oral cavity (composed of the soft palate or velum, the posterior portion of the tongue or tongue dorsum, the oro-naso-pharynx, and the glottis). In addition, structures that are often discussed while addressing the anatomic restructuring of the vocal tract include the descents of the larynx, hyoid bone, epiglottis, and more recently mandibular length and depth (Lieberman et al. 2001; Sasaki, Levine, Laitman, & Crelin, 1977; Vorperian et al., 2005; Westhorpe, 1987).

As already noted, a concept that is inherent to the notion of anatomic restructuring is that different vocal tract structures have different growth rates or growth patterns where two-thirds of the mature adult size may be achieved early during childhood, or later, during adolescence. This is not surprising if one considers the fact that the vocal tract structures are housed in the head and neck region and thus have to follow the major growth pattern that the head follows (Farkas, Posnick, & Hreczko, 1992a, 1992b). The cranium follows the neural growth curve, which is characterized by a period of rapid growth from birth until some variable time in early childhood, where the structure reaches two-thirds of its adult size, followed by a period of very slow growth until maturity (Scammon, 1930). The face, on the other hand, follows the somatic growth curve, which is characterized again by a period of rapid growth during early childhood, but the structure in this period barely reaches over a quarter of its adult size; this is followed by a period of steady growth from early childhood until the age of maturity, where growth is predominantly slow, except during puberty, when the growth rate is more rapid (Scammon, 1930). Such differences in growth curves for proximal structures are possible because of the spheno-occipital synchondrosis (a cartilaginous growth center) at the base of the cranium or basicranium (Bosma, 1976; Crelin, 1973; Kent & Vorperian, 1995; Laitman & Crelin, 1976; Powell & Brodie, 1964). The development of vocal tract length appears to follows a combined neural and somatic growth curve, but its various structures appear to follow the neural, the somatic, or the combined neural and somatic growth curves depending on their orientation with respect to the cranium or the face (Lieberman et al., 2001; Vorperian et al., 2005). Thus, for example, the hard palate and mandibular length run parallel to the cranial base and appear to follow the neural growth curve, whereas laryngeal descent and pharyngeal length run parallel to the face and appears to follow the somatic growth curve.

The development of the vocal tract is due to the growth of each of its structures irrespective of type of growth curve. Although the literature generally suggests that vocal tract lengthening and anatomic restructuring are predominantly due to changes in the posterior region of the vocal tract, namely, the descent of the larynx, epiglottis, and tongue, recent findings indicate that, particularly before age 2 years, there is as much growth in the anterior or oral portion of the vocal tract as there is in the posterior or pharyngeal region of the vocal tract (Vorperian et al., 2005). This concept of anterior versus posterior growth is schematically presented in Fig. 2.1, which displays the growth, in a male subject from infancy to young childhood, of the length and depth of the mandible (top), the anterior and posterior portions of the tongue (middle), and the hard and soft palates (bottom). This figure also captures the earlier comment on the differences in the growth curves followed by different structures, including the different portions of a given structure (e.g., mandibular length vs. depth). Furthermore, this figure lends support to the notion of coordinated growth of select structures, specifically the mandible, the tongue, and the palate (Vorperian, Kent, Gentry, & Yandell, 1999). Whether there is coordinated growth of all functionally related structures, both hard and soft tissue structures, remains to be examined. Such findings will undoubtedly have significant implications toward our understanding of the nature of motor control of the vocal tract and the development of motor maps for speech production.

To conclude, the maturation of the infant and child vocal tract structures entails changes in size and shape as well as changes in the relational size and position of the different hard and soft tissue structures. Despite the differences in the growth trajectories of the different vocal tract tissues and the wide age range where the mature size is reached, there appears to be a trend of coordinated growth of functionally related structures. The extent of coordinated growth remains to be documented however. Such knowledge on the typical anatomic development of the speech apparatus will shape our understanding of speech motor control development.

Molecular Biology of Speech

Human craniofacial muscles are specialized in their genetic, developmental, functional, and phenotypical properties (Mootoosamy & Dietrich, 2002; Sciote, Horton, Rowlerson, & Link, 2003; Shuler & Dalrymple, 2001; Yu, Stål, Thornell, & Larson, 2002). As reviewed in Kent (2004a, 2004 b). The specialization of these muscles seems well adapted to the requirements of phonation and articulation. A major part of adaptation is the heterogeneity of muscle fiber types within and across craniofacial muscles. The myosin molecule, the primary motor protein, is composed of two heavy (MyHC) and two light chains (MyLC), which work together with adenosine triphosphate (ATPase) to determine the functional characteristics of the muscle fiber. Both MyHC and MyLC present different isoforms that can appear either as a single isoform in a fiber or as a coexpression of different forms (hybrid fibers). Individual craniofacial muscles often contain several muscle fiber types, including pure isoforms and hybrids. The combinations of fibers are different from those in limb and trunk muscles,

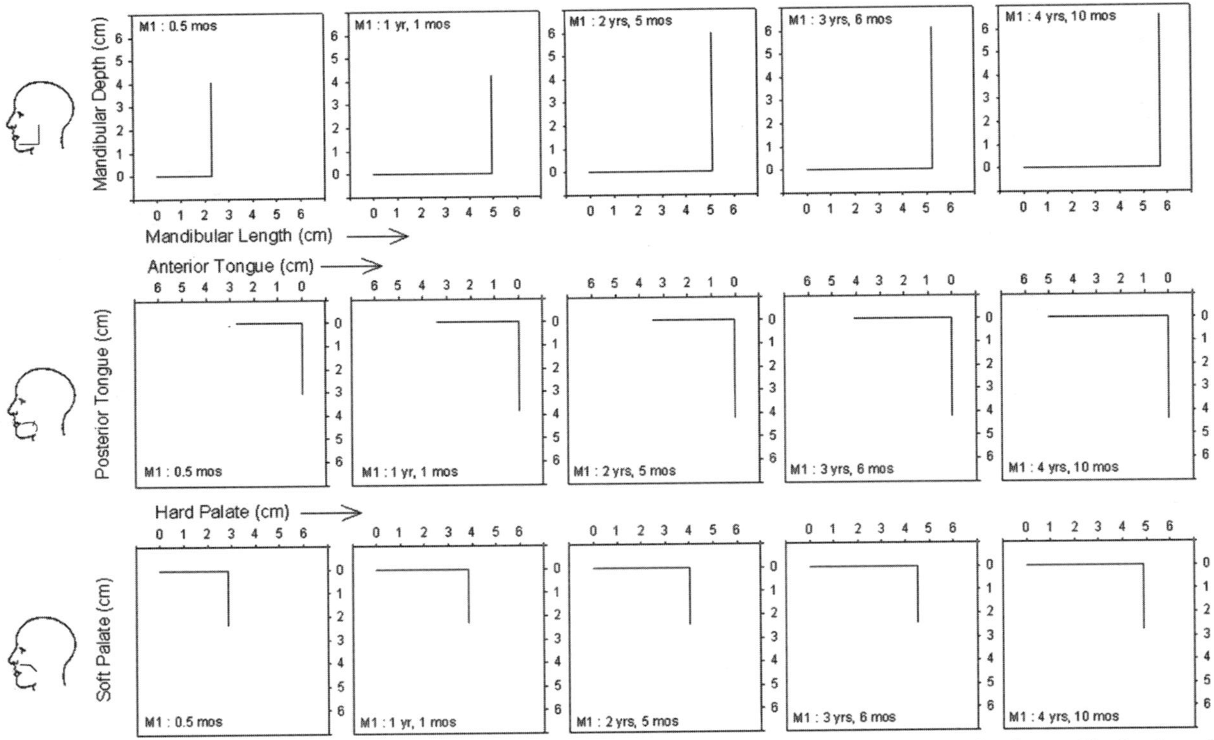

FIG. 2.1. Schematic representation of a male subject's growth, from infancy to young childhood, of mandibular length and depth (top row), the tongue (middle row), and the palates of a male (bottom row). The tongue was arbitrarily divided into an anterior or oral region and a posterior or pharyngeal region using the junction of the hard and soft palate as the dividing point. The development of mandibular length and hard palate length reflects a neural growth trajectory; mandibular depth and soft palate length a somatic growth trajectory; and the tongue a combined neural and somatic growth trajectory. Measurements were made from the magnetic resonance images of a male subject called M1. See text.

and sometimes different from those in homologous muscles in animals. The craniofacial muscles also differ from limb muscles with respect to muscle spindles, in both their form and their distribution. Muscle spindles are situated within the belly of muscles and run in parallel with the main muscle fibers. The spindle senses muscle length and changes in length. Sensory nerve terminals in the spindle increase their discharge rate as the sensory ending is stretched.

Table 2.1 summarizes several craniofacial muscles with respect to their general functional properties, muscle fiber types, and presence of muscle spindles. Human craniofacial muscles are quite different from limb and trunk muscles, and the differences are relevant in understanding how these muscles perform their specialized roles, how they develop, and how they respond to use and to aging.

The growing information on muscle fibers and muscle spindles contributes to a view of speech production that invites reappraisal of the proposition that "speech is special." Traditionally, this proposition has been examined with respect to speech perception (Liberman, 1998; Liberman & Mattingly, 1985), gross anatomy of the vocal tract (Lieberman, 1984), or behaviors such as vocal imitation (Hauser, Chomsky, & Fitch, 2002). Molecular biology has been considered less frequently as a way of informing the "speech is special" argument. There is mounting evidence that human craniofacial muscles (a) are distinct from human trunk and limb muscles, (b) can differ from homologous muscles in animals, including primates, (c) frequently differ from one another in ways that relate to function, and (d) are heterogeneous along their lengths, bellies, or zones (Kent, 2004a, in press-b). What this means for understanding children's speech development is that the craniofacial muscles are perhaps uniquely adapted to phonation and articulation. The complexity of this system at the level of molecular biology may be one key to unlocking the human capacity for the production of complex vocal sequences.

Development of Speech Motor Function

It is often assumed that the motor patterns for speech are derived from those for chewing and swallowing. The frame-then-content theory of MacNeilage and Davis (2000, 2001) is one of the most recent formal theories to build on this idea. However, there is contrary evidence, especially from studies showing task specificity in infants for movements in speech, chewing, and lip protrusion (Moore & Ruark, 1996; Ruark & Moore, 1997). These studies indicate there is an early distinction between speech-like movements and the movements for nonspeech behaviors. If, in fact, speech proceeds from a distinct motor substrate, then the development of speech motor control is better viewed as occurring in parallel with the develop-

TABLE 2.1
Summary of Craniofacial Muscle Groups, Their Fiber Types, and Their Spindle-Type Receptors

Muscle Group—Comments	*Muscle Fiber Types*	*Muscle Spindles*
Masticatory muscles—jaw elevators; these muscles operate on the only bilateral hinge joint in the human body and they serve spatial as well as mechanical goals (Koolstra, 2002).	Large proportion of hybrid muscle fibers, with up to five different MyHC isoforms in the same fiber (Korphage, Brugman, & Van Euden, 2000; Sciote, Rowlerson, Hopper, & Hunt, 1994; Yu et al., 2002).	Present in masseter, temporalis, and internal pterygoid (Korphage et al., 2000; Kubota & Masegi, 1977; Ericksson & Thornell, 1987); large number of spindles in deep portion of masseter, associated with type I muscle fibers (Ericksson & Thornell, 1987).
Masticatory muscles—jaw depressors; see comments for jaw elevators.	Compared to elevators, fewer hybrid fibers and fewer fibers expressing MyHC-I, MyHC-fetal & MyHC-cardiac alpha; but more fibers expressing MyHC-IIA (Korphage et al, 2000).	Small number in external pterygoid (arguably a depressor).
Lingual muscles—anterior; these muscles are capable of producing fast and flexible movements; best modeled as a muscular hydrostat (Hiiemae & Palmer, 2003).	Predominance of small type IIA fibers (Stål, Marklund, Thornell, De Paul, & Erickson, 2003).	Present in intrinsic and extrinsic muscles (Kubota, Negishi, & Masegi, 1975).
Lingual muscles—intrinsic; see comments for lingual muscles—anterior.	Combination of type I, IIA, and IM/IIC fibers in longitudinal, vertical, and transverse muscles, which are likely innervated in discrete regions by separate branches of the lingual nerve (Stål et al., 2003).	Present in intrinsic and extrinsic muscles (Kubota et al., 1975).

(continued on next page)

TABLE 2.1 *(continued)*

Muscle Group—Comments	*Muscle Fiber Types*	*Muscle Spindles*
Lingual muscles—posterior	Predominance of large type I and type IM/IIC fibers (Stål et al., 2003).	Present in intrinsic and extrinsic muscles (Kubota et al., 1975).
Labial muscles.	Predominance of type IIA fibers (Stål et al., 1990).	Absence of spindles in perioral tissues (Stål et al., 1990).
Palatal muscles—elevators.	Predominance of type I fibers (Stål & Lindman, 2000).	Present in tensor veli palatini (Kuehn, Templeton, & Maynard, 1990) and levator veli palatini (Liss, 1990).
Palatal muscles—depressors.	Predominance of type II fibers (some of the highest proportions ever observed in human muscle) (Stal & Lindman, 2000).	Present in palatoglossus (Kuehn et al., 1990; Liss, 1990).
Laryngeal muscles—adductors; thyroarytenoid (TA) and lateral cricoarytenoid (LCA).	Predominance of fast-type MyHCs and slow tonic muscle fibers; hybrid fibers commonly present (D'Antona et al., 2002; Li, Lehar, Nakagawa, Hoh, & Flint, 2004; Sciote, Morris, Brandon, Horton, & Rosen, 2002; Shiotani et al., 1999).	Present in all muscles (Baken & Noback, 1971); abundant in superior medial quadrant of thyroarytenoid (Shiotani, Westra, & Flint, 1999); sparse or absent in other compartments of this muscle (Tellis et al., 2004).
Laryngeal muscles—adductors: interarytenoids (IA)	Type I and types IIA and IIX (Tellis et al., 2004).	Present (Tellis et al., 2004).
Laryngeal muscles—abductor: posterior cricoarytenoid (PCA).	Abundance of mixed fast–slow type MyHCs (Shiotani et al., 1999); IIA and slow MyHCs present (Li et al., 2004); 4:1 ratio of Type I to Type II in horizontal belly but nearly equal proportion in vertical belly (Brandon et al., 2003).	Present (Grim, 1967).

ment of nonspeech motor functions, rather than derivative from those functions. This issue awaits further research for a definitive answer. But supporting data come from a study of mouth asymmetry in babies aged between 5 and 12 months (Holowka & Pettito, 2002). It was determined that the degree of mouth asymmetry differed among babbles, nonbabbles, and smiles, with the strongest right mouth asymmetry being observed for babbles. Assuming that the right mouth asymmetry reflects a dominant motor control by the left hemisphere, it follows that babbling reflects a different neural organization than nonbabble or smiling.

Phonemic mastery is one measure of speech maturation. It is typically judged by a statistical criterion, such as 75% correct production of a given sound. By this index, speech maturation continues until 7 or 8 years for most children (Sander, 1972; Smit, Hand, Frelinger, Bernthal, & Byrd, 1990). However, acoustic and physiologic measures demonstrate that motor refinements for speech continue until at least puberty (Kent & Forner, 1980) and perhaps to as late as 16 years of age in both boys and girls (Smith & Goffman, 2004). Even by a conservative criterion, the maturation of speech as a motor skill requires at least 12 years, despite the fact that speech is one of the most frequently practiced motor skills in the child's repertoire. Smith and Goffman (2004, p. 204) commented that "the late maturation of articulatory motor processes is driven primarily by interaction of speech motor systems with co-developing cognitive-linguistic systems, which are also not adult-like until this late period of development."

Summary

The maturation of speech motor control is a protracted process that continues until at least the age of puberty and perhaps well into adolescence. This process is likely multifactorial in its character, reflecting the way in which motor functions are tied to macro- and microanatomic changes, sensory refinements, and language development. Some basic questions about speech motor development await a definitive answer. Particularly important is whether speech motor control is derived from nonspeech functions such as chewing and swallowing, or whether speech motor control takes its own course early in development. A clearer picture of speech development is likely to emerge as work continues on the anatomy and molecular biology of speech, speech motor control in children and adults, and acoustic–phonetic studies of speech maturation.

SENSORIMOTOR MAPS

Sensory and motor maps must be connected if they are to be unified to achieve the goal of perception–action linkage. The connection can be accomplished in different ways, including neuronal mirror neurons, combination maps, global maps, and internal models. Possibly, all of these participate in a lifelong process in which humans continuously adapt to changing sensory information and motor capabilities.

Mirror Neurons

The name *mirror neurons* was first given to neurons in the rostral part of monkey inferior area 6 (area F5). These neurons were observed to discharge during active movements of the hand, mouth, or both (Kurata & Tanji, 1986; Rizzolatti et al., 1988), but they also discharged when the monkey observed the experimenter performing a comparable action (Fadiga, Fogassi, Gallese, & Rizzolatti, 2000; Rizzolatti, Fadiga, Gallese, & Fogassi, 1996). Rizzolatti and Arbib (1998) concluded, "These neurons (mirror neurons) appear to represent a system that matches observed events to similar, internally generated actions, and in this way forms a link between the observer and the actor" (p. 152). Neurons in visual cortex are of several different types, as shown in Fig. 2.2 (see Rizzolatti & Craighero, 2004, for an excellent summary of the mirror-neuron system). Canonical neurons respond to the presentation of objects, whereas mirror neurons respond to object-related actions. Within the general class of visuomotor mirror neurons, a subclass that holds particular relevance to speech is mouth mirror neurons, which respond in both seeing mouth movements and performing those move-

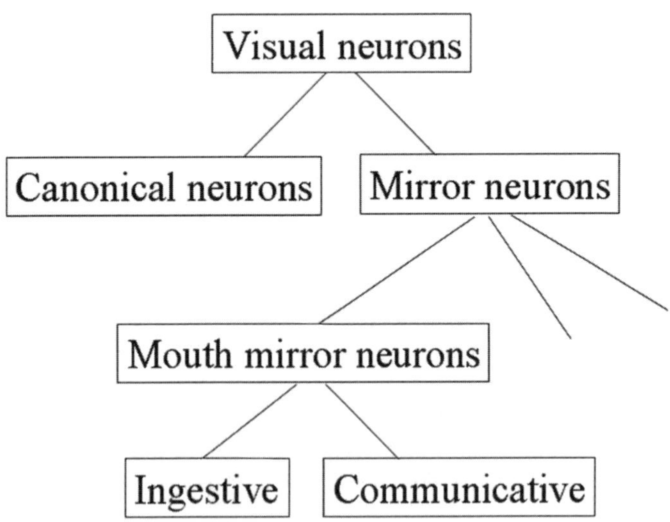

FIG. 2.2. Types of neurons in visual cortex. Ingestive and communicative neurons are subtypes of mouth mirror neurons.

ments. Mouth mirror neurons are of two types, ingestive (which respond to the observation of actions related to food intake) and communicative (which respond to the observation of communicative gestures such as lip smacking). The potential relevance of communicative mouth mirror neurons to learning speech is obvious, assuming, of course, that mirror neurons are found in humans (discussed later in this section). A conception of auditory neurons might be as shown in Fig. 2.3. Canonical neurons respond to hearing a particular environmental sound, whereas mirror neurons respond both to hearing a sound produced by an action and to actually producing that sound. Echo neurons respond in a kind of motoric resonance when an individual listens to verbal material. These neurons are discussed in more detail in the following consideration of evidence for mirror neurons and echo neurons in humans.

Evidence for mirror neuron systems in humans has come from studies using transcranial magnetic stimulation (Fadiga, Fogassi, Pavesi, & Rizzolatti, 1995), positron emission tomography (Grafton, Arbib, Fadiga, & Rizzolatti, 1996; Rizzolatti, Fadiga, Gallese, & Fogassi, 1996; Rizzolatti, Fadiga, Matelli, Bettinardi, Paulesu, Perani, & Fazio, 1996), functional magnetic resonance imaging (Binkofski et al., 2000), and neuromagnetic recordings (Jarvelainen, Schurmann, Avikainen, & Hari, 2001; Nishitani, & Hari, 2000). Broca's area appears to be part of this system (Buccino, Binkovski, & Riggio, 2004; Hamzei et al., 2003; Nishitani & Hari, 2000). It also has been demonstrated with electroencephalographic recording (EEG) during finger movements that observation and execution of movement share the same cortical network (Cochin, Barthelmy, Roux, & Martineau, 1999). Wohlschlager and Bekkering (2002) concluded that "imitation emerged from C, the mirror-neurone system of the common ancestor of monkeys and humans" (p. 335).

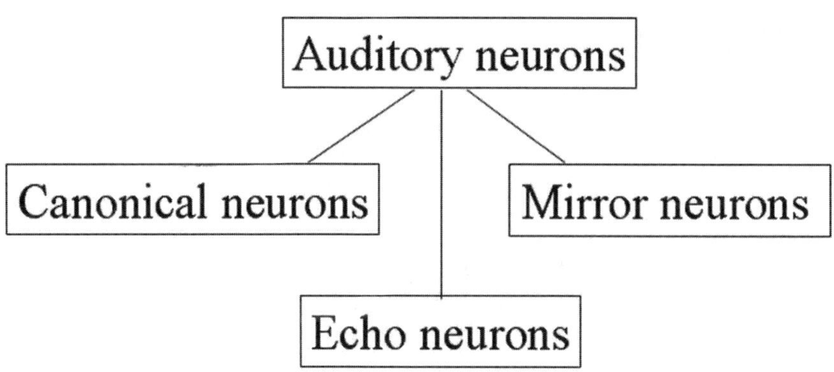

FIG. 2.3. Types of neurons in auditory cortex.

As noted earlier, echo neurons respond in a kind of motoric resonance when an individual listens to verbal material (Rizzolatti & Craighero, 2004). Evidence for an echo-neuron system in humans has been reported by Fadiga et al. (2002) and Watkins, Strafella, and Paus (2003). Briefly, these studies demonstrated that speech-related motor areas are activated when a subject listens to verbal stimuli. This is a type of action–perception linkage. In the case of speech, it would be particularly important to demonstrate that mirror neurons connect action with both visual and auditory patterns. Such appears to be the case. Keysers et al. (2003) described a population of neurons in the preventral motor cortex of monkey that discharge both when the animal performs an action and when it hears or sees that action performed by another individual. These neurons, termed *audiovisual mirror neurons,* could be the neural substrate by which motor actions are associated with auditory and visual information. Furthermore, mirror neurons may be particularly tuned to communicative functions. Studies in monkey have shown that the most effective visual stimuli for mouth mirror neurons are communicative mouth gestures (Ferrari, Gallese, Rizzolatti, & Fogassi, 2003).

As a final comment, it should be noted that there are no reports of single-neuron recordings from supposed mirror-neuron areas in humans. Therefore, the evidence for mirror neurons is only indirect at this time.

One way of explaining the coexistence of motor and sensory properties in the same neurons is that the motor system is responsible not only for executing actions but also for the internal representation (Fadiga et al., 2000). The specificity of this representation is becoming clear. Jarvelainen et al. (2001) reported that the mirror neuron system in humans differentiates natural (live) as opposed to artificially presented (videotaped) movements. There is evidence that common neural resources are deployed for observing, imagining, and performing a movement. Studies have shown that motor imagery and motor performance have similar neural substrates (Binkofski et al., 2000; Grafton et al., 1996; Kosslyn, Ganis, & Thompson, 2001; Lotze et al., 1999). The shared neural resources for these different tasks lend unity and efficiency to motor behavior.

Evidence for Sensorimotor Maps in Speech

When does auditory input begin to influence patterns in infants' sound productions? An answer to this question would help to establish when auditory maps are first formed and how they develop with experience. Experiments involving short-term exposure to audiovisual vowel stimuli indicate an influence of sensory input by the age of 12 weeks (Kuhl & Meltzoff, 1996). Similarly, experiments using social shaping demonstrate that 8-month-old infants alter their babbling patterns in response to contingent maternal behavior (Goldstein, King, & West, 2003). Supporting data come from studies that determine the effect of hearing impairment on infant vocalizations. These studies show that sound productions of hearing-impaired infants differ from those of normal-hearing infants by the age of 8 to 10 months of life (Kent, Netsell, Osberger, & Hustedde, 1987; Oller & Eilers, 1988; Stoel-Gammon & Otomo, 1986).

Another type of evidence for auditory–motor interaction is the influence of the ambient language on phonetic patterns in babbling and other early vocalizations. However, the evidence is not easily interpreted. One set of reports indicates a relatively early effect of ambient language on infant sound productions. In various studies, these early effects were noted by 2 months (Ruzza, Rocca, Boero, & Lenti, 2003), 6 months (Boysson-Bardies, Sagart, & Durand, 1984), 9 months (Boysson-Bardies et al., 1992), 10 months (Boysson-Bardies, Halle, Sagart, & Durand, 1989; Boysson-Bardies, Sagart, Halle, & Durand, 1986), and 12 months (Chen & Kent, 2005). In contrast, another set of studies found no reliable auditory classification by ambient language even by the ages of 17 or 18 months (Atkinson, MacWhinney, & Stoel, 1968; Engstrand, Williams, & Lacerda, 2003). Despite the variance in results, it seems reasonable to conclude that some aspects of infant sound production can be affected by auditory input by the age of at least 8 months. This can be taken as the age by which some kind of auditory-motor map is established, at least in some general form.

Hickok and Poeppel (2004) proposed that the early stages of speech perception are located in auditory fields in the superior temporal gyrus bilaterally (although not necessarily symmetrically). The system then diverges into ventral and dorsal streams. The ventral stream maps sound onto meaning, and the dorsal stream maps sound onto articulatory-based representations (i.e., an auditory–motor map).

If speech is served by mirror neurons, then we would expect to find one or more neural areas that are activated both by hearing a speech pattern, by seeing the associated facial movements, by producing that pattern as a motor act, or even by imagining the pattern. This possibility is supported by a number of studies showing action–perception linkages. For example, listening to speech specifically modulates the excitability of tongue muscles (Fadiga, Craighero, Buccino, & Rizzollatti, 2002), Brodmann areas 44 and 45 (supposedly speech production regions) are bilaterally activated during the observation of silent speech (Campbell, 1998; Campbell et al., 2001; Ryding, Bradvik, & Ingvar, 1996), and listening to speech activates cortical regions associated with speech production (Wilson, Saygin, Sereno, & Iacoboni, 2004).

Summary

Sensorimotor maps are proposed as a critical substrate for perception–action linkage. These maps, once an abstract conception, are coming to a more definitive reality though investigations of mirror neurons. Although much remains to be done to demonstrate that humans actually have mirror neurons, converging evidence points promisingly in that direction. It is clearly the case that speech is associated with action–perception linkages, and these linkages are important to understanding the development of speech in children. A main argument of this section is that mirror neurons would guide the establishment of a system that yokes speech perception and speech production, very likely in the formation of internal models that represent speech motor capability and its sensory consequences.

IMPLICATIONS FOR SPEECH DEVELOPMENT

Chapman (2000) has advanced an interactionist perspective of language development in which language learning is viewed as an integration of learning in multiple domains. In similar fashion, speech development can be viewed as an integration of sensorimotor processes. A critical pairing is the relationship between motor act and its sensory consequence. The development coupling between speech motor processes and their sensory consequences has been modeled by Callan, Kent, Guenther, and Vorperian (2000) and by Westerman and Miranda (2004). Both of these efforts proceed from the babbling stage of development and demonstrate how sensorimotor coupling can foster the development of speech. Figure 2.4 is a simplified model

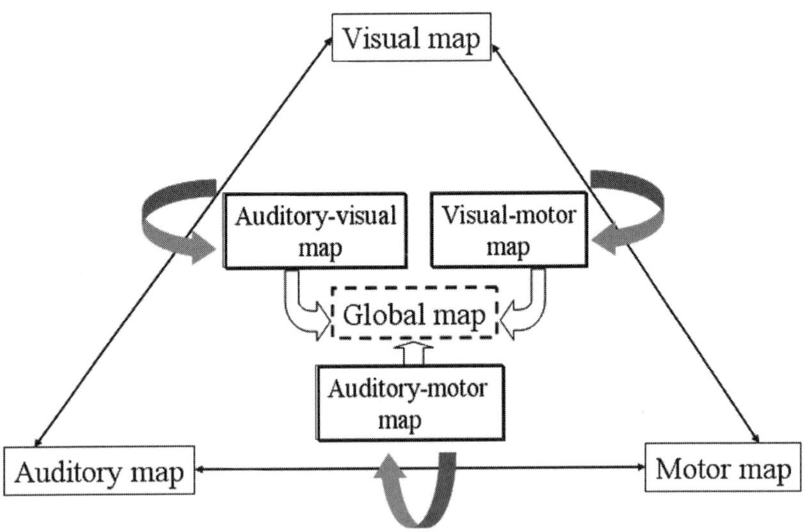

FIG. 2.4. Model of single maps, combination maps, and global maps that could contribute to speech development. See text.

of sensory and motor maps in speech production. The connection between the auditory map and motor map would include mirror neurons that assist a child in learning the associations between speech sounds and their underlying motor patterns. Miall (2003) suggests that mirror neurons serve as a general guide to motor performance, meaning that they do not provide the kind of specificity needed to perform highly accurate motor control. Greater accuracy can be achieved though other mechanisms, such as internal models. But it should be noted that mirror neurons vary in the degree of congruence between perceived action and motor response. Gallese et al. (1996) classified mirror neurons into "strictly congruent" and "broadly congruent." The former have a high correspondence between observed and executed actions, sharing, for example, the goal and the means for achieving that goal. In contrast, "broadly congruent" mirror neurons have a weaker correspondence between observed and executed actions. We might conjecture that both kinds of mirror neurons may contribute to speech development, with the broadly congruent types helping to establish general relationships and the strictly congruent types leading to more specific linkages.

Mirror neurons may have an important developmental function in that they could establish initial action–perception linkages that would be subject to refinement through experience and practice. In this way, the auditory–motor map for speech would be modified so that it can provide the kind of specificity required by internal models. With reference to Fig. 2.3, mirror neurons can be thought to operate on the lines forming the triangle (i.e., on the lines connecting auditory map with motor map, auditory map with visual map, and visual map with motor map). The perception–motion linkages and perception–perception linkages developed by these mirror neurons would facilitate the formation of the auditory–motor, visual–motor, and auditory–visual maps shown within the triangle. The global map shown in the center represents a convergence of all three combination maps and therefore reflects a high degree of sensorimotor integration.

CONCLUSION

Speech development in children draws on a number of anatomic, motor, sensory, and cognitive resources. Ultimately, these various factors need to be integrated to account for a child's progress toward the faculty of speech. This chapter has described some of the foundation stones on which a biological model of speech development can be constructed. Although the data are incomplete in many areas, recent advances hold the promise of a biological model that is relevant to the study of both typical and atypical speech development. The challenge is to synthesize the various types of information into a model that summarizes the typical developmental course and affords an understanding of the atypical patterns seen in children's speech disorders.

ACKNOWLEDGMENTS

This work was supported in part by NIDCD Research Grants R03 DC4362 (Anatomic Development of the Vocal Tract: MRI Procedures), R01 DC6282 (MRI and CT Studies of the Developing Vocal Tract), and R01 DC00319 (Intelligibility Studies of Dysarthria).

We thank Reid Durtschi for assistance with graph preparation.

REFERENCES

Allen, P., & Wightman, F. (1992). Spectral pattern discrimination by children. *Journal of Speech and Hearing Research, 35,* 222–233.

Allen, P., Wightman, F., Kistler, D., & Dolan, T. (1989). Frequency resolution in children. *Journal of Speech and Hearing Research, 32,* 317–322.

Anderson, J. L., Morgan, J. L., & White, K. S. (2003). A statistical basis for speech sound discrimination. *Language & Speech, 46,* 155–182.

Atkinson, K., MacWhinney, B., & Stoel, C. (1968). *An experiment on the recognition of babbling*. Language Behavior Research Laboratory Working Paper, University of California, Berkeley.

Baken, R. J., & Noback, C. R. (1971). Neuromuscular spindles in intrinsic muscles of a human larynx. *Journal of Speech and Hearing Research, 14,* 513–518.

Binkofski, F., Amunts, K., Stephan, K. M., Posse, S., Schormann, T., Freund, H. J., Zilles, K., & Seitz, R. J. (2000). Broca's region subserves imagery of motion: A combined cytoarchitectonic and fMRI study. *Human Brain Mapping, 11,* 273–285.

Bosma, J. F. (1975). Anatomic and physiologic development of the speech apparatus. In D. B. Tower (Ed.), *The nervous system: Human communication and its disorders* (pp. 469–481). New York: Raven Press.

Bosma, J. F. (1976). Disussion of the paper, "Postnatal development of the basicranium and vocal tract in man" by J. T. Laitman & E. S. Crelin. In J. Bosma (Ed.), *Symposium on the development of the basicranium* (pp. 219–220). Bethesda, MD: DHEW Publication No. 76–989, PHS-NIH.

Bosma, J. F. (1985). Postnatal ontogeny of performance of the pharynx, larynx, and mouth. *American Review of Respiratory Disease, 131,* S10–S15.

Boysson-Bardies, B., Halle, P., Sagart, L., & Durand, C. (1989). A crosslinguistic investigation of vowel formants in babbling. *Journal of Child Language, 16,* 1–18.

Boysson-Bardies, B., Sagart, L., & Durand, C. (1984). Discernible differences in the babbling of infants according to target language. *Journal of Child Language, 11,* 1–15.

Boysson-Bardies, B., Sagart, L., Halle, P., & Durand, C. (1986). Acoustic investigation of crosslinguistic variability in babbling. In B. Lindblom & R. Zetterstrom (Eds.), *Precursors of early speech* (pp. 113–126). New York: Stockton Press.

Boysson-Bardies, B., Vihman, M. M., Roug-Hellichius, L., Durand, C., Landberg, I., & Arao, F. (1992). Material evidence of infant selection from the target language:

a cross-linguistic phonetic study. In C. Ferguson, L. Menn, & C. Stoel-Gammon (Eds.), *Phonological development: Models, research, implications* (pp. 369–391). Timonium, MD: York Press.

Brandon, C. A., Rosen, C., Georgelis, G., Horton, J. J., Mooney, M. P., & Sciote, J. J. (2003). Muscle fiber type composition and effects of vocal fold immobilization on the two compartments of the human posterior cricoarytenoid: A case study of four patients. *Journal of Voice, 17,* 63–75.

Buccino, G., Binkofski, F., & Riggio, L. (2004). The mirror neuron system and action recognition. *Brain & Language, 89,* 370–376.

Callan, D. E., Kent, R. D., Guenther, F. H., & Vorperian, H. K. (2000). An auditory-feedback-based neural network model of speech production that is robust to developmental changes in the size and shape of the articulatory system. *Journal of Speech, Language, & Hearing Research, 43,* 721–736.

Campbell, R. (1998). Speech reading: Advances in understanding its cortical bases and implications for deafness and speech rehabilitation. *Scandinavian Audiology, 27,* 80–86.

Campbell, R., MacSweeney, M., Surguladze, S., Calvert, G., McGuire, P., Suckling, J., Brammer, M. J., & David, A. S. (2001). Cortical substrates for the perception of face actions: An fMRI study of the specificity of activation for seen speech and for meaningless lower-face acts (gurning). *Cognitive Brain Research, 12,* 233–243.

Chambers, K. E., Onishi, K. H., & Fisher, C. (2003). Infants learn phonotactic regularities from brief auditory experience. *Cognition, 87,* B69–B77.

Chapman, R. S. (2000). Children's language learning: an interactionist perspective. *Journal of Child Psychology & Psychiatry, 41,* 33–54.

Chen, L.-M., & Kent, R. D. (2005). Consonant–vowel co-occurrence patterns in Mandarin-learning infants. *Journal of Child Language, 32,* 507–534.

Cochin, S., Barthelmy, C., Roux, S., & Martineau, J. (1999). Observation and execution of movement: similarities demonstrated by quantified electroencephalography. *European Journal of Neuroscience, 11,* 1839–1842.

Crelin, E. S. (1973). *Functional anatomy of the newborn.* New Haven, CT: Yale University Press.

Crelin, E. S. (1976). Development of the upper respiratory system. *Clinical Symposia, 28,* 1–30.

D'Antona, G., Megighian, A., Bortolotto, S., Pellegrino, M. A., Marchese-Ragona, R., Staffieri, A., Bottinelli, R., & Reggiani, C. (2002). Contractile properties and myosin heavy chain isoform composition in single fibre of human laryngeal muscles. *Journal of Muscle Research and Cell Motility, 23,* 187–195.

Eguchi, S. (1976). Difference limens for the formant frequencies: normal adult values and their development in children. *Journal of the American Audiology Society, 1,* 145–149.

Engstrand, O., Williams, K., & Lacerda, F. (2003). Does babbling sound native? Listener responses to vocalizations produced by Swedish and American 12- and 18-month-olds. *Phonetica, 60,* 17–44.

Erickson, P., & Thornell, L. (1987). Relation of extra-fusal fiber type to muscle spindle structure and location in the human masseter muscle. *Archives of Oral Biology, 32,* 483–491.

Fadiga, L., Buccino, G., Craighero, L., Fadiga, L., Craighero, L., Buccino, G., & Rizzolatti, G. (2002). Speech listening specifically modulates the excitability of tongue muscles: A TMS study. *European Journal of Neuroscience, 15,* 399–402.

Fadiga, L., Fogassi, L., Gallese, V., & Rizzolatti, G. (2000). Visuomotor neurons: Ambiguity of the discharge or "motor" perception? *International Journal of Psychophysiology, 35,* 165–177.

Fadiga, L., Fogassi, L., Pavesi, G., & Rizzolatti, G. (1995). Motor facilitation during action observation: A magnetic stimulation study. *Journal of Neurophysiology, 73,* 2608–2611.

Fant, G. (1960). *Acoustic theory of speech production.* The Hague: Mouton.

Farkas, L. G., Posnick, J. C., & Hreczko, T. M. (1992a). Anthropometric growth study of the head. *Cleft Palate-Craniofacial Journal, 29,* 303–308.

Farkas, L. G., Posnick, J. C., & Hreczko, T. M. (1992b). Growth and development of regional units in the head and face based on anthropometric measurements. *Cleft Palate-Craniofacial Journal, 29,* 301–302.

Ferrari, P. F., Gallese, V., Rizzolatti, G., & Fogassi, L. (2003). Mirror neurons responding to observation of ingestive and communicative mouth actions in the monkey ventral premotor cortex. *European Journal of Neuroscience, 17,* 1703–1714.

Fitch, W. T., & Giedd, J. (1999). Morphology and development of the human vocal tract: A study using magnetic resonance imaging. *Journal of the Acoustical Society of America, 106,* 1511–1522.

Fried, M. P., Kelly, J. H., & Strome, M. (1982). Comparison of the adult and infant larynx. *Journal of Family Practice, 15,* 557–561.

Gallese, V., Fadiga, L., Fogassi, L., & Rozolatti, G. (1996). Action recognition in the premotor cortex. *Brain, 19,* 593–609.

Goldstein, M. H., King, A. P., & West, M. J. (2003). Social interaction shapes babbling: testing parallels between birdsong and speech. *Proceedings of the National Academy of Sciences, 100, USA,* 8030–8035.

Grafton, S. T., Arbib, M. A., Fadiga, L., & Rizzolatti, G. (1996). Localization of grasp representations in humans by positron emission tomography. 2: Observation compared with imagination. *Experimental Brain Research, 112,* 103–111.

Grim, M. (1967). Muscle spindles in the posterior cricoarytenoid muscle. *Folia Morphologica, 15,* 124–131.

Guenther, F. H., Husain, F. T., Cohen, M. A., & Shinn-Cunningham, B. G. (1999). Effects of categorization and discrimination on auditory perceptual space. *Journal of the Acoustical Society of America, 106,* 2900–2912.

Hamzei, F., Rijntjes, M., Dettmers, C., Glauche, V., Weiller, C., & Buchel, C. (2003). The human action recognition system and its relationship to Broca's area: An fMRI study. *Neuroimage, 19,* 637–644.

Hartley, D. E., Hill, P. R., & Moore, D. R. (2003). The auditory basis of language impairments: Temporal processing versus processing efficiency hypothesis. *International Journal of Pediatric Otorhinolaryngology, 67*(Suppl. 1), S137–S142.

Hauser, M. D., Chomsky, N., & Fitch, W. T. (2002). The faculty of language: What is it, who has it, and how did it evolve? *Science, 298,* 1565–1566.

Helmholtz, H. L. F. (1954). *On the sensations of tone as a physiological basis for the theory of music* (2nd English trans. from the 4th German edition of 1877 by A. S. Ellis). New York: Dover.

Hickok, G., & Poeppel, D. (2004). Dorsal and ventral streams: A framework for understandings aspects of the functional anatomy of language. *Cognition, 92,* 67–99.

Hiiemae, K. M., & Palmer, J. B. (2003). Tongue movements in feeding and speech. *Critical Reviews in Oral Biology and Medicine, 14,* 413–429.

Holowka, S., & Pettito, L. A. (2002). Left hemisphere cerebral specialization for babies while babbling. *Science, 297,* 1515.

Jarvelainen, J., Schurmann, M., Avikainen, S., & Hari, R. (2001). Stronger reactivity of the human primary motor cortex during observation of live rather than video motor acts. *Neuroreport, 12,* 3493–3495.

Kent, R. D. (1981). Articulatory-acoustic perspectives on speech development. In R. Stark (Ed.), *Language behavior in infancy and early childhood* (pp. 105–239). Amsterdam: Elsevier.

Kent, R. D. (2004a). The uniqueness of speech among motor systems. *Clinical Linguistics & Phonetics, 18,* 495–505.

Kent, R. D. (2004b). Development, pathology, and remediation of speech. In J. Slifka, S. Manuel, & M. Matthies (Eds.), *From sound to sense: 50+ years of discoveries in speech communication* (pp. B148–B163). Cambridge, MA: Research Laboratory of Electronics, Massachusetts Institute of Technology.

Kent, R. D., & Forner, L. L. (1980). Speech segment durations in sentence repetitions by children and adults. *Journal of Phonetics, 8,* 157–168.

Kent, R. D., Netsell, R., Osberger, M. J., & Hustedde, C. G. (1987). Phonetic development in twins who differ in auditory function. *Journal of Speech and Hearing Disorders, 52,* 64–75.

Kent, R. D., & Vorperian, H. K. (1995). Anatomic development of the craniofacial–oral–laryngeal systems: A review. *Journal of Medical Speech-Language Pathology, 3,* 145–190.

Keysers, C., Kohler, E., Umilta, M. A., Nanetti, L., Fogassi, L., & Gallese, V. (2003). Audiovisual mirror neurons and action recognition. *Experimental Brain Research, 153,* 628–636.

Knightley, L. M., Jun, S. A., Oh, J. S., & Au, T. K. (2003). Production benefits of childhood overhearing. *Journal of the Acoustical Society of America, 114,* 465–474.

Koolstra, J. (2002). Dynamics of the human masticatory system. *Critical Reviews in Oral Biology and Medicine, 13,* 366–376.

Korphage, J. A., Brugman, P., & Van Euden, T. M. (2000). Intermuscular and intramuscular differences in myosin heavy chain composition of the human masticatory muscles. *Journal of Neurological Sciences, 178,* 95–106.

Kosslyn, S. M., Ganis, G., & Thompson, W. L. (2001). Neural foundations of imagery. *Nature Reviews Neuroscience, 2,* 635–642.

Kubota, K., & Masegi, T. (1977). Muscle spindle supply of the human jaw muscle. *Journal of Dental Research, 56,* 901–909.

Kubota, K., Negishi, T., & Masegi, T. (1975). Topological distribution of muscle spindles in the human tongue and its significance in proprioception. *Bulletin of the Tokyo Medical and Dental University, 22,* 235–242.

Kuehn, D., P., Templeton, P. J., & Maynard, J. A. (1990). Muscle spindles in the velopharyngeal musculature of humans. *Journal of Speech & Hearing Research, 33,* 488–493.

Kuhl, P. K., & Meltzoff, A. N. (1996). Infant vocalizations in response to speech—vocal imitation and developmental change. *Journal of the Acoustical Society of America, 100,* 2425–2438.

Kurata, K., & Tanji, J. (1986). Premotor cortex neurons in macaques: activity before distal and proximal forelimb movements. *Journal of Neuroscience, 6,* 403–411.

Laitman, J. T., & Crelin, E. S. (1976). Postnatal development of the basicranium and vocal tract region in man. In J. Bosma (Ed.), *Symposium on the development of the basicranium* (pp. 206–220). Bethesda, MD: DHEW Publication No. 76-989, PHS-NIH.

Li, Z. B., Lehar, M., Nakagawa, H., Hoh, J. F., & Flint, P. W. (2004). Differential expression of myosin heavy chain isoforms between abductor and adductor muscles in the human larynx. *Otolaryngology—Head & Neck Surgery, 130,* 217–222.

Liberman, A. M. (1998). When theories of speech meet the real world. *Journal of Psycholinguistic Research, 27,* 111–122.

Liberman, A. M., & Mattingly, I. G. (1985). The motor theory of speech perception revisited. *Cognition, 21,* 1–36.

Lieberman, P. (1977). *Speech physiology and acoustic phonetics.* New York: Macmillan.

Lieberman, P. (1984). *The biology and evolution of language.* Cambridge, MA: Harvard University Press.

Lieberman, P., Klatt, D. H., & Wilson, W. H. (1969). Vocal tract limitations on the vowel repertoires of rhesus monkey and other nonhuman primates. *Science, 164,* 1185–1187.

Lieberman, P., Laitman, J. T., Reidenberg, J. S., & Gannon, P. S. (1992). The anatomy, physiology, acoustics, and perception of speech: Essential elements in analysis of the evolution of human speech. *Journal of Human Evolution, 23,* 447–467.

Lieberman, D. E., McCarthy, R. C., Hiiemae, K. M., & Palmer, J. B. (2001). Ontogeny of postnatal hyoid and larynx descent in humans. *Archives of Oral Biology, 46,* 117–128.

Liss, J. M. (1990). Muscle spindles in the human levator palatini and palatoglossus muscle. *Journal of Speech & Hearing Research, 33,* 736–746.

Lotze, M., Montoya, P., Erb, M., Hulsmann, E., Flor, H., Klose, U., Birbaumer, N., & Grodd, W. (1999). Activation of cortical and cerebellar motor areas during executed and imagined hand movements: An fMRI study. *Journal of Cognitive Neuroscience, 11,* 491–501.

Macaluso, F., George, N., Dolan, R., Spence, C., & Driver, J. (2004). Spatial and temporal factors during processing of audiovisual speech: A PET study. *Neuroimage, 21,* 725–732.

MacNeilage, P. F., & Davis, B. L. (2000). On the origin of internal structure of word forms. *Science, 288,* 527–551.

MacNeilage, P. F., & Davis, B. L. (2001). Motor mechanisms in speech ontogeny: Phylogenetic, neurobiological and linguistic implications. *Current Opinion in Neurobiology, 11,* 696–700.

Maxon, A. B., & Hochberg, I. (1982). Development of psychoacoustic behavior: sensitivity and discrimination. *Ear and Hearing, 3,* 301–308.

Meltzoff, A. N., & Moore, M. K. (1977). Imitation of facial and manual gestures by human neonates. *Science, 198,* 75–78.

Meltzoff, A. N., & Moore, M. K. (1983). Newborn infants imitate adult facial gestures. *Child Development, 54,* 702–709.

Miall, R. C. (2003). Connecting mirror neurons and forward models. *Neuroreport, 14,* 2135–2137.

Moore, C. A., & Ruark, J. L. (1996). Does speech emerge from earlier appearing motor behaviors? *Journal of Speech and Hearing Research, 39,* 1034–1047.

Moore, J. K. (2002). Maturation of human auditory cortex: Implications for speech perception. *Annals of Otology, Rhinology, & Laryngology, Suppl., 189,* 7–10.

Mootoosamy, R. C., & Dietrich, S. (2002). Distinct regulatory cascades for head and trunk myogenesis. *Development, 129,* 573–583.

Nishitani, N., & Hari, R. (2000). Temporal dynamics of cortical representation for action. *Proceedings of the National Academy of Sciences, USA, 97,* 913–918.

Oller, D. K., & Eilers, R. E. (1988). The role of audition in babbling. *Child Development, 59,* 441–449.

Petkov, C. I., Kang, X., Alho, K., Bertrand, O., Yund, E. W., & Woods, D. L. (2004). Attentional modulation of human auditory cortex. *Natural Neuroscience, 7,* 658–663.

Pierrehumbert, J. B. (2003). Phonetic diversity, statistical learning, and acquisition of phonology. *Language & Speech, 46,* 115–154.

Powell, T. V., & Brodie, A. G. (1964). Closure of the spheno-occipital synchondrosis. *Anatomical Record, 147,* 15–23.

Purhonen, M., Kilpelainen-Lees, R., Valkonen-Korhonen, M., Karhu, J., & Lehtonen, J. (2004). Cerebral processing of mother's voice compared to unfamiliar voice in 4-month-old infants. *International Journal of Psychophysiology, 52,* 257–266.

Rizzolatti, G., & Arbib, M. A. (1998). From grasping to speech: imitation might provide a missing link—Reply [Letter]. *Trends in Neurosciences, 22,* 152.

Rizzolatti, G., Camarda, R., Fogassi, L., Gentilucci, M., Luppino, G., & Matelli, M. (1988). Functional organization of inferior area 6 in the macaque monkey. II: Area F5 and the control of distal movements. *Experimental Brain Research, 71,* 491–507.

Rizzolatti, G., & Craighero, L. (2004). The mirror-neuron system. *Annual Reviews in Neuroscience, 27,* 169–192.

Rizzolatti, G., Fadiga, L., Gallese, V., & Fogassi, L. (1996). Premotor cortex and the recognition of motor actions. *Cognitive Brain Research, 3,* 131–141.

Rizzolatti, G., Fadiga, L., Matelli, M., Bettinardi, V., Paulesu, E., Perani, C., & Fazio, F. (1996). Localization of grasp representation in humans by PET: 1. Observation versus execution. *Experimental Brain Research, 111,* 246–252.

Rizzolatti, G., Fogassi, L., & Gallese, V. (2002). Motor and cognitive functions of the ventral premotor cortex. *Current Opinion in Neurobiology, 12,* 149–154.

Rosenblum, L. D., Schmuckler, M. A., & Johnson, J. A. (1997). The McGurk effect in infants. *Perception & Psychophysics, 59,* 347–357.

Ruark, J. L., & Moore, C. A. (1997). Coordination of lip muscle activity by 2-year-old children during speech and nonspeech tasks. *Journal of Speech, Language, and Hearing Research, 40,* 1373–385.

Ruzza, B., Rocca, F., Boero, D. L., & Lenti, C. (2003). Investigating the musical quality of early infant sounds. *Annals of the New York Academy of Sciences, 999,* 527–529.

Ryding, E., Bradvik, B., & Ingvar, D. H. (1996). Silent speech activates prefrontal cortical regions asymmetrically, as well as speech-related areas in the dominant hemisphere. *Brain & Language, 52,* 435–451.

Saffran, J. R., & Thiessen, E. D. (2003). Pattern induction by infant language learners. *Developmental Psychology, 39,* 484–494.

Sander, R. K. (1972). When are speech sounds learned? *Journal of Speech and Hearing Research, 37,* 55–63.

Sasaki, C. T., Levine, P. A., Laitman, J. T., & Crelin, E. S. (1977). Postnatal descent of the epiglottis in man. *Archives of Otolaryngology, 103,* 169–171.

Scammon, R. E. (1930). The measurement of the body in childhood. In J. A. Harris, C. M. Jackson, D. G. Patterson, & R. E. Scammon (Eds.), *The measurement of man* (pp. 173–215). Minneapolis: University of Minnesota Press.

Sciote, J. J., Horton, M. J., Rowlerson, A. M., & Link, J. (2003). Specialized cranial muscles: How different are they from limb and abdominal muscles? *Cells, Tissues, Organs, 174,* 73–86.

Sciote, J. J., Morris, T. J., Brandon, C. A., Horton, M. J., & Rosen, C. (2002). Unloaded shortening velocity and myosin heavy chain variations in human laryngeal muscle fibers. *Annals of Otology, Rhinology, & Laryngology, 111,* 120–127.

Sciote, J. J., Rowlerson, A. M., Hopper, C., & Hunt, N. P. (1994). Fibre type classification and myosin isoforms in the human masseter muscle. *Journal of Neurological Sciences, 126,* 15–24.

Shiotani, A., Westra, W. H., & Flint, P. W. (1999). Myosin heavy chain composition in human laryngeal muscles. *Laryngoscope, 109,* 1521–1524.

Shuler, C. R., & Dalrymple, K. R. (2001). Molecular regulation of tongue and craniofacial muscle differentiation. *Critical Reviews in Oral Biology and Medicine, 12,* 3–17.

Siegenthaler, B. M. (1969). Maturation of auditory abilities in children. *International Audiology, 8,* 59–71.

Smit, A., Hand, L., Frelinger, J., Bernthal, J., & Byrd, A. (1990). The Iowa articulation norms project and its Nebraska replication. *Journal of Speech and Hearing Disorders, 55,* 779–798.

Smith, A., & Goffman, L. (2004). Interaction of motor and language factors in the development of speech. In B. Maassen, R. Kent, H. Peters, P. van Lieshout, & W. Hulstijn (Eds.), *Speech motor control in normal and disordered speech* (pp. 227–252). Oxford, England: Oxford University Press.

Sowell, E. R., Peterson, B. S., Thompson, P. M., Welcome, S. E., Henkenius, A. L., & Toga, A. W. (2003). Mapping cortical change across the human life span. *Nature Neuroscience, 6,* 309–315.

Stål, P., & Lindman, R. (2000). Characterisation of human soft palate muscles with respect to fibre types, myosins and capillary supply. *Journal of Anatomy, 197,* 275–290.

Stål, P., Eriksson, P. O., Eriksson, A., & Thornell. L. E. (1990). Enzyme-histochemical and morphological characteristics of muscle fibre types in the human buccinator and orbicularis orix. *Archives of Oral Biology, 35,* 449–458.

Stål, P., Marklund, S., Thornell, L. E., De Paul, R., & Eriksson, P. O. (2003). Fibre composition of human intrinsic tongue muscles. *Cells, Tissues, Organs, 173,* 147–161.

Stoel-Gammon, C., & Otomo, K. (1986). Babbling development of hearing-impaired and normally hearing subjects. *Journal of Speech and Hearing Disorders, 51,* 33–41.

Stollman, M. H., van Velzen, E. C., Simkens, H. M., Snik, A. F., & van den Broek, P. (2004). Development of auditory processing in 6–12-year-old children: A longitudinal study. *International Journal of Audiology, 43,* 34–44.

Swingley, D. (2003). Phonetic detail in the developing lexicon. *Language & Speech, 46,* 265–294.

Tellis, C., Rosen, C., Thekdi, A., & Sciote, J. (2004). Anatomy and fiber type composition of human interarytenoid muscle. *Annals of Otology, Rhinology, and Laryngology, 113,* 97–107.

Thierry, G., Vihman, M., & Roberts, M. (2003). Familiar words capture the attention of 11-month-olds in less than 250 ms. *Neuroreport, 14,* 2307–2310.

Vorperian, H. K. (2000). *Anatomic development of the vocal tract structures as visualized by MRI.* Unpublished doctoral dissertation, University of Wisconsin–Madison.

Vorperian, H. K., Kent, R. D., Gentry, L. R., & Yandell, B. S. (1999). Magnetic resonance imaging procedures to study the concurrent anatomic development of the vocal tract structures: Preliminary results. *International Journal of Pediatric Otorhinolaryngology, 49,* 197–206.

Vorperian, H. K., Kent, R. D., Lindstrom, M. J., Kalina, C. M., Gentry, L. R., & Yandell, B. S. (2005). Development of vocal tract length during early childhood: A magnetic resonance imaging study. *Journal of the Acoustical Society of America.*

Watkins, K. E., Strafella, A. P., & Paus, T. (2003). Seeing and hearing speech excites the motor system involved in speech production. *Neuropsychologia, 41,* 989–994.

Werker, J. F., & Pegg, J. E. (1992). Infant speech and phonological acquisition. In C. A. Ferguson, L. Menn, & C. Stoel-Gammon (Eds.), *Phonological development: Models, research, implications* (pp. 285–311). Timonium, MD: York Press.

Werker, J. F., & Tees, R. C. (1984). Cross-language speech perception: Evidence for the perceptual reorganization during the first year of life. *Infant Behavior and Development, 7,* 49–63.

Westerman, G., & Miranda, E. R. (1994). A new model of sensorimotor coupling in the development of speech. *Brain and Language, 89,* 393–400.

Westhorpe, R. N. (1987). The position of the larynx in children and its relationship to the ease of intubation. *Anaesthesia and Intensive Care, 15,* 384–388.

Wightman, F., Allen, P., Dolan, T., Kistler, D., & Jamieson, D. (1989). Temporal resolution in children. *Child Development, 60,* 611–624.

Wilson, S. M., Saygin, A. P., Sereno, M. I., & Iacoboni, M. (2004). Listening to speech activates motor areas involved in speech production. *Nature Neuroscience, 7,* 701–702.

Wohlschlager, W., & Bekkering, H. (2002). Is human imitation based on a mirror-neurone system? Some behavioural evidence. *Experimental Brain Research, 143,* 335–341.

Yu, F., Stål, P, Thornell, L. E., & Larson, L. (2002). Human single masseter muscle fibers contain unique combinations of myosin and myosin binding protein C isoforms. *Journal of Muscle Research and Cell Motility, 23,* 317–326.

3

Typical Talkers, Late Talkers, and Children With Specific Language Impairment: A Language Endowment Spectrum?

Susan Ellis Weismer
Department of Communicative Disorders, Waisman Center, University of Wisconsin–Madison

The influence of developmental perspectives on research in the field of communicative disorders is particularly evident in the study of late talkers. Since the late 1980s numerous empirical investigations of late talkers have appeared in the literature. The impetus for studying late talkers arises from an interest in examining variability in the rate and patterns of typical language development, as well as from an interest in identifying toddlers who may be at risk for later language impairment. The late talker topic has also received attention in the popular press with books authored by parents of late talkers, including two books by Thomas Sowell, *Late Talking Children* (1997) and *The Einstein Syndrome* (2001), that paint a very optimistic picture and a book by Agin, Geng, and Nicholl, *The Late Talker: What to Do If Your*

Child Isn't Talking Yet (2003), that focuses primarily on treatment issues for severe speech-language delay.

Late talkers typically have been identified on the basis of late onset of productive language abilities. Varying criteria and cut points have been used by researchers who are interested in late talking from the perspective of subsequent language impairment (Paul, 1991; Rescorla, 1989, 1991; Thal & Bates, 1988; Whitehurst et al., 1991). The age at which late talkers are identified has also proven to be an important consideration in studying these children because samples of very young toddlers (18 months or younger) are more likely than somewhat older samples to include a higher proportion of late bloomers who get a slow start but catch up to their peers. The terminology used to describe children who are late to talk reflects differing underlying assumptions about the nature of the phenomenon. In contrast to earlier terms such as *expressive language delay* (ELD) (Fischel, Whitehurst, Caulfield, & DeBaryshe, 1989) or *expressive specific language impairment* (SLI-E) (Rescorla & Goossens, 1992), the term *late talker* provides a descriptive, developmental characterization that does not carry connotations regarding clinical language delay or impairment (see discussions of this point by Ellis Weismer, Murray-Branch, & Miller, 1994; Rescorla & Roberts, 2002). A report based on a National Institutes of Health (NIH) workshop that focused on defining the phenotype for specific language impairment (SLI) concluded that young children at risk for SLI (few words, no word combinations) could be identified before age 3 and that SLI could be identified between 3 and 5 years (Tager-Flusberg & Cooper, 1999). However, Rescorla and Lee (2000) have advocated an even more conservative approach to diagnosis of specific language impairment. They recommend 2 to 4 years as the developmental range for use of the term late talker, with the designation of SLI being reserved for children over 4 years of age.

Research on late talkers and investigations of SLI have proceeded, to a certain extent, as separate lines of inquiry even though there are compelling theoretical and clinical reasons to better understand the nature of the relation between these groups. Rescorla and colleagues (Rescorla, 2000, 2002; Rescorla & Roberts, 2002) argue against considering late talkers and preschoolers with SLI to be distinct groups. They suggest that this distinction may have evolved from an overly optimistic view of outcomes for late talkers (Rescorla & Roberts, 2002). Although the vast majority of late talkers perform within normal range on clinical measures of language ability by kindergarten (Paul, 1996; Rescorla & Lee, 2000; Whitehurst & Fischel, 1994), these children continue to manifest poorer language skills than comparison groups (matched on SES and nonverbal cognition) throughout elementary school and into early adolescence (Rescorla, 2000, 2002). Building on the normal distribution account of SLI (Leonard, 1987, 1991), Rescorla and colleagues propose that late talkers and children with SLI can both be conceptualized in terms of a "language endowment spectrum." That is, a spectrum of language ability is proposed, with the continuum ranging from children with typical language development to late bloomers who start late but catch up quickly to late talkers with more persistent delays to children with specific language impairment. According to this view, there is not a single factor (such as a grammatical deficit) that is hypothesized to account for lower language abilities; instead, weaknesses in various skills that subserve language (such as auditory processing, working memory, motor planning) can result in poorer language endowment. This assumption is similar to the claims that others have made regarding multiple underlying factors in SLI that are likely to differ across individual children (Ellis Weismer & Thordardottir, 2002; Johnston, 2004).

This chapter provides a summary of a longitudinal investigation of late talkers, with a focus on considering the notion of a language endowment spectrum. In addition to the specific issues addressed by each study within this project, the overarching question is the following: What is the extent of overlap or distinction between typical language development, late talking, and specific language impairment?

PROJECT SUMMARY

In the Early Language Learning Project (Ellis Weismer, Evans, & Chapman, co-principal investigators), language skills of late talkers were compared to those of typically developing toddlers throughout the preschool period. In total, 106 children, 53 late talkers and 53 normal language controls matched on age, nonverbal cognition, sex, and socioeconomic status (SES), participated in this longitudinal project. A summary of participant characteristics for the two groups is provided in Table 3.1. Late talkers were identified at 2

TABLE 3.1
Summary of Participant Characteristics in the Early Language Learning Project

	NL Group	*LT Group*
CA[a]	30.45 (1.12)	30.03 (.39)
Cognition[b]	7.89 (1.42)	7.49 (1.94)
SES[c]	15.45 (2.04)	15.41 (1.95)
Sex	37 M/16 F	37 M/16 F
Heritage	46 White/6 African American/ 1 Asian American	46 White/7 African American

[a]Chronological age in months.
[b]Nonverbal items from the Bayley Scales of Infant Development (Bayley, 1993).
[c]Socioeconomic status, as indexed by number of years of maternal education.

years of age as scoring in the lowest 10th percentile for productive vocabulary on a parent report measure of language development. All children were seen for annual assessments at 2½, 3½, 4½, and 5½ years. A subset of children also participated in a microgenetic study of novel word learning at 2 years, 9 months of age.

A primary aim of this project was to further investigate the link between late onset of talking and subsequent specific language impairment (SLI). Measures that have revealed deficits in the SLI population were adapted for use with late talkers to determine the extent to which early language delay predicts subsequent language impairment. Additionally, patterns of linguistic growth were compared across late talkers and typical talkers, and mechanisms of language learning and development, including fast mapping processes and lexical–grammatical continuity, were explored.

Initial Identification of Late Talkers

In this project, late talkers were first identified on the basis of reported limitations in early language use. The MacArthur Communicative Development Inventory (MCDI), a parent report measure of early lexical and grammatical skills, has been used extensively to study language development in typically developing toddlers (Bates et al., 1994; Bauer, Goldfield, & Reznick, 2002; Dale, Dionne, Eley, & Plomin, 2000; Marchman & Bates, 1994), as well as young children with delayed language development (Hick, Joseph, Conti-Ramsden, Serratrice, & Faragher, 2002; Thal, O'Hanlon, Clemmons, & Fralin, 1999). Nevertheless, concern has been raised about the MCDI's ability to identify early language delay given the extent of variation in linguistic abilities during this early period of language development (see Feldman et al., 2000, and response by Fenson et al., 2000). That is, the question arises as to whether this measure constitutes a valid indicator of "late talking" in light of the considerable variation in reported language abilities. Given this controversy, we sought to examine the validity of this parent report measure for our particular sample in two studies (Ellis Weismer, Evans, Hollar, & Jones, 2001; Heilmann, Ellis Weismer, Evans, & Hollar, 2005). One study investigated the concurrent validity of the MCDI for a group of 38 late talkers at 2½ years of age. Three subsections of the MCDI were evaluated: total productive vocabulary, mean of three longest utterances, and complexity. Each subsection of the MCDI was compared with direct language assessment measures including the expressive language assessment of a standardized test and measures derived from examiner–child and parent–child language samples. Significant, moderate correlations were found between each section of the MCDI and each of the direct assessment measures. In a second study, likelihood ratio analysis (Sackett, Haynes, Guyatt, & Tugwell, 1991) was used to determine how well the MCDI distinguished 39 late talkers from 62 children with normal language development as identified by direct assessment measures. The MCDI did an excellent job of distinguishing late talkers who scored up to the 11th percentile and in distinguishing toddlers with normal language who scored above the 49th percentile but was somewhat less effective within the intermediate percentiles. Taken together, these two studies demonstrated the MCDI's utility in characterizing the language skills of late talking toddlers.

Lexical Processing and Early Prediction of Outcomes

Delayed onset of vocabulary is a defining characteristic of late talkers; therefore, understanding the mechanisms involved in early word learning is crucial for understanding late talkers' language delay. A process referred to as "fast mapping" putatively enables young children to quickly construct lexical representations for unfamiliar words given minimal exposure and has been hypothesized to account for rapid gains in vocabulary. Children with SLI have been observed to have deficits in fast mapping processes involved in novel word learning (Dollaghan, 1987; Ellis Weismer & Hesketh, 1996, 1998; Rice, Buhr, & Oetting, 1992).

In the current project, we investigated fast mapping in 30 late talkers and 30 typical talkers at 2½ years of age (Ellis Weismer, 2002a; Ellis Weismer & Evans, 2002). Children were exposed to novel object labels in the context of a puppet game and were then asked to name the objects (to measure novel word production) or identify the objects given the verbal label (to measure of novel word comprehension). Late talkers performed significantly more poorly on the production, but not the comprehension, of novel words. Modest, significant correlations were observed within each group between novel word production and performance on standardized language measures, and novel word production/comprehension at 2½ was a significant predictor of mean length of utterance (MLU) at 3½ years ($R^2 = .36$). When standardized language measures (MCDI, PLS-3) were added to novel word production at 2½, the ability to predict MLU at 3½ was increased, with these combined variables accounting for 65% of the variance ($R^2 = .65$). In addition, typical talkers manifested sensitivity to the novel words' resemblance to real words (i.e., the novel words' neighborhood density), but late talkers, as a group, appeared not to be sensitive to this. However, those late talkers who were sensitive at 2½ to the novel words' neighborhood density had significantly higher MLUs at 3½ than late talkers who did not show the typical pattern of sensitivity to neighborhood density.

Lexical Microgenetic Study

In addition to investigating fast mapping (i.e., the initial stage of acquisition after very limited exposure to a novel word), we have investigated the rate and pattern of mastery of novel words over multiple sessions, using microgenetic methods (Ellis Weismer, Evans, Jones, Horton-Ikard, & Hollar, in preparation). Microgenetic methods allow for fine-grained analysis of change within a delimited time period; they have been used to study cognitive, linguistic, and motor development, including children's grammatical morpheme acquisition and narrative skill development (Chen & Siegler, 2000; Daehler, 2000; McKeough & Sanderson, 1996; Peters & Menn, 1993; Siegler, 1996; Thelen & Corbetta, 2002). In our microgenetic study of early word learning, 23 late talkers and 26 typical talkers who were 2 years, 9 months of age participated in 6 sessions occurring within a 2-week period. Comprehension and production of both novel and familiar words were compared in a high-script or a low-script context. Scripts can be thought of as mental representations of routines that are established on the basis of real world experiences; they have a clear temporal sequence, with predictable actors and props (Nelson, 1986). Scripts are the centerpiece of script-based interventions for children with language disorders (Ellis Weismer, 2000; Robertson & Ellis Weismer, 1999). In the high-script condition, late talkers performed more poorly than normal language controls on both comprehension and production, but there were no group differences in the low-script condition—perhaps because the high-script condition involved following a specific sequence and was more heavily adult-directed. Growth curve analysis examined changes in the two groups' MLU for utterances containing the novel words. Although the rate of increase in MLU across the six sessions was similar for LT and NL groups in the low-script condition, in the high-script condition the rate of increase in MLU was significantly greater for typical talkers than late talkers.

Relation Between Lexical and Grammatical Skills in Late Talkers

It has been proposed that early acquisition of grammar is dependent on lexical development, such that advances in grammar occur once vocabulary has reached a "critical mass" (Bates & Goodman, 2001; Marchman & Bates, 1994). In an initial study (Ellis Weismer, Marchman, & Evans, 2001) we explored the continuity of lexical and grammatical development in late talking toddlers (24 months) compared to age-matched controls and younger vocabulary-matched controls (16 months) with normal language development. Language abilities of the three groups (N = 60, 20 per group) were assessed using the MacArthur Communicative Development Inventory (MCDI). The findings indicated that late talkers did not display selective delays in the acquisition of verbs, which are often assumed to play a special role in grammatical development (late talkers had the same proportion of verbs in their lexicon as younger children matched on vocabulary size). In addition to verb growth, the late talkers generally displayed typical patterns of lexical–grammatical relationships during this early period. One notable exception was that they appeared to have a weaker relationship between vocabulary and MLU (mean length of utterance) as compared to typically developing peers. At 24 months, late-talking toddlers were less likely to combine words than younger, vocabulary-matched controls. That is, late talkers demonstrated later entrance into syntax with the same lexical building blocks.

A subsequent longitudinal investigation (Jones, Ellis Weismer, Evans, & Hollar, 2003) extended the earlier study by exploring lexical–grammatical continuity for late talkers and typical talkers from 2 to 5½ years. Language measures included the MCDI (words produced, mean of 3 longest utterances, complexity score) and lexical and grammatical subtests from two standardized language measures (Preschool Language Scale-3, PLS-3, Zimmerman, Steiner, & Pond, 1992; Test of Language Development-Primary:3, TOLD-P:3, Newcomer & Hammill, 1997). Cross-lagged correlations performed across adjacent time points examined the directionality between lexical and grammatical development. Different patterns were observed for the LT and NL groups. For the NL group, bidirectional influences of lexical and grammatical development were observed between 2 and 3½ years, but no significant influences in either direction were observed between 3½ and 5½ years. These findings support those of Dionne, Dale, Boivin, and Plomin (2003), who also found evidence for both lexical and grammatical bootstrapping in typically developing toddlers between 2 and 3 years. In contrast to typical talkers, late talkers in our study exhibited a unidirectional influence of lexical development on later grammatical development between 2½ and 5½ years. This result corroborates our (Ellis Weismer, Marchman, & Evans, 2001) earlier observation that, at least in some respects, late talkers' grammatical skills are less developed than would be expected based on their lexical development. Further analysis involving growth curve modeling and hierarchical clustering analysis (Jones, 2004) has revealed that (a) late talkers as a group exhibited similar patterns of lexical and grammatical growth as typical talkers despite the late talkers' reduced levels of skills and (b) late talkers formed two distinct clusters—late bloomers who caught up with the typically development group in lexical and grammatical skills, and late talkers whose performance remained relatively lower in both areas.

Relation between Comprehension and Production

According to the criteria used to initially identify late talkers, all late talkers in our project had delayed onset of productive vocabulary. At 2½ years of age only a small proportion of the LT group (6/53 or 11%) exhibited clinically significant delays in comprehension based on performance more than one standard deviation below the mean on the auditory comprehension scale of the PLS-3. However, it should be noted that Wisconsin children in the current sample scored much higher overall than the national normative sample for the PLS-3. Few toddlers with comprehension delays participated in this project, even though we had made every attempt to include these children in the sample. We had reasoned that some prior investigations of late talkers had not included the full array of children who were likely to exhibit persistent language delay (SLI) because children with receptive–expressive difficulties were excluded intentionally (to focus on expressive language delay only) or inadvertently through the inclusion of verbal items on cognitive measures (see discussion of this point by Ellis Weismer, 2000). In an attempt to minimize bias toward eliminating toddlers with comprehension problems, only the nonverbal items from the Mental Scale of the Bayley Scales of Infant Development (Bayley, 1993) were used to match groups in the current project (see Paul, 2000; Spitz, Tallal, Flax, & Benasich, 1997). Nevertheless, the vast majority of toddlers who met selection criteria (including normal range nonverbal cognition) exhibited a profile of expressive language delay, with only a few children also displaying substantial lags in comprehension skills.

The gap between comprehension and production that characterized the early period of development for the LT group narrowed and approached that of the NL group, with comprehension skills remaining somewhat higher than production throughout the preschool period. Prior studies have found that the size of the comprehension–production gap in late talkers was related to language advances and language outcomes (Olswang & Bain, 1996; Thal, Tobias, & Morrison, 1991). In our project, there was a significant positive correlation between performance on the comprehension and production scales of the PLS-3 and TOLD-P:3 at each age point for the sample as a whole (ranging from .40 to .64). Both the LT and NL group showed similar patterns of relationship, with the strongest associations between comprehension and production occurring at the early points in development even though some late talkers had considerable comprehension-production gaps at 2 years. This finding should be viewed with caution with respect to its developmental significance because it was not possible to use the same measure of language skills throughout the entire period; therefore, it is also feasible that this result reflects differences in the relation between the receptive and expressive scales of the two test instruments. For both groups, comprehension skills at 4½ were quite strongly correlated with comprehension at 5½ and production at 4½ was strongly correlated with production at 5½, indicating similar patterns of stability.

Short-Term Outcomes at Age 3½

There has been considerable debate surrounding the need for intervention with late talkers (Ellis Weismer, 2000; Paul, 2000), and predictors of outcomes for individual children have been elusive. In the current project, short-term outcomes of late talking toddlers were explored by systematically examining factors that classified children according to language and treatment status outcomes at 3½ years (Ellis Weismer, 2002b). Participants included 40 toddlers who had been identified as late talkers at 2 years based on restricted productive vocabulary. The following findings were noted: (a) 35% of the late talkers had been enrolled in speech-language treatment by 3;6 (3 years, 6 months); (b) 25% were late bloomers who exhibited normal range language skills by 3;6 without treatment; (c) a combination of socioeconomic (SES) and nonverbal IQ, expressive language, and articulation skills at 2½ correctly identified 81% of the late talkers who had been enrolled in speech-language treatment by 3½; and (d) a combination of nonverbal IQ, expressive language, and novel word comprehension at 2½ correctly identified 90% of the late talkers who achieved normal range language skills by 3½ and correctly rejected 91% who did not achieve normal range language skills by 3½. Thus, a model in which early linguistic processing abilities (fast mapping scores) were combined with traditional language and cognitive assessment measures resulted in excellent sensitivity and specificity with respect to short-term outcomes.

Longer Term Outcomes at Age 5½

Eighty-three of the 106 participants (81%) enrolled in this longitudinal project completed the final assessment at 5½, including 40 children who were identified as late talkers as toddlers and 43 who were identified as typically developing talkers at 2 years. Using performance on a standardized measure of language comprehension and production (TOLD:P-3) as the criterion measure to assess outcome, only 3/40 (7.5%) late talkers scored at least one standard deviation (*SD*) below the mean according to the national norms for the speaking quotient of the TOLD:P-3 and none scored beyond normal range (–1 SD) for the listening quotient. Thus, very few late talkers scored low enough on a standardized language measure to qualify them for a clinical diagnosis of SLI at 5½ years of age. This finding is consistent with results from prior longitudinal studies indicating that most late talkers exhibit normal range language skills by 5 years (Paul, 1996; Rescorla & Lee, 2000; Whitehurst & Fischel, 1994). Despite their relatively good performance on the TOLD:P-3, 15 of the 40 LTs (37.5%) were receiving services from a speech-language clinician at 5½, whereas none of the 43 children in the NL group were receiving speech-language treatment at kindergarten. This apparent discrepancy between these standardized test scores and clinical services could be partly, but not completely, accounted for by the fact that about half of the children enrolled in therapy had speech production problems. Although intervention focused exclusively on speech production for 8 of the children (6 articulation, 1 oral–motor/dyspraxia, and 1 fluency), 7 children were receiving services that targeted both language and speech goals. Whitehurst and colleagues (1991), among others, have similarly reported persistent articulation difficulties in late talkers.

Although most late talkers moved into normal range, they continued to perform substantially more poorly than the comparison sample (who had been matched on SES and nonverbal cognition) on various language measures. This same phenomenon has also been reported in previous investigations (Paul, 1996; Rescorla, 2000, 2002; Thal & Katich, 1996). The pattern of group differences was statistically equivalent whether the entire LT group was compared to the NL group or the 3 late talkers who scored within clinical range were removed from the LT group and only the performance of the remaining children was considered. At 5½, late talkers (minus the 3 late talkers who did not score within normal range on the TOLD-P:3) scored significantly worse than the NL group on the listening and speaking quotients of the TOLD-P:3, on nonword repetition, and on a verbal working memory measure. The largest between-group differences occurred on the sentence imitation (partial eta squared = .19) subtest of the TOLD-P:3, and percentage of phonemes correct (PPC) on the nonword repetition task (partial eta squared = .23). Examination of individual scores revealed that 10 late talkers scored more than 2 *SD*s below the mean of the NL group for both the sentence imitation subtest and the overall spoken quotient of the TOLD-P:3, and 17 late talkers scored below 2 *SD*s on the nonword repetition task. Although the late talker group had lower mean scores than the typically developing group, the two groups did not differ significantly on MLU or narrative comprehension/retell. On both of these measures there was considerable variability in performance in both groups.

Mixed results have been reported in the literature with respect to narrative skills of children with a history of late talking (Paul, Hernandez, & Taylor, 1996; Manhardt & Rescorla, 2002). The findings related to sentence imitation and nonword repetition are consistent with patterns of performance that have been reported for children with SLI. A number of investigations have documented that children with SLI are less proficient at nonword repetition than normal-language peers (Bishop, North, & Donlan, 1996; Dollaghan & Campbell, 1998; Edwards & Lahey, 1998; Ellis Weismer et al., 2000). Conti-Ramsden (2001) examined various psycholinguistic markers of specific language impairment, including nonword repetition and sentence repetition; she reported that sentence repetition was a particularly useful marker of SLI. In a subsequent study of "risk markers" for SLI, Conti-Ramsden and Hesketh (2003) concluded that poor nonword repetition performance in young children (under 5 years) with slow language development is a potential indicator of SLI risk.

As a group, late talkers remained less linguistically proficient than children without a history of late onset of language development despite the fact that they maintained equivalent nonverbal cognitive skills at 5½ (compared to the NL group to whom they were matched at 2½ years on nonverbal cognition). Performance on the Leiter visualization and memory composites at 5½ were very similar (LT $M = 118.66$, $SD = 7.11$; NL $M = 119.56$; $SD = 8.84$). Findings from this sample did not support the notion that late talkers in general exhibit an "Einstein syndrome" (Sowell, 2001); instead, this group displayed a range of cognitive abilities at 2½ years and throughout the study. Both groups were comprised of a small subset of children with exceptionally high cognitive abilities, with 9 children in the NL group and 9 children in the LT group scoring more than two standard deviations above the mean (standard score of greater than 130) on one of the two composite measures from the Leiter at 5½ years of age. Group differences in social communication skills did not account for the lower language performance by the LT group. Children who exhibited social difficulties or were suspected of having a pervasive developmental disorder were not enrolled in this study. At the completion of the study, parents were asked to complete the Social Communication Questionnaire (Berument, Rutter, Lord, Pickles, & Bailey, 1999). The scores on this measure were very similar for the two groups (NL $M = 5.59$, $SD = 4.26$; LT $M = 5.57$, $SD = 3.07$). One of the typical talkers met the cutoff criteria (15), suggesting possible concern regarding autism spectrum disorder (ASD), but none of the late talkers displayed social communication difficulties.

It is important to note that although the late talkers, as a group, demonstrated less proficient language skills than the typical talkers, this was not the case for all late talkers. Ten out of 40 children in the LT group (25%) displayed normal or above normal range language skills across all of the standardized and nonstandardized language measures at 5½ years. Therefore, it is certainly possible to get a late start at talking but to truly "catch up" to the proficiency level of your peers. The children who present this profile, however, appear to be in the minority. Although we are continuing to examine possible predictors of language outcome, preliminary results indicated that four 2½ year measures—the comprehension scale on the PLS-3, expressive scale on the PLS-3, productive vocabulary from the MCDI, and nonverbal items on the Bayley—significantly predicted ($R^2 = .52$) expressive language abilities at 5½ as measured by the TOLD-P:3. Comprehension at 2½ was the strongest single predictor of language production at 5½ (accounting for 41% of the variance). In the preliminary analysis, these same four variables provided the best prediction model for both the late talkers and typical talkers when the groups were considered separately; however, the ability to predict language outcomes for late talkers ($R^2 = .51$) was greater than for typical talkers ($R^2 = .35$). Even though only a few children in the LT group had demonstrated early comprehension skills that fell below normal range, those with relatively lower comprehension abilities at 2½ tended to have lower productive language skills at 5½ years of age. Findings from prior late talker investigations have been mixed with respect to the role of early comprehension abilities in subsequent language outcomes. Thal and colleagues reported that comprehension abilities at 18 to 28 months were a significant predictor of language skills in late talkers in a 1-year follow-up study (Thal et al., 1991). Further examination of that late talker sample indicated that toddlers who had both comprehension and production delays at 2 years demonstrated poorer productive language abilities at 3 years than those with only early expressive delays (Thal, Reilly, Seibert, Jeffries, & Fenson, 2004). On the other hand, Paul (1991, 2000) did not find that comprehension was a significant predictor of early school-age outcomes, although this may have been due to the fact that a parent report measure of comprehension was used rather than direct assessment of early receptive language.

Summary of Patterns of Language Development

As a group, late talkers displayed many similarities to the children with typical language development with respect to patterns of linguistic growth and mechanisms of language learning, though there were also some differences. At 24 months of age, the proportion of verbs in late talkers' vocabularies was similar to that of younger children matched on total vocabulary level. Thus, there was no early evidence for a special restriction in verbs, which are assumed to play a key role in grammatical development and have been observed to be a weakness for children with SLI (see review by Leonard, 1998). This result is consistent with related findings by Rescorla and Roberts (2002), who found no selective deficit in verbal morpheme use compared to nominal morphemes for 3- and 4-year-old late talkers. For the most part, late talkers in the present sample displayed typical patterns of lexical–grammatical relationships despite the early lag in development. However, late talkers were slower to combine words than typical talkers with the same number of words in their vocabulary and exhibited unidirectional influences of lexical development on later grammatical development throughout the preschool period (i.e., they failed to show evidence of grammatical bootstrapping that was observed for the typical talkers). Despite the early gap between comprehension and production skills that characterized the language profiles of the late talkers, they displayed considerable overlap with the typical talkers in terms of the pattern of association between comprehension and production across development. With regard to language learning mechanisms, late talkers demonstrated fast mapping comprehension abilities similar to those of typical talkers but, similar to children with SLI, were less proficient in producing novel words. Microgenetic analyses revealed that late talkers were as skilled as typical talkers at using newly learned novel words within spontaneous utterances under certain contexts (low script condition) but not others (high script conditions) where performance demands were apparently greater. In this regard, the late talkers also appear to be similar to children with SLI who have been shown to exhibit limitations in more demanding contexts.

CONCLUSIONS AND FUTURE DIRECTIONS

Many of the findings from the current project support Rescorla's notion of a language endowment spectrum (Rescorla, 2000; Rescorla & Roberts, 2002). That is, there is considerable overlap in patterns and mechanisms of language development for typical talkers and late talkers, as well as certain similarities between aspects of the late talker's skills and those previously reported for children with SLI. However, future research is needed to explain factors underlying differential trajectories of late talkers who truly catch up to the proficiency level of the comparison group versus those with consistently lower language endowment. Language development appears to proceed in a dynamic fashion, perhaps triggered by changes in skills subserving language that lead to shifts in language proficiency. Conceptualizing the relationship between differing levels of linguistic proficiency exhibited by children with SLI, late talkers, late bloomers, and typical talkers in terms of global severity levels (Rescorla & Roberts, 2002) may not be an adequate characterization; this notion deserves further consideration. Another issue that warrants additional scrutiny involves the apparent mismatch between the percentage of late talkers who exhibit clinical language impairment at 5 years and the percentage of kindergarten children with SLI (estimated to be approximately 7% according to findings of Tomblin et al., 1997). Although it is problematic to make comparisons across population-based samples and convenience samples, it might be assumed that samples of late talkers would consist of a substantially higher proportion of children at risk for SLI than the proportion within the population at large. Given the relatively low proportion of late talkers who display clinical language impairment at school entry, we must continue to ask where those 7% of kindergarten children with SLI come from if not from the ranks of late talkers.

The notion of a language endowment spectrum as it applies to late talkers also relates to broader theoretical debates in the literature regarding continuous versus dichotomous characterizations of various language based skills. For example, specific language impairment can be conceptualized within a dimensional account in terms of overlap with the lower end of normal range language skills or overlap with other disorders entailing language and communication deficits, such as autism spectrum disorders (see discussion of this point by Gernsbacher, Geye, & Ellis Weismer, 2005). Recently, a number of investigations have explored dimensional versus distinct category accounts of SLI (Dollaghan, 2004; Zhang & Tomblin, in preparation) as well as dyslexia (Bishop & Snowling, 2005; Whitehurst & Fischel, 2000). Although there is some evidence to suggest to that dyslexia should be viewed as a distinct category, the findings to date do not seem to uphold this view for spoken language impairment. In fact, investigations of language processing and language development across various clinical populations (Bates, 2004; Thal et al., 2004) reveal more similarities than differences. Viewed through a developmental lens, overlaps often become apparent across populations that have traditionally been regarded as dichotomous groups.

ACKNOWLEDGMENT

Funding for this research was provided by the National Institutes of Health (NIH), National Institute of Deafness and Other Communication Disorders (NIDCD) grant 5 R01 DC0371, "Linguistic Processing in Specific Language Delay," awarded to S. Ellis Weismer, J. L. Evans, and R. S. Chapman.

REFERENCES

Agin, M., Geng, L., & Nicholl, M. (2003). *The late talker: What to do if your child isn't talking yet.* New York: St. Martin's Press.

Bates, E. (2004). Explaining and interpreting deficits in language development across clinical groups: Where do we go from here? *Brain and Language, 88,* 248–253.

Bates, E., & Goodman, J. (2001). On the inseparability of grammar and the lexicon: Evidence from acquisition. In M. Tomasello & E. Bates (Eds.), *Language development: The essential readings* (pp. 134–162). Malden, MA: Blackwell.

Bates, E., Marchman, V., Thal, D., Fenson, L., Dale, P., Reznick, J., et al. (1994). Developmental and stylistic variation in the composition of early vocabulary. *Journal of Child Language, 21,* 85–123.

Bauer, D., Goldfield, B., & Reznick, J. (2002). Alternative approaches to analyzing individual differences in the rate of early vocabulary development. *Applied Psycholinguistics, 23,* 313–315.

Bayley, N. (1993). *Scales of Infant Development.* New York: Cambridge University Press.

Berument, S., Rutter, M., Lord, C., Pickles, A., & Bailey, A. (1999). Autism screening questionnaire: Diagnostic validity. *British Journal of Psychiatry, 175,* 444–451.

Bishop, D. V. M., North, T., & Donlan, C. (1996). Nonword repetition as a behavioral marker for inherited language impairment: Evidence from a twin study. *Journal of Child Psychology and Psychiatry, 36,* 1–13.

Bishop, D. V. M., & Snowling, M. (2004). Developmental dyslexia and specific language impairment: Same or different? *Psychological Bulletin, 130,* 858–886.

Chen, Z., & Sielger, R. (2000). Across the great divide: Bridging the gap between understanding of toddlers' and older children's thinking. *Monographs of the Society for Research in Child Development, 65,* v–96.

Conti-Ramsden, G. (2001). Psycholinguistic markers for specific language impairment (SLI). *Journal of Child Psychology and Psychiatry, 42,* 741–748.

Conti-Ramsden, G., & Hesketh, A. (2003). Risk-markers for SLI: A study of young language-learning children. *International Journal of Language and Communication Disorders, 38,* 251–263.

Daehler, M. (2000). Commentary: A key bridge to understanding the development of thinking and problem solving. *Monographs of the Society for Research in Child Development, 65*(Serial No. 261), 97–105.

Dale, P., Dionne, G., Eley, T., & Plomin, R. (2000). Lexical and grammatical development: A behavioural genetic perspective. *Journal of Child Language, 27,* 619–642.

Dionne, G., Dale, P., Boivin, M., & Plomin, R. (2003). Genetic evidence for bidirectional effects of early lexical and grammatical development. *Child Development, 74,* 394–412.

Dollaghan, C. (1987). Fast mapping in normal and language-impaired children. *Journal of Speech and Hearing Disorders, 52,* 218–222.

Dollaghan, C. (2004). Taxometric analyses of specific language impairment in 3- and 4-year-old children. *Journal of Speech, Language, and Hearing Research, 47,* 464–475.

Dollaghan, C., & Campbell, T. (1998). Nonword repetition and child language impairment. *Journal of Speech, Language, and Hearing Research, 41,* 1136–1146.

Edwards, J., & Lahey, M. (1998). Nonword repetitions of children with specific language impairment: Exploration of some explanations for their inaccuracies. *Applied Psycholinguistics, 19,* 279–309.

Ellis Weismer, S. (2000). Language intervention for children with developmental language delay. In D. Bishop & L. Leonard (Eds.), *Speech and language impairments: From theory to practice* (pp. 157–176). Hove, England: Psychology Press.

Ellis Weismer, S. (2002a, July). *Fast mapping in late talking and typically developing toddlers.* Paper presented at Symposium on Lexical Processing in Children with Typical and Disordered Language Development at the joint conference of the International Congress for the Study of Child Language and the Symposium on Research in Child Language Disorders, Madison, WI.

Ellis Weismer, S. (2002b, September). *Examination of short-term language and treatment status outcomes of late talking toddlers.* Poster presented at the Treatment Efficacy Conference for People with Communication Disorders, City University of London.

Ellis Weismer, S., & Evans, J. (2002). The role of processing limitations in early identification of specific language impairment. *Topics in Language Disorders, 22,* 15–29.

Ellis Weismer, S., Evans, J., Hollar, C., & Jones, M. (2001, April). *Concurrent validity of the CDI at 30 months for toddlers with early language delay.* Poster presented at the biennial meeting of the Society for Research in Child Development, Minneapolis, MN.

Ellis Weismer, Evans, J., Jones, M., Horton-Ikard, R., & Hollar, C. (in preparation). *A microgenetic study of novel word learning in late talking and typically developing toddlers.*

Ellis Weismer, S., & Hesketh, L. (1996). Lexical learning by children with specific language impairment: Effects of linguistic input presented at varying speaking rates. *Journal of Speech and Hearing Research, 39,* 177–190.

Ellis Weismer, S., & Hesketh, L. (1998). The impact of emphatic stress in novel word learning by children with specific language impairment. *Journal of Speech, Language and Hearing Research, 41,* 1444–1458.

Ellis Weismer, S., Marchman, V., & Evans, J. (2001, December). Continuity of lexical–grammatical development in typical and late talking toddlers. *Proceedings of the Early Lexicon Acquisition Conference* (pp. 69–70). Lyon, France.

Ellis Weismer, S., Murray-Branch, J., & Miller, J. (1994). A prospective longitudinal study of language development in late talkers. *Journal of Speech and Hearing Research, 37,* 852–867.

Ellis Weismer, S., & Thordardottir, E. T. (2002). Cognition and language. In P. Accardo, A. Capute, & B. Rogers (Eds.), *Disorders of language development* (pp. 21–37). Timonium, MD: York.

Ellis Weismer, S., Tomblin, J. B., Zhang, X., Buckwalter, P., Chynoweth, J. G., & Jones, M. (2000). Nonword repetition performance in school-age children with and without language impairment. *Journal of Speech, Language, and Hearing Research, 43,* 865–878.

Feldman, H., Dollaghan, C., Campbell, T., Jurs Lasky, M., Janosky, J., & Paradis, J. (2000). Measurement properties of the MacArthur Communicative Development Inventories at ages one and two years. *Child Development, 71,* 310–322.

Fenson, L., Bates, E., Dale, P., Goodman, J., Reznick, J. S., & Thal, D. (2000). Measuring variability in early child language: Don't shoot the messenger. *Child Development, 71,* 323–328.

Fischel, J., Whitehurst, G., Caulfield, M., & DeBaryshe, B. (1989). Language growth in children with expressive language delay. *Pediatrics, 82,* 218–227.

Gernsbacher, M. A., Geye, H. M., & Ellis Weismer, S. (2005). The role of language and communication impairments within autism. In P. Fletcher & J. Miller (Eds.), *Language disorders and developmental theory* (pp. 73–93). Philadelphia: John Benjamins.

Heilmann, J., Ellis Weismer, S., Evans, J., & Hollar, C. (2005). Utility of the MacArthur Communicative Development Inventory in identifying children's language level. *American Journal of Speech-Language Pathology, 14,* 40–51.

Hick, R., Joseph, K., Conti-Ramsden, G., Serratrice, L., & Faragher, B. (2002). Vocabulary profiles of children with specific language impairment. *Child Language Teaching and Therapy, 18,* 165–180.

Johnston, J. (2004, June). *Fearless and bold in following ideas wherever they lead: The Elizabeth Bates memorial lecture.* Paper presented at 25th Symposium on Research in Child Language Disorders, Madison, WI.

Jones, M. (2004). *Longitudinal relationships between lexical and grammatical development in typical and late-talking children.* Unpublished doctoral dissertation, University of Wisconsin–Madison.

Jones, M., Ellis Weismer, S., Evans, J., & Hollar, C. (2003, July). *Lexical–grammatical development in typical and late-talking children.* Poster presented at the American Speech-Language-Hearing Association Annual Convention, Chicago.

Leonard, L. B. (1987). Is specific language impairment a useful construct? In S. Rosenberg (Ed.), *Advances in applied psycholinguistics* (pp. 1–39). New York: Cambridge University Press.

Leonard, L. B. (1991). Specific language impairment as a clinical category. *Language, Speech, and Hearing Services in the Schools, 22,* 66–68.

Leonard, L. B. (1998). *Children with specific language impairment.* Cambridge, MA: MIT Press.

Manhardt, J., & Rescorla, L. (2002). Narrative outcomes in late talkers. *Applied Psycholinguistics, 23,* 1–21.

Marchman, V., & Bates, E. (1994). Continuity in lexical and morphological development: A test of the critical mass hypothesis. *Journal of Child Language, 21,* 339–366.

McKeough, A., & Sanderson, A. (1996). Teaching storytelling: A microgenetic analysis of developing narrative structure. *Journal of Narrative and Life History, 6,* 157–192.

Nelson, K. (1986). *Event knowledge: Structure and function in development.* Hillsdale, NJ: Lawrence Erlbaum Associates.

Newcomer, P., & Hammill, D. (1997). *Test of Language Development–3 (Primary).* Austin, TX: Pro-Ed.

Olswang, L., & Bain, B. (1996). Assessment information for predicting upcoming change in language production. *Journal of Speech and Hearing Research, 39,* 414–423.

Paul, R. (1991). Profiles of toddlers with slow expressive language development. *Topics in Language Disorders, 11,* 1–13.

Paul, R. (1996). Clinical implications of the natural history of slow expressive language development. *American Journal of Speech-Language Pathology, 5,* 5–21.

Paul, R. (2000). Predicting outcomes of early expressive language delay: Ethical implications. In D. Bishop & L. Leonard (Eds.), *Speech and language impairments in children* (pp. 195–209). Hove, England: Psychology Press.

Paul, R., Hernandez, R., & Taylor, L. Narrative development in late talkers: Early school age. *Journal of Speech and Hearing Research, 39,* 1295–1303.

Peters, A., & Menn, L. (1993). False starts and filler syllables: Ways to learn grammatical morphemes. *Language, 69,* 742–777.

Rescorla, L. (1989). The Language Development Survey: A screening tool for delayed language in toddlers. *Journal of Speech and Hearing Disorders, 54,* 587–599.

Rescorla, L. (1991). Identifying expressive delay at age two. *Topics in Language Disorders, 11,* 14–20.

Rescorla, L. (2000). Do late-talking toddlers turn out to have reading difficulties a decade later? *Annals of Dyslexia, 50,* 87–102.

Rescorla, L. (2002). Language and reading outcomes to age 9 in late-talking toddlers. *Journal of Speech, Language, and Hearing Research, 45,* 360–371.

Rescorla, L., & Goossens, M. (1992). Symbolic play development in toddlers with expressive specific language impairment. *Journal of Speech and Hearing Research, 35,* 1290–1302.

Rescorla, L., & Lee, E. (2000). Language impairments in young children. In T. Layton & L. Watson (Eds.), *Handbook of early language impairment in children: Vol I. Nature* (pp. 1–38). New York: Delmar.

Rescorla, L., & Roberts, J. (2002). Nominal versus verbal morpheme use in late talkers at ages 3 and 4. *Journal of Speech, Language, and Hearing Research, 45,* 1219–1231.

Rice, M., Buhr, J., & Oetting, J. (1992). Specific-language-impaired children's quick incidental learning of words: The effect of a pause. *Journal of Speech and Hearing Research, 35,* 1040–1048.

Robertson, S., & Ellis Weismer, S. (1999). Effects of treatment on linguistic and social skills in toddlers with delayed language. *Journal of Speech, Language and Hearing Research, 42,* 1234–1248.

Sackett, D., Haynes, R., Guyatt, G., & Tugwell, P. (1991). *Clinical epidemiology: A basic science for clinical medicine.* Boston: Little, Brown.

Siegler, R. (1996). *Emerging minds.* Oxford, England: Oxford University Press.

Sowell, T. (1997). *Late-talking children.* New York: Basic Books.

Sowell, T. (2001). *The Einstein Syndrome: Bright children who talk late.* New York: Basic Books.

Spitz, R., Tallal, P., Flax, J., & Benasich, A. (1997). Look who's talking: A prospective study of familial transmission of language impairments. *Journal of Speech, Language, and Hearing Research, 40,* 990–1001.

Tager-Flusberg, H., & Cooper, J. (1999). Present and future possibilities for defining a phenotype for specific language impairment. *Journal of Speech, Language, & Hearing Research, 42,* 1275–1278.

Thal, D., & Bates, E. (1988). Language and gesture in late talkers. *Journal of Speech and Hearing Research, 34,* 604–612.

Thal, D., & Katich, J. (1996). Predicaments in early identification of specific language impairment: Does the early bird always catch the worm? In P. S. Dale (Ed.), *Assessment of communication and language: Vol. 6. Communication and language intervention series* (pp. 1–28). Baltimore, MD: Paul H. Brookes.

Thal, D., O'Hanlon, L., Clemmons, M., & Fralin, L. (1999). Validity of a parent report measure of vocabulary and syntax for preschool children with language impairment. *Journal of Speech, Language, and Hearing Research, 42,* 482–496.

Thal, D., Reilly, J., Seibert, L., Jeffries, R., & Fenson, J. (2004). Language development in children at risk for language impairment: Cross-population comparisons. *Brain and Language, 88,* 167–179.

Thal, D., Tobias, S., & Morrison, D. (1991). Language and gesture in late talkers: A one year follow-up. *Journal of Speech and Hearing Disorders, 34,* 604–612.

Thelen, E., & Corbetta, D. (2002). Microdevelopment and dynamic systems: Applications to infant motor development. In N. Granott & J. Parziale (Eds.), *Microdevelopment: Transition processes in development and learning: Cambridge studies in cognitive perceptual development* (pp. 59–79). New York: Cambridge University Press.

Tomblin, J. B., Records, N., Buckwalter, P., Zhang, X., Smith, E., & O'Brien, M. (1997). The prevalence of specific language impairment in kindergarten children. *Journal of Speech, Language, and Hearing Research, 40,* 1245–1260.

Whitehurst, G., & Fischel, J. (1994). Early developmental language delay: What, if anything, should the clinician do about it? *Journal of Child Psychology and Psychiatry, 35,* 613–648.

Whitehurst, G., & Fischel, J. (2000). Reading and language impairments in conditions of poverty. In D. Bishop & L. Leonard (Eds.), *Speech and language impairments in children* (pp. 53–71). Hove, England: Psychology Press.

Whitehurst, G., Fischel, J., Lonigan, C., Valdez-Menchaca, M., Arnold, D., & Smith, M. (1991). Treatment of early expressive language delay. *Topics in Language Disorders, 11,* 55–68.

Zhang, X., & Tomblin, J. B. (in preparation). *Developmental language disorder: A categorical or dimensional construct?*

Zimmerman, I., Steiner, V., & Pond, R. (1992). *Preschool Language Scale–3.* Chicago: Psychological Corporation.

4

Utterance Length and Lexical Diversity in American- and British-English Speaking Children: What is the Evidence for a Clinical Marker of SLI?

Thomas Klee
University of Newcastle upon Tyne, Newcastle upon Tyne, UK

William J. Gavin
Colorado State University, Fort Collins, Colorado, USA

Stephanie F. Stokes
University of Newcastle upon Tyne, Newcastle upon Tyne, UK

The search for possible genetic underpinnings of specific language impairment (SLI) has led researchers to consider more carefully what the key behavioral features of the disorder are, with the eventual goal being the establishment of a widely agreed behavioral phenotype of the condition (McCardle, Cooper, & Freund, 2005; Mervis & Robinson, 2005). In considering what features might be relevant to the construction of a phenotype, one obvious place to start is the literature on normal language development. Although work on normal development has provided the foundation on which research in developmental language disorders has been built, the direction of that relationship has by no means been one way. For example, many of the measurement tools in child language used today were spawned by researchers who had a joint interest in child language development and disorders and who saw the value of having one field inform the other.

Someone who has exemplified this dual approach to discovery throughout her career is Robin Chapman. She and Jon Miller, her colleague of many years at the University of Wisconsin–Madison, jointly published what has become one of the most widely cited measurement studies in the field (Miller & Chapman, 1981). Together, they also pioneered the use of language sample analysis as a clinical assessment procedure (e.g., Miller, 1981), with their protocols still used by clinicians and researchers today, and developed the first computerized language sample analysis (Miller & Chapman, 1981–2004), changing forever the face of research involving children's spontaneously produced language. The present chapter owes heavily to the work they have done. This chapter considers whether two measures that had their origins in the study of normal language development, one based on utterance length and the other on lexical diversity, can be used to differentiate children with and without SLI, and critically examines the usefulness of these and other measures as potential clinical markers of SLI.

We begin by reviewing the literature on clinical markers of specific language impairment (SLI) by focusing on linguistic markers (as opposed to processing markers) that have been proposed for children under the age of 5 years. The focus on young children is driven by our long-term aim of wanting to be able to reliably identify children with language difficulties from as early an age as possible (Gavin, Klee, & Membrino, 1993; Klee, 1992; Klee, Carson, Gavin, Hall, Kent, & Reece, 1998; Klee, Pearce, & Carson, 2000; Stokes, 1997). Most clinical marker research to date has focused on children from the age of 4 or 5 onward because the certainty of diagnosis increases as children get older; however, our interest is primarily in children as young as 2–3 years of age and in whether a reliable marker can be identified in children of this age. Most linguistic markers that have so far been proposed appear to be language specific; that is, application of the marker is only possible in languages with similar linguistic properties to the language from which the marker was originally derived. A second aim of this research is to find a language-neutral linguistic marker because such a marker would facilitate the cross-linguistic study of SLI and ensure greater consistency of sampling children with SLI from different language backgrounds.

Although language impairment in children can be secondary to any number of readily identifiable primary conditions (e.g., hearing impairment, cognitive delay, head injury), SLI by definition is not associated with concomitant conditions. A common profile of children with SLI involves language ability that in some respects resembles that of younger, typically developing children but in other respects is more severely compromised. Thus the language skills, particularly those involving grammar and the lexicon, of children with SLI generally resemble those of younger typically developing children (Leonard, 1998). This characterization yields a profile of a child who falls at the lower end of a continuum of language abilities (e.g., Leonard, 1987). Such a view might suggest that there is nothing special about the condition and that efforts to identify the etiology of such disorders are misplaced.

However, recent research points to a possible genetic basis for (some forms of) SLI in that children with affected family members are at greater risk of developing SLI than children without a family history of the condition (see Bishop, 2002, for a recent summary). This finding has provided renewed motivation for the hunt for causal factors of the condition, but this is not what concerns us here. Research into the etiology of SLI has refocused the spotlight on a longstanding issue, the identification of SLI. Accurate identification of SLI is critical to the conduct of research into the nature of the condition and ultimately the provision of clinical services. Although the diagnosis of SLI is made by excluding factors known to negatively affect language development (e.g., hearing impairment, general nonverbal cognitive difficulties, neurological abnormalities, environmental deprivation), in tandem with low performance on standardized language measures, research over the past decade has focused on a search for "clinical markers" of the condition capable of differentiating children with and without the condition with a high degree of accuracy.

Two kinds of clinical markers have so far been proposed. These fall broadly into what might be called processing markers, such as children's performance on tests of working memory (e.g., Dollaghan & Campbell, 1998; Gathercole & Baddeley, 1990; Hoffman & Gillam, 2004) and linguistic markers, such as the deployment of various verb and noun constructions in conversational speech (e.g., Bedore & Leonard, 1998; Gavin et al., 1993; Rice & Wexler, 1996). It is the latter that concerns us here, because it is the lack of language skills that first alerts parents and health care workers to the presence of a problem (Stokes, 1997). Although most of the research has focused on English, the search for linguistic markers has also begun in other languages, such as Italian (Bortolini, Caselli, Deevy, & Leonard, 2002) and Cantonese (Klee, Stokes, Wong, Fletcher, & Gavin, 2004).

A review of the evidence base for making claims about clinical markers is one of the thrusts of this chapter. The research on clinical markers has employed two different statistical approaches to evaluating the evidence. One approach is based on tests of group mean differences (e.g., *t*-tests or analyses of variance [ANOVAs]) in which an SLI group is compared to an age-matched (AM) control group of unaffected children, and in some cases, a language-matched (LM) control group of younger children without language impairment as well. A second approach employs discriminant analysis, which, in addition to examining whether diagnostic groups can be differentiated with respect to specific linguistic features, is also concerned with how accurately the proposed marker classifies individual children into their respective diagnostic groups. Studies employing discriminant analysis usually also report the percentage of children with SLI who tested positive on the marker (sensitivity) and the percentage of children without SLI who tested negative on the marker (specificity). Several representative studies from each approach are reviewed next.

STUDIES EMPLOYING TESTS OF GROUP MEAN DIFFERENCES

For the past 40 years, researchers (e.g., Lee, 1966; Menyuk, 1964) and clinicians have identified children as language impaired if they demonstrated language skills, whether assessed by standardized tests or language samples, that were below those expected for their age. However, with the search for a genotype of SLI, some researchers have asserted that children with SLI must perform significantly below both age-matched peers (AM) and younger typically developing children matched in some way on language ability (LM), thereby demonstrating different rather than delayed development (e.g., Rice, 1997). An interesting outcome is that the difference turns out to be a higher frequency of error patterns, such as higher omission rates of the third-person singular inflection, rather than a different pattern altogether (e.g., *they walks home*) (Leonard, 1998). That is, a clinical marker that is comprised of a composite score derived from several linguistic features identifies a quantitative difference between children with SLI and both AM and LM children, rather than a qualitative difference. Next, we briefly review some representative studies to illustrate how thinking on clinical markers has evolved.

English-speaking children with SLI have long been known to have specific difficulty with grammatical markers of tense (see Leonard, 1998, for a review). Rice and colleagues (Rice, 2003, Rice & Wexler, 1996; Rice, Wexler, & Cleave, 1995) proposed a "composite tense" measure on which children with SLI perform significantly poorer than typically developing age-matched (AM) peers and children 2 years younger. This measure is based on the average of scores on grammatical morpheme use in obligatory contexts centered around the "third person singular *-s,* regular past tense *-ed,* *Be* copula and auxiliary in statements and questions, and *Do* auxiliary in questions" (Rice, 1997, p. 73). The error forms of target sentences are comprised of nonfinite root clauses wherein obligatory morphosyntactic inflections or morphemes are omitted. The resulting structure (an unmarked bare verb stem) is also described as a root infinitive (e.g., Paradis & Crago, 2001). Examples 1–5 (from Rice, 1997) illustrate the nature of the problem, where an asterisk indicates an ungrammatical sentence structure and parenthesized material represents morphemes omitted from obligatory contexts:

1. a. Patsy *walks.*
   b. *Patsy *walk(s).*
2. a. Yesterday Patsy *walked* home after work.
   b. *Yesterday Patsy *walk(ed)* home after work.
3. a. Patsy *is* walking.
   b. *Patsy *(is)* walking.
4. a. Patsy *is* happy.
   b. *Patsy *(is)* happy.
5. a. Patsy *did* not work today/ *does* Patsy work today?
   b. *Patsy *(did)* not work today/ *(does)* Patsy work today?

Younger, typically developing (TD-Y) children and children with SLI tend to use the errors exemplified in sentences 1b–5b inconsistently, interspersed with correct productions, in both conversational speech and elicited probes. Three-year-old TD-Y children use the correct forms about 60% of the time they are obligatory, children with SLI use them about 30% of the time, and TD-AM peers use them about 95% of the time (Rice, 1997). This inconsistent use suggested to the authors that children conceptualize these forms as optional markers ("optional infinitives") due to an "incomplete specification of grammatical tense in the children's underlying grammatical representations" (Rice, Wexler, & Hershberger, 1998, p. 1413). When the representations become robust, conversational use of the forms becomes consistently correct, or adult-like. Children with SLI tend to use the error forms for a much longer period of time than typically developing children, and the term *extended optional infinitive* (EOI) has been used to describe this process.

The optional infinitive stage has been identified in several languages other than English, including Dutch (de Jong, 1999), French (Paradis & Crago, 2001), German (Rice, Noll, & Grimm, 1997) and Swedish (Hansson, 1997). Rice and colleagues attribute the cause to a deficit in the child's underlying grammar; other researchers have also proposed limitations in linguistic knowledge (e.g., Clahsen, 1989; Gopnik, 1990; van der Lely, 1994).

STUDIES EMPLOYING DISCRIMINANT ANALYSIS

Researchers have begun to acknowledge that simply showing that there are significant differences between children with and without SLI on a particular linguistic or processing feature is insufficient for demonstrating the presence of a marker (for an excellent review of the issues, see Dollaghan, 2004a). Any proposed marker should also demonstrate high sensitivity (the percentage of individuals with the target disorder who have positive results) and specificity (the percentage of individuals without the target disorder who have negative test results) (Sackett, Haynes, Guyatt, & Tugwell, 1991; Sackett, Straus, Richardson, Rosenberg, & Haynes, 2000). Two other indices that are also informative are positive predictive value (the percentage of individuals with positive test results who actually have the disorder) and negative predictive value (the percentage of individuals with negative test results without the disorder), although computing these on small samples can be misleading because they are affected by the prevalence of those having the condition (i.e., the pretest probability) in the sample. In addition, the marker should also demonstrate a high positive likelihood ratio and low negative likelihood ratio. Likelihood ratios have the advantage of being independent of prevalence, and knowledge of them can inform us of the probability that *a particular individual* has the condition compared to individuals who do not have the condition (Attia, 2003). We return to these later.

One of the earliest mentions of the term *linguistic marker* was made by Gavin et al. (1993), in a study that set out to "determine which aspects of language production ... differentiate children diagnosed with a specific language impairment from children without language impairment" and to "isolate specific characteristics of the grammar that might serve as linguistic markers of language impairment" (p. 193). This work was an extension of an earlier study by Fletcher and Peters (1984), and we review their study before returning to Gavin et al. (1993).

Fletcher and Peters (1984) posed the question of "what constitutes language impairment" (p. 34) in a study of 9 children with SLI (mean age 5;2) and 20 typically developing, age-matched (AM) children (mean age 5;1), by analyzing 200 utterances collected from each child in conversation, play, and picture description for the presence of 65 grammatical and lexical categories. The groups were significantly different on 23 of the categories. Ten of these were selected for inclusion in a stepwise multiple regression that served as a semidiscriminant analysis (coordination, subordination within object and adverbial clause elements, full progressive auxiliary, *do*-support, modal, unmarked verb forms, regular past tense, word types, and verb types). Their analysis revealed that two of the variables, unmarked verb forms and verb types, jointly accounted for 49% of the variance between groups and discriminated the groups with 90% accuracy overall, with 89% of the children in the SLI group (sensitivity) and 90% of the children in the AM control group (specificity) being correctly classified. Table 4.1 provides a summary of these values, and their associated confidence intervals, for this study and the ones to follow.[1] Fletcher and Peters concluded that reduced lexical (verb) diversity and a higher number of unmarked verb forms (i.e., lexical verbs unmarked by auxiliaries or inflections) were indicative of language impairment. One child in the SLI group and two in the AM group were misclassified by the discriminant function.

Following this study, Gavin et al. (1993) examined a mean of 200 utterances of conversational speech per child in a sample of 23 children with SLI and 24 AM children (mean age 36.2 and 37.8 months, respectively) for clause, phrase, and word structures based on the LARSP clinical analysis (Crystal, Fletcher, & Garman, 1989). The original 200 LARSP categories were collapsed into 26 composite variables, in addition to age, for inclusion in a discriminant analysis. Three linguistic variables, in conjunction with age, were found to differentiate children with and without SLI in this age range with a high degree of accuracy. The children with SLI were found to use proportionally more single-word utterances composed solely of nouns or verbs, had higher rates of errors associated with verbs (e.g., copula and auxiliary omissions), and had fewer elaborated noun phrases (NP) and prepositional phrases (PP) (e.g., DAdjN, Adj Adj N, and PrDN). These variables jointly accounted for 59% of the variance between groups and discriminated the groups with 92% accuracy overall, with 91% of the children in the SLI group and 92% of the children in the AM control group being correctly classified (see Table 4.1). In order to demonstrate the predictive validity of these key linguistic features, the procedure was repeated in a second, independent sample involving 37 new children (22 SLI and 15 AM; aged 2;1–4;1) and found 86.5% accuracy when compared with the clinical diagnosis. Based on this study, and Fletcher and Peters's earlier study, there was evidence that linguistic features associated with SLI could be identified using discriminant analysis and were likely to include a higher use of single-word utterances and unmarked verb forms, reduced lexical diversity (at least insofar as verbs were concerned), and less elaborated NPs and PPs.

In addition to these studies of specific linguistic features, there was also evidence that children with SLI differed from typically developing children on more general quantitative language sample measures having to do with utterance length and lexical diversity. Building on the finding that age and

[1]The figures in Table 4.1 were computed using the "stats calculator" on the Web site of the Centre for Evidence-Based Medicine at the University of Toronto (2004b). It should be noted that in some instances the sensitivity and specificity values differ slightly from those reported in the original studies, because the CEBM's calculations are adjusted by adding 0.5 to each cell when any cell is zero (Paul Glasziou, personal communication, November 12, 2004).

TABLE 4.1
Sensitivity, Specificity, and Positive and Negative Likelihood Ratios (With 95% Confidence Intervals) of Candidate Linguistic Markers of SLI in English

Features	*Sensitivity*	*Specificity*	*LR+*	*LR–*	*Sample*[a] *(N; age)*	*Source*
Unmarked verb forms + verb types	88.9% (56–99%)	90.0% (70–97%)	8.89 (2.34–33.78)	0.12 (0.02–0.79)	9 SLI, 20 AM; age 3;4–6;11	Fletcher and Peters (1984, p. 46)
Major single-word utterances + 3-element NPs and PPs + VP errors + Age	91.3% (73–98%)	91.7% (74–98%)	10.96 (2.89–41.55)	0.10 (0.02–0.36)	23 SLI, 24 AM; age 2;0–4;2	Gavin et al. (1993, pp. 197–198)
Percent structural errors + MLU + Age	96.5% (93–98%)	48.8% (34–64%)	1.88 (1.40–2.54)	0.07 (0.03–0.16)	201 SLI; 41 AM; age 2;6–6;11	Dunn et al. (1996, p. 650)
Noun + Verb + MLU	89.5% (69–97%)	94.7% (75–100%)	17.0 (2.51–115.26)	0.11 (0.03–0.41)	19 SLI, 19 AM; age 3;7–5;9	Bedore and Leonard (1998, p. 1189)
Noun + MLU	87.5% (67–96%)	97.5% (80–100%)	35.0 (2.26–543.13)	0.13 (0.04–0.41)	As above	As above
Verb + MLU	94.7% (75–100%)	94.7% (75–100%)	18.0 (2.66–121.64)	0.06 (0.01–0.38)	As above	As above
Noun + Verb (same for Verb alone)	82.5% (61–93%)	97.5% (80–100%)	33.0 (2.12–513.34)	0.18 (0.07–0.47)	As above	As above

Noun	77.5% (56–90%)	97.5% (80–100%)	31.0 (1.99–483.55)	0.23 (0.10–0.52)	As above	As above
MLU	94.7% (75–100%)	89.5% (69–97%)	9.0 (2.42–33.53)	0.06 (0.01–0.40)	As above	As above
Past tense, based on 25th percentile	71.4% (50–86%)	90.6% (76–97%)	7.62 (2.51–23.14)	0.32 (0.16–0.63)	21 SLI; 32 AM; age 4;2–5;10	Conti-Ramsden (2003, p. 1033)
Past tense, based on discriminant function	81.0% (60–92%)	81.0% (65–91%)	4.32 (2.04–9.14)	0.23 (0.10–0.58)	As above	As above
Plural, based on 25th percentile	16.7% (8–33%)	98.5% (87–100%)	11.0 (0.63–191.05)	0.85 (0.72–0.99)	32 SLI; 32 AM; age 4;2–5;10	Conti-Ramsden (2003, p. 1033)

Note. Indices were computed from raw data reported in original study using the stats calculator on the Web site of the Centre for Evidence-Based Medicine at the University of Toronto (2004b). Sensitivity and specificity calculations may differ from those reported in the original study in cases where the frequency of one or more cells in the 2 × 2 table was zero. LRs were derived from the sensitivity and specificity figures reported on p. 650 of Dunn et al. (1996) because cell frequencies were not reported.
[a]AM, age-matched control group.

MLU (mean length of utterance in morphemes) were highly correlated in typically developing children (Miller & Chapman, 1981), MLU was also found to have a strong association with age in children with SLI, although MLU was significantly reduced in comparison to typically developing children (Klee, Schaffer, May, Membrino, & Mougey, 1989). This same pattern held when a general measure of lexical diversity based on the number of different words (NDW) occurring in language samples controlled for the number of utterances was examined. NDW was highly correlated with age in typically developing children (Miller, 1991) as well as in children with SLI (Klee, 1992; Watkins, Kelly, Harbers, & Hollis, 1995), although as with MLU, the NDW of children with SLI was significantly reduced in comparison to that of typically developing age peers. These studies, then, suggested that general measures of utterance length and lexical diversity could serve as distinctive features of SLI in young children.

Subsequently, Dunn, Flax, Sliwinski, and Aram (1996) compared 201 children with SLI (aged 2;10–6;11) with 41 controls (aged 2;6–6;6) and found that age, MLU, and the percent of structural errors (reduced grammatical complexity, predominantly involving morphology) discriminated the two groups of children with about 88% overall accuracy, with 96% of the children in the SLI group being correctly classified (see Table 4.1). However, there was a high proportion of false negatives, as only 49% of the children in the AM control group were correctly classified.

In a study of 19 children with SLI and 19 AM controls, aged 3;7 to 5;9, Bedore and Leonard (1998) used a series of discriminant analyses to examine three possible linguistic markers alone and in combination. The first represented a finite verb morpheme composite that included regular past-tense inflections, regular third-person singular inflections, and copula and auxiliary *be* forms. The second pertained to noun morphology and included the genitive and plural inflections and articles. The third proposed marker was MLU in morphemes. The sensitivity and specificity of each of the three candidate markers, and combinations of markers, are summarized in Table 4.1.

In the final study to be examined here, Conti-Ramsden (2003) provided a direct comparison of various candidate markers on the same sample of children. Two processing marker tasks, involving digit recall (Elliott, Murray, & Pearson, 1983) and nonword repetition (Gathercole & Baddeley, 1996), and two linguistic marker tasks, involving past tense (based on Marchman, Wulfeck, & Ellis Weismer, 1999) and plurals (based on Oetting & Rice, 1993), were administered to 32 children with SLI (4;4–5;10) and 32 AM children (4;4–5;8). In contrast to the studies reviewed earlier, each of the markers evaluated by Conti-Ramsden was evaluated using elicitation tasks rather than language sampling. The sensitivity of the linguistic marker tasks ranged from 17 to 81% depending on the task and the cutoff level used, with the specificity ranging from 81 to 98%. It should be noted that only 21 of the children in the SLI group were able to complete the past-tense task.

Because sensitivity and specificity reflect how a diagnostic measure functions in the population, they do not easily translate to predicting outcomes for individuals (Attia, 2003). Likelihood ratios provide a practical way of doing this, in that they allow us to use an individual's results to narrow down the possibility of a diagnosis. A likelihood ratio (LR) expresses the likelihood, or odds, that a given result (e.g., the presence of a positive marker) would be expected in an individual with the target disorder (e.g., SLI) compared with the likelihood that the same result would be expected in an individual without the disorder (Sackett et al., 2000). Positive likelihood ratios (LR+) indicate the likelihood of having the condition given a positive test result, whereas negative likelihood ratios (LR–) indicate the likelihood of having the condition given a negative test result. The larger the LR+ the more likely an individual is to have the condition, given a positive test result. The smaller the LR–, the less likely an individual is to have the condition, given a negative test result (Attia, 2003). Because LRs are based on a ratio of sensitivity and specificity, they are less susceptible to changes in prevalence than sensitivity and specificity, such as when the mix of mild and severely affected individuals with the target disorder changes from one setting, or study, to another (Sackett et al., 1991).

Table 5.1 summarizes the positive and negative likelihood ratios, along with their associated confidence intervals, for each of the proposed clinical markers reviewed earlier that have been assessed using discriminant analysis. It should be noted that LRs were not reported in any of the original studies; rather, they were computed here so that the diagnostic potential of the various candidate markers could be compared. As was done for the sensitivity and specificity values in this table, likelihood ratios were computed using the "stats calculator" on the Web site of the Centre for Evidence-Based Medicine at the University of Toronto (2004b). Although there are no absolutes regarding the interpretation of LRs, LR+ values greater than 10 are considered to be "high" and "indicate that the test, sign or symptom can be used to rule in the [condition]" (Centre for Evidence-Based Medicine, 2004a). They also indicate a "large and often conclusive increase in the likelihood of a [condition]" (Ebell, 1999) and that "an individual ... is very likely to have the target condition" (Dollaghan, 2004a, p. 397). Dollaghan (2004a) suggests that "when LR+ is 20 or more, [the] individual is virtually certain to have the condition" (p. 397). It is important that LR+ values are viewed in conjunction with the measure's LR– value, because the diagnostic value of a measure improves as LR+ increases and LR– decreases. Dollaghan (2004a) suggests that "when a measure has an LR– value lower than 0.20, an individual scoring within the unaffected range is very likely to be free of the target condition; when LR–

is 0.10 or lower such an individual is virtually certain to be free of the condition" (p. 397).

Based on these interpretations, if we adopt the admittedly arbitrary criterion that a candidate marker must have an LR+ ≥ 10 and LR– ≤ 0.20 in order to be of practical use, 6 of the 13 proposed markers in Table 5.1 meet that standard. These include the composite measure proposed by Gavin et al. (1993) and the following composites examined by Bedore and Leonard (1998): Verb, Noun + Verb, Noun + MLU, Verb + MLU, Noun + Verb + MLU. Three other measures approach, but fall just short of, this threshold: the separate Noun and MLU measures examined by Bedore and Leonard, and Fletcher and Peters's (1984) composite measure. If we adopt a more stringent criterion of LR+ ≥ 20 and LR– ≤ 0.10, then none of the proposed markers in the table meets the standard; however, two of Bedore and Leonard's measures approach this level: Noun + MLU and Verb + MLU.

Up to this point, we have examined several statistical properties of various linguistic markers of SLI that have been mooted. These properties give an indication of how accurate the marker was in correctly identifying children with and without SLI in the sample data of the research study. Their associated confidence intervals, listed in Table 4.1, provide an indication of the degree to which the measures could potentially vary in other samples and the range within which the population value is likely to fall. The wider the confidence interval, the less faith can be put in the sample value as being reflective of the true population value, and hence, the less convincing is its value as a clinical marker. In each case the purported clinical marker's confidence interval is unacceptably wide, reflecting in part the modest sample sizes of the studies on which the markers were examined.

Leonard (1998) stated that "the Achilles' heel of most of these accounts is that their predictions hold for only a limited range of languages" (p. 235), as did Johnston (2004), who observed that "the nature of SLI differs according to the demands of the particular language." It may be time to search for a clinical marker that will not only highlight differences between children with SLI and typically developing children, but will also suggest similarities in children with SLI cross-linguistically. Is there a linguistic marker that has the potential for universal applicability that may in turn lead to a cross-linguistic account of the disorder?

Children with SLI differ from typically developing children in terms of the average length of their spoken utterances, their lexical development, and their deployment of specific grammatical morphemes. Their language abilities resemble those of younger children, although there are some pockets of performance that are not commensurate with those of even younger children. Armed with the knowledge that the pockets are likely to be in language-specific features, and that methodology has moved on from that used up until 1993, we reappraise the role of MLU, lexical diversity and age as clinical markers of SLI. Age appears to be worthy of investigation, as researchers have found that inclusion of age as a variable increases the likelihood of the correct classification of impairment (e.g., Dunn et al., 1996; Gavin et al., 1993). Indeed, clinicians often look to the child's age in determining the need for clinical services, and for this reason, the role of age as a variable requires further investigation (Bortolini et al., 2002). Lexical diversity deserves a reappraisal due not only to historical findings (e.g., Fletcher & Peters, 1984), but also to the fact that "the emergence of first vocabulary items may function much like a clinical marker in affected children, although whether or not vocabulary status retains this marker function for older children remains to be seen" (Rice, 2000, p. 28).

In our previous study of Cantonese-speaking children in Hong Kong (Klee et al., 2004), we presented data showing that two summary measures based on the utterance length (MLU) and lexical diversity (*D*; Malvern, Richards, Chipere, & Durán, 2004) of children's conversational language were significantly related to age. MLU increased linearly ($R = .44$), whereas *D* showed a curvilinear increase ($R = .73$), between the ages of 2;3 and 5;8. We also presented data showing that MLU and D could be used in conjunction with age to accurately differentiate 4-year-old children with SLI from both age-matched peers and younger children matched on language comprehension. In that study, we proposed that the measures could be used jointly as a clinical marker of SLI in Cantonese because they differentiated the groups with a high degree of accuracy (98% overall), but that further study was needed to validate this. The joint measures demonstrated sensitivity of 97%, specificity of 91%, LR+ of 10.33, and LR– of 0.03. Because the measures are computable in any language, we went on to suggest the advantages of employing a common marker across languages in the cross-linguistic study of SLI.

The current investigation further explores the potential value of a joint measure based on utterance length (MLU), lexical diversity (*D*), and age in differentiating children with and without SLI, following the methodology employed in our earlier study of Cantonese-speaking children (Klee et al., 2004). However, it differs from that study both in the language examined and in the age range studied. Before doing that, we present the findings of a cross-sectional study of young British- and American-English speaking children, focusing on the developmental characteristics of each of the constituent measures.

STUDY 1

In the first study we examine the relation between age and measures of utterance length (MLU) and lexical diversity (*D*) in young, typically developing children learning English as their first language. We also examine whether the two measures are correlated with each other independently of age.

Data Collection and Transcription

Language samples from a total of 152 children between the ages of 24 and 48 months served as the data for this study. Half the children ($n = 76$) lived in or around two locations in the United States (Nashville, TN, and Laramie, WY) and half lived in or around Newcastle upon Tyne in the United Kingdom; 50% of the children were girls. The data for this study come from a variety of sources, some of which have been previously reported in the literature (Gavin & Giles, 1996; Gavin et al., 1993; Klee, 1992; Klee et al., 1989, 1998).

All the language samples were collected and transcribed in one of three laboratory or clinical settings following a common protocol. The U.S. samples were recorded in purpose-built Child Language Laboratories at Vanderbilt University and the University of Wyoming. The UK samples were recorded in the Paediatric Speech and Language Clinic at the University of Newcastle upon Tyne as part of a project funded by the Nuffield Foundation. The manner in which the language samples were collected was similar across all children, in that they were based on parent–child, free-play interactions, each lasting 20 min. A common set of age-appropriate toys was used in each setting during the play sessions, and children were left to interact with one parent while being recorded. No outside observer was present in the room, although parents and possibly the children were aware of being observed from an adjacent room separated by a one-way mirror. The dyadic interactions were recorded on audiotape using a combination of FM radio microphones and wall-mounted microphones. Most of the data collected at the U.S. sites was video-recorded as well.

The language samples were transcribed from audiotape by teams of student research assistants trained by the first two authors. Transcription conventions originally developed for the SALT computer program by Jon Miller and Robin Chapman of the University of Wisconsin–Madison (Miller & Chapman, 1985–2004), and later extended by the first two authors, were used in coding all language samples. Utterance segmentation criteria, developed by Paul Fletcher and Michael Garman at the University of Reading (Fletcher & Garman, 1988; Garman, 1989a, 1989b), were employed for all language samples to insure consistency across the entire database. Interobserver transcription agreement and/or reliability was calculated on various subsamples of the data as new transcribers joined the team and was found to be consistently high.

For the current study, the 152 SALT transcripts were converted to CHAT transcription format so that the *vocd* program of CLAN (MacWhinney, 2003) could be used to generate *D* values.[2] For consistency, the MLU values

[2]A step-by-step guide for how this was done is available from the authors.

used in this study were also generated by CLAN. Incomplete (i.e., abandoned) and interrupted utterances were coded in the CHAT transcripts with the postcodes [+inc] and [+int], respectively, and symbolic noise was coded with the @ code. Utterances containing these postcodes, and segments marked as symbolic noise, were then excluded from the calculation of MLU using the following command:

```
MLU +t*CHI –s"[+ inc]" –s"[+ int]" –s"*@*" *.cha
```

MLU values, then, were based on all complete and intelligible utterances occurring in the transcript and excluded words occurring in retracings (mazes). To test the integrity of converting the transcripts from SALT to CHAT format, MLU values (in morphemes) were computed on each language sample using the SALT and CLAN computer programs. MLU values generated by the two programs were identical to two decimal places in the case of 122/152 transcripts (80%) and differed by 0.01 morpheme on 21 transcripts (14%), by 0.02 morphemes on 5 transcripts (3%), by 0.03 morphemes on 3 transcripts (2%), and by 0.04 morphemes on 1 transcript (< 1%).

The calculation of *D* was based on all intelligible words, including those occurring in incomplete or partly intelligible utterances, as the presence of a lexical item in any context was taken as evidence of the word being present in the child's lexicon. Unintelligible words were excluded (by default) from the calculation of *D* as were words occurring in retracings (using the +r6 switch). *D* was calculated using the follow CLAN command:

```
VOCD +t*CHI +r6 –s"*@*" *.cha
```

Data Summary

Summary statistics for MLU and *D* for the group as a whole, as well as for sub-groups broken down by gender and nationality, are presented in Table 5.2, along with the number of utterances, word tokens, and word types in the 20-min language samples. The children produced an average of 164 complete and fully intelligible utterances (*SD* = 50), 524 intelligible word tokens (*SD* = 227) and 139 word types (*SD* = 45) (e.g., *go, goes,* and *going* counted as one word type).

Effects of Gender and Nationality on MLU and *D*

Before deciding whether to treat the entire data set as representing a single sample of children learning English, we explored the effects of gender and nationality on the two variables of interest (MLU and *D*). We did this after removing the effect of age, because previous studies have shown that age correlates highly with both MLU (e.g., Klee et al., 1989; Miller & Chapman,

TABLE 4.2
Sample Size (*n*), Age, and Language Scores (Mean, Standard Deviation) of Each Group of Typically Developing Children and of the Full Group

Group	*n*	*Age (months)*	*Number of CI utterances*[a]	*Total number of words*[b]	*Number of different words*[b]	*MLU*[c]	*D*[b]
U.S.	76	35.8 (7.0)	173.7 (54.0)	518.4 (226.9)	131.4 (40.4)	2.72 (0.74)	43.3 (14.7)
UK	76	34.5 (7.0)	154.6 (43.5)	529.0 (229.2)	146.7 (47.7)	2.92 (0.78)	48.8 (15.3)
Boys	76	35.6 (7.2)	156.7 (48.4)	483.1 (221.0)	133.1 (46.2)	2.72 (0.81)	44.3 (15.1)
Girls	76	34.7 (6.8)	171.5 (50.4)	564.2 (227.8)	145.0 (42.6)	2.92 (0.70)	47.8 (15.2)
Total	152	35.2 (7.0)	164.1 (49.8)	523.7 (227.4)	139.0 (44.7)	2.82 (0.77)	46.0 (15.2)

Note. MLU, mean length of utterance; *D*, lexical diversity score.
[a]CI, complete and intelligible utterances.
[b]Based on all utterances, excluding mazes.
[c]Based on CI utterances.

1981) and *D* (e.g., Malvern et al., 2004) in English. Two separate 2 × 2 analyses of covariance (ANCOVA) were conducted, with MLU as the dependent variable in one analysis and *D* as the dependent variable in the other. The independent variables were gender and nationality and the covariate was age calculated in months.

Table 4.2 displays the unadjusted means of the variables for each group. As expected, the main effect of the age covariate was statistically significant for both MLU ($F(1, 147) = 109.09, p < .0005$, partial $\eta^2 = .43$) and *D* ($F(1, 147) = 165.80, p < .0005$, partial $\eta^2 = .53$). After removing the effect of age, the main effect for gender was significant both in the case of MLU ($F(1, 147) = 7.84, p = .006$, partial $\eta^2 = .05$) and *D* ($F(1, 147) = 8.39, p = .004$, partial $\eta^2 = .05$). The adjusted mean MLU of the girls was 0.26 morphemes higher than that of the boys, and the adjusted *D* of the girls was 4.86 points higher than that of the boys. Similarly, the main effect for nationality was significant when holding age constant, both for MLU ($F(1, 147) = 9.33$, $p = .003$, partial $\eta^2 = .06$) and *D* ($F(1, 147) = 19.45, p < .0005$, partial $\eta^2 = .12$). The adjusted mean MLU of the UK sample exceeded that of the U.S. sample by 0.29 morphemes, and the adjusted mean *D* of the UK sample was 7.41 points higher than that of the U.S. sample. The gender-by-nationality interaction was not significant for either measure.

Although in our sample of 152 children, girls differed from boys and British children differed from American children in terms of both average utterance length (measured by MLU) and lexical diversity (measured by *D*), the effect sizes associated with gender (partial η^2 of .05 for MLU and *D*) and nationality (.06 for MLU and .12 for *D*) were small. Therefore, in the analyses that follow that examine the relationship between the language measures and age, we have taken these findings into account by including gender as a factor in the regression analyses and computing separate regression equations for the UK and U.S. samples.[3]

Relation between MLU and Age

Regression analyses were conducted to determine the degree to which MLU and age were related in the U.S. and British samples separately as well as in

[3]Although these findings reveal nationality differences in our sample, caution is warranted in generalizing the findings to the population. The small but significant difference in the average utterance length and lexical diversity of the UK and U.S. samples may not be due to real differences in grammatical or vocabulary usage of children in those countries. Rather, it may be due to variation in the SES composition (e.g., parental education level) of the two research samples or to undetected differences in the way the samples were collected or transcribed in the two countries. Every effort was made to insure that the language samples were collected in a similar manner and that the transcription teams in both countries were working to the same set of transcription criteria. These possibilities cannot be ruled out at this stage and need to be explored further before suggesting that there may be differences in the language abilities that these measures estimate.

the combined sample of 152 children. Data are presented separately for each country so that researchers and clinicians can make practical use of the data for children in their respective countries. For each country, regression analyses were first run using age in months as the criterion (dependent) variable and MLU and gender as predictor (independent) variables. They were then repeated using MLU as the criterion variable and age and gender as the predictor variables. All analyses were conducted with SPSS (2001). Figure 4.1 displays two graphs of the age–MLU relationship. In the first graph, the difference between the UK and U.S. samples is portrayed. The second illustrates the difference between boys and girls on this measure.

U.S. Sample. In the U.S. sample, the multiple correlation between age and the variables of MLU and gender was .66 with 43% of the variance in age accounted for by its linear relationship with MLU and gender ($F(2, 73) = 28.04$, $p < .0005$). The change in the amount of variance accounted for by fitting a quadratic function of MLU was not significant. The resulting equations for (a) predicting a child's age in months given the child's MLU and gender (where boys =1 and girls = 2) and (b) predicting a child's MLU given age in months and gender are:

$$\text{Predicted Age} = (6.23 \times \text{MLU}) + (-1.67 \times \text{Gender}) + 21.36$$

$$\text{Predicted MLU} = (0.07 \times \text{Age}) + (0.20 \times \text{Gender}) - 0.07$$

UK Sample. Similar results were found in the British sample. The multiple correlation between age and the variables of MLU and gender was .65 with approximately 42% of the variance in age accounted for by its linear relationship with these two variables ($F(2, 73) = 26.84$, $p < .0005$), with no significant additional variance accounted for by a quadratic fit of MLU. The resulting regression equations for the British data are:

$$\text{Predicted Age} = (5.84 \times \text{MLU}) + (-2.54 \times \text{Gender}) + 21.30$$

$$\text{Predicted MLU} = (0.07 \times \text{Age}) + (0.32 \times \text{Gender}) - 0.05$$

Relation Between *D* and Age

The same procedures were used to examine the relationship between *D* and the variables of age and gender in the U.S. and British samples. Figure 4.2 displays plots of age and *D* broken down by national groups and by gender.

U.S. Sample. In the U.S. sample, the multiple correlation between age and the variables of *D* and gender was .70 with approximately 48% of the variance in age accounted for by its linear relationship with *D* and gender

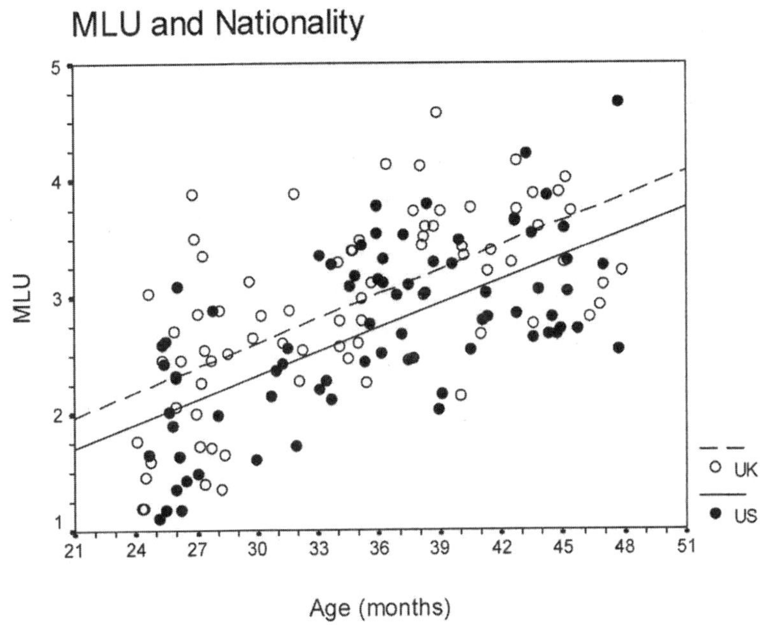

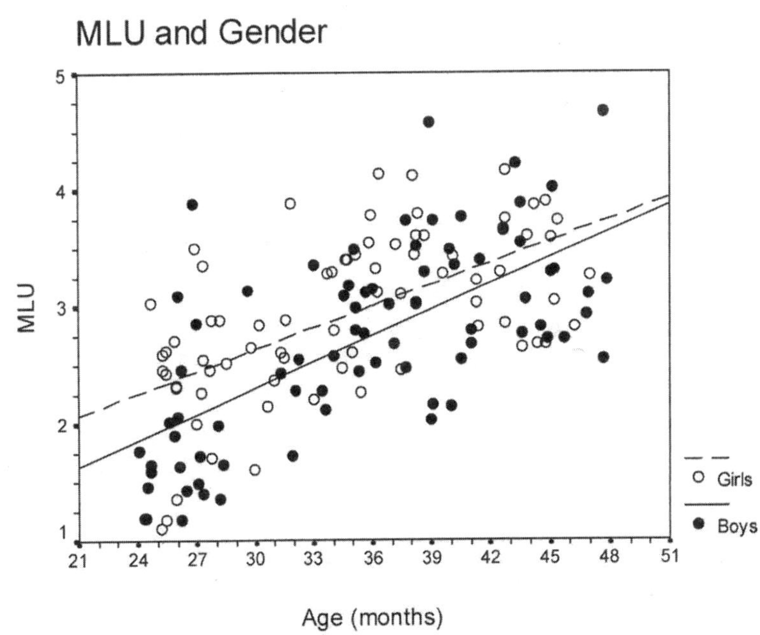

FIG. 4.1. Scatterplots of age and MLU, with linear regression lines, for the UK and U.S. samples (upper graph) and for boys and girls (lower graph) ($n = 152$).

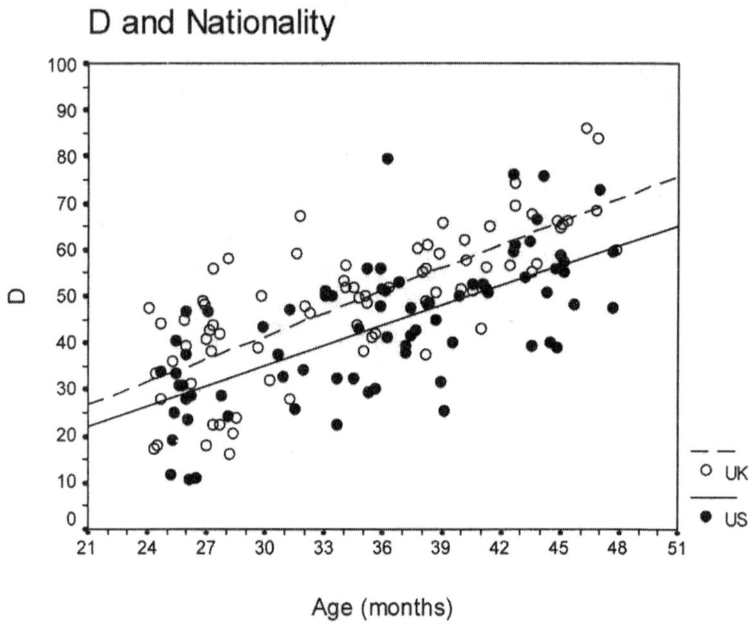

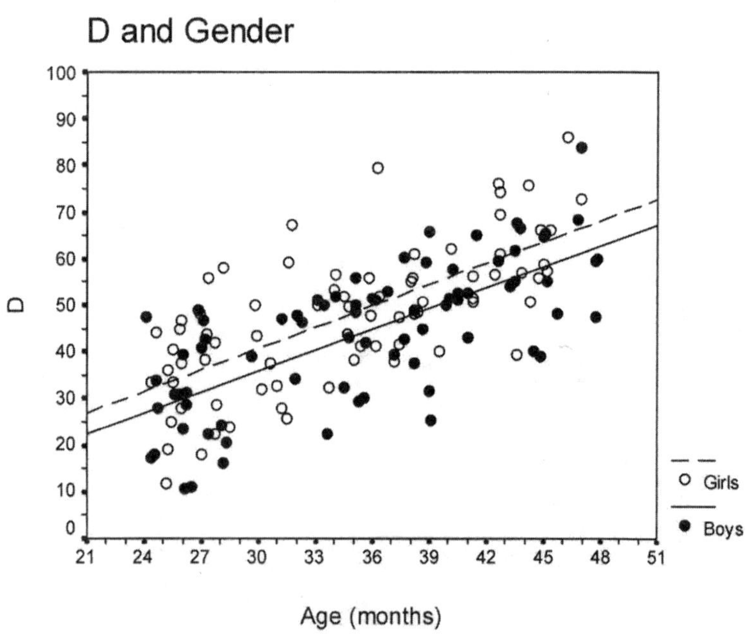

FIG. 4.2. Scatterplots of age and *D*, with linear regression lines, for the UK and U.S. samples (upper graph) and for boys and girls (lower graph) ($n = 152$).

($F(2,73) = 34.02, p < .0005$). Fitting a quadratic curve for *D* to the data did not significantly account for any additional variance. The resulting equations for (a) predicting a child's age in months given the child's *D* score and gender, where boys = 1 and girls = 2, and (b) predicting a child's *D* score given age in months and gender are:

$$\text{Predicted Age} = (0.33 \times D) + (-2.17 \times \text{Gender}) + 24.69$$

$$\text{Predicted } D = (1.45 \times \text{Age}) + (5.44 \times \text{Gender}) - 16.76$$

UK Sample. The multiple correlation between age and the variables *D* and gender in the UK sample was .76 with approximately 58% of the variance in age accounted for by its linear relationship with *D* and gender ($F(2, 73) = 50.84, p < .0005$). No significant additional variance could be accounted for by fitting a quadratic curve of *D* to the data. The resulting regression equations for the British data are:

$$\text{Predicted Age} = (0.35 \times D) + (-1.98 \times \text{Gender}) + 20.47$$

$$\text{Predicted } D = (1.66 \times \text{Age}) + (4.32 \times \text{Gender}) - 15.03$$

Relation between MLU and *D*

The relation between MLU and *D* was examined using correlation procedures. Based on the findings of our Cantonese study, and the findings of earlier studies examining the relation between vocabulary size and grammatical complexity, we anticipated that the correlation between MLU and *D* would be in a positive direction; hence, one-tailed tests were used. In the full sample of 152 children, MLU and *D* were strongly correlated with each other ($r(150) = .65, p < .0005$, one-tailed). However, because they were each also highly correlated with age, the partial correlation between MLU and *D* was computed after removing the effect of age. The partial correlation provides an idea of the association between utterance length and lexical diversity when the effects of age are held constant. The partial correlation dropped but was still significant ($r(149) = .40, p < .0005$, one-tailed).

Joint Contribution of MLU and *D* in Predicting Age

The final analysis of Study 1 involved performing hierarchical multiple regression analyses using MLU and *D* as predictor variables in order to determine the joint contribution of the two measures in predicting age and to establish whether MLU and *D* contributed any unique variance beyond that contributed by the other measure. Given that children's language abilities change with age, age was used as a proxy for general language development for this analysis. Jointly, MLU and *D* were significantly related to age, $R = .72$ ($F(2, 149) = 79.35$, $p < .0005$) and accounted for approximately 52% of the variance in age (see Table 4.3). When MLU was entered first, it accounted for about 38% of the variance in age ($F(1, 150) = 91.39$, $p < .0005$), with *D* accounting for an additional 14% above that contributed by MLU ($F(1, 149) = 42.20$, $p < .0005$). When *D* was entered first, the lexical diversity measure accounted for approximately 47% of the variance in age ($F(1, 150) = 130.40$, $p < .0005$), with MLU accounting for an additional 5% of the variance above that already accounted for by *D* ($F(1, 149) = 15.60$, $p < .0005$). Table 4.4 shows the interrelationship of the variables. Examination of the beta weights for MLU and *D* (.30 and .49, respectively) reveals that each accounts for a significant amount of variance in age ($p < .0005$), with the relative contribution of *D* accounting for more of the variance than MLU.

STUDY 2

In the second study, we examine whether the combination of MLU, *D*, and age can be used as a clinical marker to differentiate young English-speaking

TABLE 4.3
Multiple Correlation (*R*), Variance Accounted for (R^2), Change in R^2, and Significance of Change (*p*) for Two Hierarchical Regression Analyses ($n = 152$)

Step	*Predictors*	*R*	R^2	R^2 *change*	*p*
1	MLU	.62	.38	.38	< .0005
2	MLU, D	.72	.52	.14	< .0005
1	D	.68	.47	.47	< .0005
2	D, MLU	.72	.52	.05	< .0005

TABLE 4.4
Unstandardized Coefficient (*B*), Standardized Coefficient (b), Significance of Language Measure in Predicting Age, Zero-Order Correlation With Age, and Partial Correlation With Age After Removing the Effect of the Other Measure ($n = 152$)

Predictor	*B*	*b*	*p*	*Zero-order correlation*	*Partial correlation*
D	.22	.49	< .0005	.68	.47
MLU	2.71	.30	< .0005	.62	.31

children with and without SLI, as we found they did in our study of older Cantonese-speaking children (Klee et al., 2004). More importantly, this study begins to address the issue of whether children with language difficulties can be reliably detected before the age of four using this set of simple measures.

Some investigators have suggested that it is not possible to reliably diagnosis SLI before the age of 4. While this may be the case, we agree with Locke's (1994) premise that SLI is a developmental condition present from the earliest stages. That is, the language of these children does not start off on a normal developmental trajectory, only for the condition to arise at some later point in childhood. Assuming this, if a diagnosis can be made by the age of 4 with a fair degree of certainty, there are bound to be indicators, linguistic or otherwise, present in the behavior of younger children that would lead to a diagnosis of SLI earlier in life.

One of the reasons some researchers and clinicians do not feel confident in making such a diagnosis in young children may be due to the research that has been done on clinical markers of the condition. As Table 4.1 shows, most of this research has focused on *grammatical* features that are not fully developed even in 4-year-old typically developing children (Balason & Dollaghan, 2002). With few exceptions in the research on clinical markers (e.g., Conti-Ramsden & Jones, 1997; Fletcher & Peters, 1984), studies have focused on grammar to the exclusion of the lexicon. In any case, the children who have been classified as SLI in this study represented a group of individuals presenting with clinically delayed language that was not the consequence of impaired hearing, nonverbal cognitive functioning, or any other obviously delayed or impaired developmental function. Moreover, intervention had been recommended for each of these children by speech-language pathologists and many of these children received treatment for their language difficulties subsequent to the evaluation reported in this study.

The data available to examine these issues in English-speaking children differed in several important ways from the Cantonese data reported in Klee et al. (2004). First, the English-speaking children with SLI were, on average, 18 months younger than their counterparts in Hong Kong. Second, because of this, the data we had available did not allow us to include a younger, language-matched group that would have permitted a three-group comparison, as was done in the Cantonese study. We were, however, able to compare the SLI group to an age-matched control group (AM). Third, the diagnosis of SLI in the English sample was more tentative than would have been the case with older children, simply because they were younger.

The Children and Their Data

Language samples from 48 children between 24 and 50 months of age were available for analysis. Twenty-four children with SLI were clinically diagnosed by ASHA-certified speech-language pathologists and matched to 24 children of similar age without language difficulties. Analyses of language sample measures based on these children have been reported previously (Klee, 1992; Klee et al., 1989). The language sample of one child in the SLI group did not contain enough word tokens to allow D to be computed and was dropped from subsequent analyses. The final sample of 47 children in this study had previously been analyzed with respect to grammatical features in a study of linguistic markers by Gavin et al. (1993).

The two groups were similar with respect to age (SLI: M = 38.0 months; AM: M = 36.5 months), gender (SLI: 19 boys, 4 girls; AM: 19 boys, 5 girls), language background (all were monolingual speakers of standard American English), and socioeconomic level (Duncan socioeconomic index, Mueller & Parcel, 1981). The groups were also similar with regard to parental education level, in that 75% of the children in each group came from families where the more educated parent had attained, at most, a high school diploma and 25% of the children had at least one parent with a university degree.

All of the children were given a clinical evaluation of language, speech, hearing, and cognitive abilities. None of the children in either group had histories of neurological, cognitive or emotional problems and all of them demonstrated normal hearing (through audiometric screening or threshold testing) and had speech that was sufficiently intelligible for orthographic transcription to be done. The clinical diagnosis of each child as either having SLI or language within normal range was based on the Sequenced Inventory of Communication Development–Revised (SICD–R; Hedrick, Prather, & Tobin 1984), a standardized test of receptive and expressive language, in conjunction with an observation of the child during a free-play interaction with the mother (or in the case of two children, the grandmother). In addition, the parent was interviewed about the child's developmental history and current level of functioning. Although each child was given the SICD–R, the clinical diagnosis was not based solely on a test score; rather, it was based on test results supported by clinical judgment, with each diagnosis being independently confirmed by a second speech-language pathologist. It is important to note that the diagnosis was not made on the basis of either of the variables of interest in this study (MLU or D), because these were not known at the time the diagnosis was made.

Table 4.5 provides a summary of each group's performance on the SICD–R. Mann–Whitney tests indicated that the SLI group scored significantly lower than the AM group on the expressive language test (p = .007) but not on the receptive test. Wilcoxon matched-pairs tests indicated that both the receptive (p < .0008) and expressive language scores (p < .00005) of the SLI group were significantly below the age level of that group and that their expressive scores were significantly below their receptive scores (p = .021).

TABLE 4.5
Summary Statistics for the SLI and Age-Matched Groups

	SLI (n = 23)		*Age-matched (n = 24)*	
Variable	*M*	*SD*	*M*	*SD*
Age (months)	38.04	7.00	36.53	7.64
SICD–R: RCA	32.87	7.90	35.50	6.70
SICD–R: ECA	30.26	7.71	36.83	8.08
Number of CI utterances[a]	160.61	68.04	153.20	54.74
Total number of words[b]	384.39	195.53	464.30	237.82
Number of different words[b]	102.61	38.61	120.80	43.12
MLU[c]	2.27	0.60	3.01	0.86
D[b]	35.84	15.32	44.60	15.07

Note. SICD–R: RCA, ECA, Sequenced Inventory of Communicative Development–Revised: Receptive and Expressive Communication Age. MLU, mean length of utterance. *D*, lexical diversity score.
[a]CI, complete and intelligible utterances.
[b]Based on all utterances, excluding mazes.
[c]Based on CI utterances.

Language Sample Measures. The language samples used in this study were elicited, transcribed, and converted to CHAT format in the same manner as was done in Study 1. For this study, MLU and *D* were computed from each language sample using the CLAN computer program. MLU in morphemes was based on all complete and fully intelligible utterances, whereas *D* was based on all intelligible words. Retracings (mazes) were excluded from the calculation of both measures.

Accuracy of MLU and *D* in Differentiating SLI and AM Children

A discriminant analysis was performed to determine whether a linear combination of age, MLU, and *D* could be used to differentiate the SLI and AM groups and if so, to determine how accurate the measures were in classifying the 47 children into their diagnostic groups. The Wilks Λ of .53 was significant (χ^2 (3, $N = 47$) = 27.54, $p < .0005$), indicating the three variables (age, MLU, and *D*) successfully differentiated the two groups of children. The within-group correlations between the variables and the discriminant function are presented in Table 4.6, along with the standardized discriminant function coefficients. As may be seen in this table, the MLU component was relatively stronger than the *D* component, while the age component was negative.

Overall, the linear combination of age, MLU, and *D* resulted in correct classification of 39/47 cases (83%). As shown in Table 4.7, 19/23 children in the SLI group and 20/24 children in the AM group were correctly classified (sensitivity = 82.6%; specificity = 83.3%). As a first step toward validating the discriminant function, the same cases were reclassified using the "leave-one-out classification" option in SPSS, resulting in 38/47 cases (81%) being correctly reclassified, one less than in the original analysis. The single discrepancy between analyses involved a child in the SLI group who was predicted to be normal by the discriminant function.

This analysis reveals that the measures were less accurate in classifying English-speaking children (83%) than they were in classifying Canton-

TABLE 4.6
Correlation of Predictor Variables With Discriminant Function (Function Structure Matrix) and Standardized Discriminant Function Coefficient ($n = 47$)

Predictor variable	*Correlation with discriminant function*	*Standardized discriminant function coefficients*
Age (months)	–.112	–1.426
MLU	.540	1.274
D	.314	.487

TABLE 4.7
Classification Analysis for 2-Year-Olds, 3-Year-Olds, and Combined Sample

	Actual Group					
	2-Year-Olds		*3-Year-Olds*		*Combined*	
Predicted Group	*SLI* ($n = 9$)	*AM* ($n = 13$)	*SLI* ($n = 14$)	*AM* ($n = 11$)	*SLI* ($n = 23$)	*AM* ($n = 24$)
Original analysis						
SLI	7	3	12	1	19	4
Age-matched	2	10	2	10	4	20
Cross-validated analysis						
SLI	6	3	12	1	18	4
Age-matched	3	10	2	10	5	20

ese-speaking children (98%). This could be due to differences between the two languages or it could be due to other differences between the studies. As was pointed out earlier, the children in the Cantonese study were an average of 18 months older than those in the present study. Because language impairment can be more reliably diagnosed the older the child is, it is possible that the predictive power of the variables increases with age. We tested this by removing the 2-year-olds from our sample and rerunning the discriminant analysis on children aged 36 months and older. The result was that 22 of 25 3-year-old children (88%) were correctly classified. As shown in Table 4.7, 12/14 children in the SLI group and 10/11 children in the AM group were correctly classified (sensitivity = 85.7%; specificity = 90.9%). Table 4.7 also displays the classification results for the 2-year-olds, where 17/22 cases (77%) were correctly classified.

DISCUSSION

Developmental Characteristics of MLU and *D* in English

The present study is an initial attempt to determine whether the hypothesized marker derived from age, MLU, and *D* behaves similarly in a language other than Cantonese. We began by examining a data set of 152 English-speaking children from the United States and the United Kingdom to evaluate the developmental functions of MLU and *D* in the two varieties of English and to determine the correspondence between the two measures. We also examined the joint contribution of the two measures and age with respect to differentiating English-speaking children with SLI from age-matched peers. A brief summary of the findings follows, along with a comparison of the results from English and Cantonese.

First, we found that for English, MLU and *D* varied according to gender and nationality, with girls having higher MLU and *D* values than boys, and children in the UK sample having higher values than children in the U.S. sample. Because of this, we analyzed the UK and U.S. data separately, while statistically controlling for the effect of gender. The relationship between age and MLU, after controlling for the effect of gender, was similar in each country. In the U.S. sample the correlation between age and MLU was .66, and in the UK sample it was .65. These values are higher than the correlation of .44 that characterized the Cantonese sample. As we reasoned in the earlier paper, this is probably due to differences in the conversational constraints of Cantonese and English, in that in Cantonese both subject and object marking are optional and context dependent, in the way that only subject marking is in English. The overall effect of this is a reduction in the absolute value of MLU relative to English, particularly as Cantonese-speaking children reach the age of 3;0. This is also a period of rapid growth in inflectional morphology for English-speaking children, which in turn affects MLU, whereas inflections do not feature in Cantonese.

The age–MLU relation found in the present study is compared with those of two other studies in Fig. 4.3, and with our sample of children with SLI. For purposes of illustration, the U.S. and UK samples in the present study were combined and are represented by a single regression line based on all 152 children. This is depicted along with the regression lines reported by Miller and Chapman (1981) for 123 typically developing American children in Madison, WI, and for 70 typically developing Chinese children in Hong Kong (Klee et al., 2004). The slope of the regression line of our sample is not as steep as that of the Madison sample, possibly reflecting a more diverse socioeconomic characteristic of our sample compared with the "predominantly middle- to upper-middle-class" community of Madison (Miller & Chapman, 1981, p. 155). That said, the differences between the two data sets are of a magnitude similar to the differences among earlier

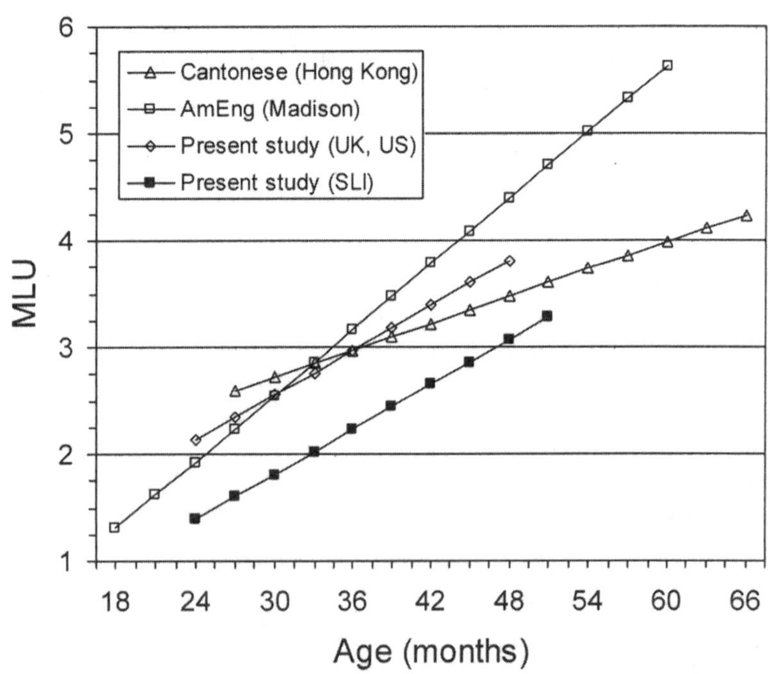

FIG. 4.3. Comparison of age/MLU regression lines from the present study with those of American-English speaking children in Madison, WI (Miller & Chapman, 1981), Cantonese-speaking children in Hong Kong (Klee et al., 2004), and American-English speaking children with SLI.

studies of children's mean length of response in words depicted by Miller and Chapman (1981, Fig. 1, p. 155).

The shallower slope of the regression line for Cantonese-speaking children relative to English-speaking children, however, suggests that several grammatical features characteristic of Cantonese may conspire to reduce the MLU of Chinese children. Several candidate constructions for why this might be so are discussed in Klee et al. (2004). This is no way implies that the grammatical abilities of Chinese children are any less advanced than those of English children at any given age, only that differences between the two languages are reflected in the MLU differences.

Figure 4.3 also depicts the regression line of the SLI group we studied. The predicted MLU of SLI group was derived from the equation MLU = (0.07 × Age) – 0.29. It can be seen that throughout the developmental period between 24 and 50 months, the predicted MLU of the children with SLI is uniformly below that of the children without SLI, as was reported in Klee et al. (1989).

Turning now to the developmental function of the lexical diversity measure, the multiple correlation between age and *D*, after controlling for the effect of gender, was .70 in the U.S. sample and .76 in the UK sample. As with MLU, the relation between *D* and age was linear across the developmental period between 2;0 and 3;11 for English. There was a similarly strong, positive correlation between age and *D* for Cantonese ($R = .73$), but because the age range of that sample extended to 5;8, the relation was curvilinear, with the acceleration in *D* appearing to slow somewhat after the age of about 4;6. There is an indication of a similar deceleration in *D* in the data reported by Malvern et al. (2004), in their longitudinal sample of children between 1;6 and 3;6 and again at age 5;0 living in Bristol, England. These data are illustrated in Fig. 4.4, along with the combined samples of the present study as well as the Cantonese data. The developmental curves are remarkably similar across the three groups of young children illustrated in the figure.

Figure 4.4 also depicts the regression line of the SLI group, which was computed using the equation $D = (1.53 \times \text{Age}) - 22.31$. It can be seen that throughout the developmental period of 24–50 months, the predicted *D* of the children with SLI is uniformly below that of the typically developing children, a finding that corroborates our earlier study of Cantonese-speaking 4-year-olds (Klee et al., 2004) and the three SLI cases illustrated by Durán, Malvern, Richards, and Chipere (2004, Fig. 3, p. 235). This finding also supports earlier studies based on lexical diversity measures that predated *D* (Klee, 1992; Watkins et al., 1995). The conclusion we can draw from these studies is that, in addition to exhibiting shorter utterances, children with SLI also exhibit less lexical diversity in their conversational language than unaffected children.

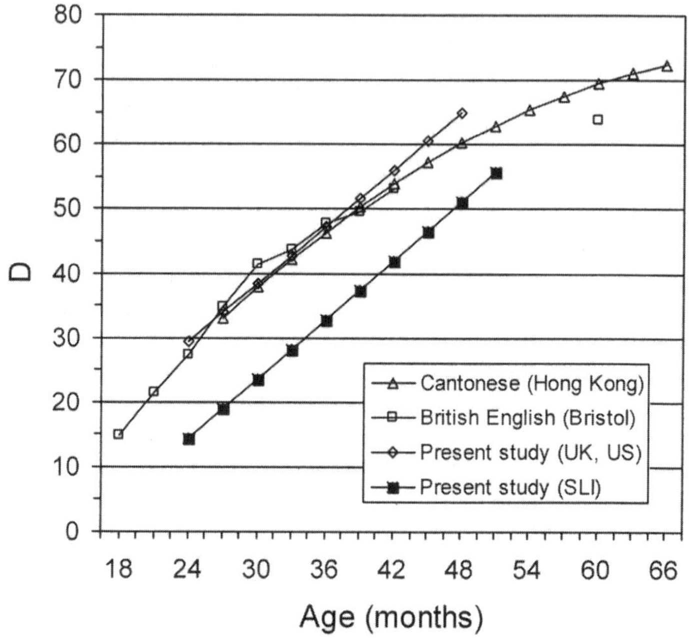

FIG. 4.4. Comparison of age/*D* regression lines from the present study with those of British-English speaking children in Bristol, England (Malvern et al., 2004), Cantonese-speaking children in Hong Kong (Klee et al., 2004), and American-English speaking children with SLI.

Relation Between MLU and *D*

Looking now at the relation between the two language measures, MLU and *D* were significantly correlated after removing the effect of age in English ($r = .40$), whereas they were not in Cantonese ($r = -.13$, $p = .135$, one-tailed). Our findings corroborate those of Malvern et al., where *D* and MLUS, an alternative measure of utterance length used by Wells (1985), were significantly correlated in 8 of 9 age groups between 1;6 and 3;6, with a median correlation across the age groups of .558 (Malvern et al., 2004, Table 5.3, p. 86). Whether or not it was because the Cantonese study included children up to age 5;8, whereas the studies of English-speaking children stopped earlier, there does appear to be a difference in the relation between utterance length and lexical diversity in these two languages.

Differentiating Children With and Without SLI

In Study 2, we asked whether the combination of age, MLU, and *D* could be used jointly to differentiate English-speaking children with and without SLI, as they did in Cantonese. A discriminant analysis based on the three measures showed that children with and without SLI were accurately classified in 83% of the cases overall, compared with 98% of the Cantonese-speaking children using the same variables. The accuracy of the discriminant function was lower overall for English, a finding that might be related to differences in what the measures reflect in each language, which if so would weaken our argument that this clinical marker could be applied cross-linguistically. However, it is also possible that the lower overall accuracy for English might be related to differences in the ages of the English and the Cantonese samples. The fact that children in the Cantonese sample were 4 years old whereas children in the English sample were younger led us to ask whether the success of the proposed marker in differentiating children with and without language difficulties might be age related rather than language related.

As a first step toward answering this question, we divided our sample into 2- and 3-year-olds and compared them with the 4-year-old children from our Cantonese study to see whether the predictive power of the proposed marker improved with age. Table 4.8 displays the sensitivity, specificity, and positive and negative likelihood ratios for the proposed clinical marker, along with their 95% confidence intervals. The figures in this table were computed using the stats calculator on the Web site of the Centre for Evidence-Based Medicine at the University of Toronto (2004b).

Sensitivity in this case refers to the percentage of children with SLI who were correctly identified by the clinical marker (i.e., the joint combination

TABLE 4.8
Sensitivity, Specificity, and Positive and Negative Likelihood Ratios (with 95% Confidence Intervals), for Discriminant Function Based on Age, MLU, and *D*

	English 2-Year-Olds	*English 3-Year-Olds*	*Cantonese 4-Year-Olds*
Sensitivity	78% (45–94%)	86% (60–96%)	97% (76–100%)
Specificity	77% (50–92%)	91% (62–100%)	91% (68–98%)
LR+	3.37 (1.18–9.65)	9.43 (1.44–61.85)	10.33 (2.25–47.53)
LR−	0.29 (0.08–1.02)	0.16 (0.04–0.58)	0.03 (0–0.53)

Note. The method of calculation outlined in Sackett et al. (1991) results in slightly better values for the 4-year-old Cantonese-speaking children: sensitivity = 100%, specificity = 93%, LR+ = 15, and LR− = 0.

of age, MLU and *D* resulting from the discriminant function analysis), with specificity referring to the percentage of children without SLI whose discriminant score was within normal range. As seen in Table 4.8, the sensitivity and specificity of the marker increased with age. If we adopt Plante and Vance's (1994) criteria for judging sensitivity and specificity levels, where 90% is considered to be *good*, 80% is considered to be *fair*, and less than 80% is considered to be *unacceptable*, the proposed clinical marker approached, but did not meet, the minimum acceptable level in the case of 2-year-old children. However, the diagnostic accuracy of the marker was *fair* to *good* with 3-year-olds and uniformly *good* with 4-year-olds.

Having determined the accuracy of the clinical marker in our sample of children, we next estimated confidence intervals (CI) for each measure to get an idea of the precision of the marker. As can be seen in Table 4.8, the CIs for the measures were fairly wide, indicating that if the marker were to be applied to other samples of children, the sensitivity and specificity values computed on those samples could fall somewhere between the minimum and maximum values of the CI. The CIs are large because the size of our samples was small. If these sensitivity and specificity levels were to hold in a larger sample of children, the corresponding CIs would be much narrower, but this requires further empirical investigation.

Table 4.8 reveals that the LR+ of the proposed marker increased with age, while the LR– decreased. So, for example, the LR+ of the marker for 4-year-old (Cantonese) children indicates that the presence of a positive marker is more than 10 times (or 15 times; see Table 4.8 note) as likely to occur in children with SLI as in children without. In the same age group, the LR– of 0.03 indicates that a child who does not have a positive marker is virtually certain to be free of SLI.

The data from our 4-year-olds suggest that the presence of the marker in a Cantonese-speaking child of this age would indicate that the likelihood of that child having SLI is very likely. The LRs for our 3-year-olds are quite similar and suggest that the marker may hold promise with this younger group as well: The LR+ approaches the arbitrary threshold of 10, indicating that a positive marker can be used to rule in SLI, while the low LR– indicates that a negative marker can be used to rule out SLI. However, the intermediate LRs for the 2-year-old group indicate that a child's diagnostic status based on the marker cannot be determined with any degree of certainty and that additional testing will need to be done to confirm the diagnosis (Dollaghan, 2004a). As we discussed earlier with regard to sensitivity and specificity, it is worth bearing in mind that the small samples we studied meant that the CIs for the likelihood ratios are fairly large, indicating the need to replicate the study on a larger sample of children before any claims about these variables functioning as a clinical marker can be made.

The value of computing likelihood ratios is that they can be used to estimate the probability that an *individual* has a condition. If the pretest probability of the condition can be estimated, and the LR is known, then the posttest probability of having the condition can be determined. For example, if a child were chosen at random from the population, there would be about a 7% chance of that child having SLI, based on the prevalence of the condition reported by Tomblin, Records, Bookwalter, Zhang, Smith and O'Brien (1997). If a language sample were then taken and the resulting discriminant score based on age, MLU, and *D* was found to be positive, the (posttest) probability of that child having SLI would increase to around 45% given an LR+ of 10, using the likelihood ratio nomogram (Sackett et al., 2000). In practice, of course, this would never be done. A more typical situation would be a child who presents in clinic with the possibility of having SLI, and the clinician or researcher wishes to verify the diagnosis. In such a situation, the pretest probability of having the condition is far greater than 7%. For the sake of argument, if we put the pretest probability at 50% (i.e., half the children with suspected language disorder we encounter in clinic do in fact have SLI[4]) and take into account the child's discriminant score and the marker's LR+, the posttest probability of SLI increases to greater than 90%.

DIRECTIONS FOR FUTURE RESEARCH

At the conclusion of our study of Cantonese-speaking children (Klee et al., 2004), we suggested that a discriminant score based on the composite of age, MLU, and *D* might serve as a clinical marker of SLI in that language. The present study has found additional support for this hypothesis by replicating the finding with a younger sample of children (3-year-olds) in another language (English); however, use of the proposed marker to reliably identify SLI in 2-year-olds cannot be supported. A reason for this might be found in the literature on late-talking toddlers. The research in this area suggests that late talkers fall into two categories, which, at present, cannot be differentiated with any degree of certainty in children as young as 2 (although see Olswang, Rodriguez, & Timler, 1998). Some of these children apparently grow out of their problem (so-called "late bloomers"), whereas others have persistent language difficulties that may take different forms over time. It is likely that some of the children in the latter group will eventually be given a diagnosis of SLI.

[4]This figure is based on two large-scale studies of the prevalence of language impairment in young children. Tomblin, Records, and Zhang (1966) estimated that 13.6% of their sample of 1,205 American Kindergarten children had a language impairment using the EpiSLI standard. Beitchman, Nair, Clegg, and Patel (1986) reported that 12.6% of their sample of 1,655 Canadian 5-year-olds exhibited a language impairment. If we divide the prevalence of SLI reported by Tomblin et al. (1997) by the average figure from these two studies, we get 7/13 = 54%.

The most pressing need at this stage in the search for clinical markers of SLI is replication. Proposed markers need to be examined on large samples of children, with likelihood ratios and their associated confidence intervals being reported as well as the more traditional measures of sensitivity and specificity. At present, the CIs for this particular marker, and other markers that have been proposed, are unacceptably large. Whether this is due to the nature of the measure (the implication being that what we have proposed will ultimately not prove useful as a marker) or simply the small sample sizes employed to date will become clear only when the measure is evaluated with a large sample of children. Related to this is the need for other empirical methods of data analysis that would lead to convergent validity (see, e.g., the promising use of taxometric analysis recently undertaken by Dollaghan, 2004b).

If subsequent research does not produce results that are as promising as these initial studies suggest, and the notion of a clinical marker based on a composite measure of utterance length and lexical diversity is ultimately rejected, then at least we will have data suggesting that the composite score can help clarify the diagnosis of SLI in 3- and 4-year-old children.

ACKNOWLEDGMENTS

This research was supported in part by a grant from the Nuffield Foundation in London (DIR/14). We are grateful for their support and for the support of all the families who gave freely of their time to participate in the research. We are also grateful to Christine Dollaghan, Paul Fletcher, and Anita Wong for commenting on an earlier draft of this chapter.

REFERENCES

Attia, J. (2003). Moving beyond sensitivity and specificity: using likelihood ratios to help interpret diagnostic tests. *Australian Prescriber, 25*(5), 111–113.

Balason, D. V., & Dollaghan, C. A. (2002). Grammatical morpheme production in 4-year-old children. *Journal of Speech, Language, and Hearing Research, 45,* 961–969.

Bedore, L. M., & Leonard, L. B. (1998). Specific language impairment and grammatical morphology: A discriminant function analysis. *Journal of Speech, Language, and Hearing Research, 41,* 1185–1192.

Beitchman, J. H., Nair, R., Clegg, M., & Patel, P. G. (1986). Prevalence of speech and language disorders in 5-year-old kindergarten children in the Ottawa-Carleton region. *Journal of Speech and Hearing Disorders, 51,* 98–110.

Bishop, D. V. M. (2002). The role of genes in the etiology of specific language impairment. *Journal of Communication Disorders, 35,* 311–328.

Bortolini, U., Caselli, M. C., Deevy, P., & Leonard, L. B. (2002). Specific language impairment in Italian: The first steps in the search for a clinical marker. *International Journal of Language & Communication Disorders, 37,* 77–93.

Centre for Evidence-Based Medicine. (2004a). *Likelihood ratios*. Retrieved November 11, 2004, from http://www.cebm.utoronto.ca/glossary/lrs.htm#top

Centre for Evidence-Based Medicine. (2004b). *Stats calculator, EBM toolbox*. Retrieved November 12, 2004, from http://www.cebm.utoronto.ca

Clahsen, H. (1989). The grammatical characterization of developmental dysphasia. *Linguistics, 27*, 897–920.

Conti-Ramsden, G. (2003). Processing and linguistic markers in young children with specific language impairment (SLI). *Journal of Speech, Language, and Hearing Research, 46*, 1029–1037.

Conti-Ramsden, G., & Jones, M. (1997). Verb use in specific language impairment. *Journal of Speech, Language, and Hearing Research, 40*, 1298–1313.

Crystal, D., Fletcher, P., & Garman, M. (1989). *Grammatical analysis of language disability* (2nd ed.). London: Whurr.

de Jong, J. (1999). *Specific language impairment in Dutch: Inflectional morphology and argument structure*. Groningen Dissertations in Linguistics 28. Groningen, the Netherlands: University of Groningen.

Dollaghan, C., & Campbell, T. F. (1998). Nonword repetition and child language impairment. *Journal of Speech, Language, and Hearing Research, 41*, 1136–1146.

Dollaghan, C. A. (2004a). Evidence-based practice in communication disorders: What do we know, and when do we know it? *Journal of Communication Disorders, 37*, 391–400.

Dollaghan, C. A. (2004b). Taxometric analyses of specific language impairment in 3- and 4-year-old children. *Journal of Speech, Language, and Hearing Research, 47*, 464–475.

Dunn, M., Flax, J., Sliwinski, M., & Aram, D. M. (1996). The use of spontaneous language measures as criteria for identifying children with specific language impairment: An attempt to reconcile clinical and research incongruence. *Journal of Speech and Hearing Research, 39*, 643–654.

Durán, P., Malvern, D. D., Richards, B. J., & Chipere, N. (2004). Developmental trends in lexical diversity. *Applied Linguistics, 25*, 220–242.

Ebell, M. H. (1999). *Likelihood ratios*. Retrieved November 18, 2004, from http://www.poems.msu.edu/EBM/Diagnosis/Diagnosis.htm

Elliott, C. D., Murray, D. J., & Pearson, L. S. (1983). *British ability scales*. Windsor: NFER-Nelson.

Fletcher, P., & Garman, M. (1988). LARSPing by numbers. *British Journal of Disorders of Communication, 23*, 309–321.

Fletcher, P., & Peters, J. (1984). Characterizing language impairment in children: an exploratory study. *Language Testing, 1*, 33–49.

Garman, M. (1989a). The role of linguistics in speech therapy: assessment and interpretation. In P. Grunwell & A. James (Eds.), *The functional evaluation of language disorders* (pp. 29–57). London: Croom Helm.

Garman, M. (1989b). Syntactic assessment of expressive language. In K. Grundy (Ed.), *Linguistics in clinical practice* (pp. 92–117). London: Taylor & Francis.

Gathercole, S. E., & Baddeley, A. D. (1990). Phonological memory deficits in language-disordered children: is there a causal connection? *Journal of Memory and Language, 29*, 336–360.

Gathercole, S. E., & Baddeley, A. D. (1996). *The Children's Test of Non-Word Repetition*. London: Psychological Corporation.

Gavin, W. J., & Giles, L. (1996). Sample size effects on temporal reliability of language sample measures of preschool children. *Journal of Speech and Hearing Research, 39,* 1258–1262.

Gavin, W. J., Klee, T., & Membrino, I. (1993). Differentiating specific language impairment from normal language development using grammatical analysis. *Clinical Linguistics & Phonetics, 7,* 191–206.

Gopnik, M. (1990). Feature-blind grammar and dysphasia. *Nature, 344,* 715.

Hansson, K. (1997). Patterns of verb usage in Swedish children with SLI: An application of recent theories. *First Language, 17,* 195–217.

Hedrick, D. L., Prather, E. M., & Tobin, A. R. (1984). *Sequenced Inventory of Communication Development–Revised*. Seattle: University of Washington Press.

Hoffman, L. M., & Gillam, R. B. (2004). Verbal and spatial information processing constraints in children with specific language impairment. *Journal of Speech, Language, and Hearing Research, 47,* 114–125.

Johnston, J. R. (2004, June). *Fearless and bold in following ideas wherever they lead: The Elizabeth Bates Memorial Lecture*. Paper presented at the 25th annual Symposium on Research in Child Language Disorders, Madison, WI.

Klee, T. (1992). Developmental and diagnostic characteristics of quantitative measures of children's language production. *Topics in Language Disorders, 12,* 28–41.

Klee, T., Carson, D. K., Gavin, W. J., Hall, L., Kent, A., & Reece, S. (1998). Concurrent and predictive validity of an early language screening program. *Journal of Speech, Language, and Hearing Research, 41,* 627–641.

Klee, T., Pearce, K., & Carson, D. K. (2000). Improving the positive predictive value of screening for developmental language disorder. *Journal of Speech, Language, and Hearing Research, 43,* 821–833.

Klee, T., Schaffer, M., May, S., Membrino, I., & Mougey, K. (1989). A comparison of the age-MLU relation in normal and specifically language-impaired preschool children. *Journal of Speech and Hearing Disorders, 54,* 226–233.

Klee, T., Stokes, S. F., Wong, A. M. Y., Fletcher, P., & Gavin, W. J. (2004). Utterance length and lexical diversity in Cantonese-speaking children with and without specific language impairment. *Journal of Speech, Language, and Hearing Research, 47,* 1396–1410.

Lee, L. L. (1966). Developmental sentence types: A method for comparing normal and deviant syntactic development. *Journal of Speech and Hearing Disorders, 31,* 311–330.

Leonard, L. B. (1987). Is specific language impairment a useful construct? In S. Rosenberg (Ed.), *Advances in applied psycholinguistics: Disorders of first-language development* (pp. 1–39). Cambridge: Cambridge University Press.

Leonard, L. B. (1998). *Children with specific language impairment*. Cambridge, MA: MIT Press.

Locke, J. L. (1994). Gradual emergence of developmental language disorders. *Journal of Speech and Hearing Research, 37,* 608–616.

MacWhinney, B. (2003). Computerized language analysis (CLAN) (Version 23, September) [Computer software]. Pittsburgh, PA.

Malvern, D., Richards, B., Chipere, N., & Durán, P. (2004). *Lexical diversity and language development: Quantification and assessment*. Basingstoke: Palgrave Macmillan.

Marchman, V. A., Wulfeck, B., & Ellis Weismer, S. (1999). Morphological productivity in children with normal language and SLI: A study of the English past tense. *Journal of Speech, Language, and Hearing Research, 42,* 206–219.

McCardle, P., Cooper, J., & Freund, L. (2005). Language and genetics: Needs and opportunities. *Applied Psycholinguistics, 26,* 129–135.

Menyuk, P. (1964). Comparison of grammar of children with functionally deviant and normal speech. *Journal of Speech and Hearing Research, 7,* 109–121.

Mervis, C. B., & Robinson, B. F. (2005). Designing measures for profiling and genotype/phenotype studies of individuals with genetic syndromes or developmental language disorders. *Applied Psycholinguistics, 26,* 41–64.

Miller, J. F. (Ed.). (1981). *Assessing language production in children: Experimental procedures*. Baltimore: University Park Press.

Miller, J. F. (1991). Quantifying productive language disorders. In J. F. Miller (Ed.), *Research on child language disorders: A decade of progress* (pp. 211–220). Austin, TX: Pro-Ed.

Miller, J. F., & Chapman, R. S. (1981). The relation between age and mean length of utterance in morphemes. *Journal of Speech and Hearing Research, 24,* 154–161.

Miller, J. F., & Chapman, R. S. (1981–2004). *Systematic analysis of language transcripts (SALT)*. Madison: Language Analysis Laboratory, Waisman Center, University of Wisconsin–Madison.

Mueller, C. W., & Parcel, T. L. (1981). Measures of socioeconomic status: Alternative and recommendations. *Child Development, 52,* 13–30.

Oetting, J. B., & Rice, M. L. (1993). Plural acquisition in children with specific language impairment. *Journal of Speech and Hearing Research, 36,* 1236–1248.

Olswang, L. B., Rodriguez, B., & Timler, G. (1998). Recommending intervention for toddlers with specific language learning difficulties: We may not have all the answers, but we know a lot. *American Journal of Speech-Language Pathology, 7*(1), 23–32.

Paradis, J., & Crago, M. B. (2001). The morphosyntax of specific language impairment in French: An extended optional default account. *Language Acquisition, 9,* 269–300.

Plante, E., & Vance, R. (1994). Selection of preschool language tests: A data-based approach. *Language, Speech, and Hearing Services in Schools, 25,* 15–24.

Rice, M. L. (1997). Specific language impairments: in search of diagnostic markers and genetic contributions. *Mental Retardation and Developmental Disabilities Research Reviews, 3,* 350–357.

Rice, M. L. (2000). Grammatical symptoms of specific language impairment. In D. V. M. Bishop & L. B. Leonard (Eds.), *Speech and language impairments in children: Causes, characteristics, intervention and outcome*. East Sussex, England: Psychology Press.

Rice, M. L. (2003). A unified model of specific and general language delay: Grammatical tense as a clinical marker of unexpected variation. In Y. Levy & J. Schaeffer

(Eds.), *Language competence across populations: toward a definition of specific language impairment* (pp. 63–95). Mahwah, NJ: Lawrence Erlbaum Associates.

Rice, M. L., Noll, K. R., & Grimm, H. (1997). An extended optional infinitive stage in German-speaking children with specific language impairment. *Language Acquisition, 6,* 255–296.

Rice, M. L., & Wexler, K. (1996). Toward tense as a clinical marker of specific language impairment in English-speaking children. *Journal of Speech and Hearing Research, 39,* 1239–1257.

Rice, M. L., Wexler, K., & Cleave, P. L. (1995). Specific language impairment as a period of extended optional infinitives. *Journal of Speech and Hearing Research, 38,* 850–863.

Rice, M. L., Wexler, K., & Hershberger, S. (1998). Tense over time: the longitudinal course of tense acquisition in children with specific language impairment. *Journal of Speech, Language, and Hearing Research, 41,* 1412–1431.

Sackett, D. L., Haynes, R. B., Guyatt, G. H., & Tugwell, P. (1991). *Clinical epidemiology: A basic science for clinical medicine* (2nd ed.). Boston: Little, Brown.

Sackett, D. L., Straus, S. E., Richardson, W. S., Rosenberg, W., & Haynes, R. B. (2000). *Evidence-based medicine: how to practice and teach EBM* (2nd ed.). Edinburgh: Churchill Livingstone.

SPSS, Inc. (2001). SPSS for Windows (Version 11.0) [Computer software]. Chicago: Author.

Stokes, S. F. (1997). Secondary prevention of paediatric language disability: A comparison of parents and nurses as screening agents. *European Journal of Disorders of Communication, 32,* 139–158.

Tomblin, J. B., Records, N. L., Bookwalter, P., Zhang, X., Smith, E., & O'Brien, M. (1997). Prevalence of specific language impairment in kindergarten children. *Journal of Speech, Language, and Hearing Research, 40,* 1245–1260.

Tomblin, J. B., Records, N. L., & Zhang, X. (1996). A system for the diagnosis of specific language impairment in kindergarten children. *Journal of Speech and Hearing Research, 39,* 1284–1294.

van der Lely, H. K. J. (1994). Canonical linking rules: Forward versus reverse linking in normally developing and specifically language-impaired children. *Cognition, 98,* 242–272.

Watkins, R. V., Kelly, D. J., Harbers, H. M., & Hollis, W. (1995). Measuring children's lexical diversity: Differentiating typical and impaired language learners. *Journal of Speech and Hearing Research, 38,* 1349–1355.

Wells, G. (1985). *Language development in the pre-school years.* Cambridge, England: Cambridge University Press.

5

Gesture Development From an Interactionist Perspective

Elizabeth Crais
University of North Carolina at Chapel Hill

Robin Chapman in earlier (Chapman et al., 1992) and more recent work (Chapman, 2000) has laid the groundwork for taking an interactionist perspective to the acquisition of language. This perspective serves to reframe the "nature versus nurture" argument into one that recognizes both "nature and nurture" as essential to language learning. Language learning is seen as the result of the integration of learning across multiple domains. The interactionist view values the interdependence of motor, social, cognitive, and learning abilities and opportunities in the developing child. From this perspective, the development of these skills can lead to learning in other areas and is seen as the precursor to the emergence of linguistic forms. Bates and Goodman (1997) similarly suggest that "language is a new machine built out of old parts" dependent on individual skills in joint attention, play, language, imitation, and perception. Chapman's earlier work (Miller, Chapman, Branston, & Reichle, 1980) link cognitive and language milestones from a Piagetian (Piaget, 1970; Werner & Kaplan, 1963) perspective, whereas later work acknowledges the effect of social scaffolding from Bruner's (1983) and Vygotsky's (1987) perspectives. In addition, the interactionist view argues that because skills develop through continual interaction with the child's environment, a broad range of individual differences across children is likely to occur. Thus the interactionist perspective takes into account genetic contributions from individuals and across groups, while also acknowledging the variations between children in environmental input.

Based on the existing literature, Chapman (2000) suggests two important generalizations about children's language learning: (a) language acquisition follows a developmental course where new meanings and communicative functions are first expressed by old means (or old forms) of behavior; and (b) new forms typically emerge to express meanings and communicative intents already in the child's repertoire. Chapman uses examples across multiple domains within language to support these premises. This chapter highlights recent findings in the development of gestures, and uses them to further support the interactionist perspective. First, an overview of gesture types is presented. Then the findings across gesture studies are used to provide additional examples of Chapman's two key generalizations, as well as to address aspects of both nurture and nature as related to gesture development. Next, the chapter looks at the importance of caregiver input to gesture development and the relationship of gesture use to language development. Finally, the degree to which gesture use and differing patterns of use in children can be predictive of communication deficits is examined.

TYPES OF GESTURES

In discussing gesture development, it is important to identify what is meant by the term *gesture*. Gestures are actions produced with the intent to communicate and are typically expressed using the fingers, hands, and arms, but can also include facial features (e.g., lip smacking for "eating") and body motions (e.g., bouncing for "horsie") (Iverson & Thal, 1998). Iverson and Thal distinguish between two primary categories of gestures: deictic and representational. *Deictic* gestures are used to establish reference by calling attention to or indicating an object or event (Bates, 1976; Bates, Benigni, Bretherton, Camaioni, & Volterra, 1979). These gestures can only be interpreted by their context, but can be used with a wide variety of objects and events (e.g., pointing to an airplane overhead, reaching for a cup) (Iverson & Thal, 1998).

The earliest deictic gestures have been reported to emerge between 7 and 9 months of age (Carpenter, Nagell, & Tomasello, 1998; Crais, Douglas, & Campbell, 2004), depending on the setting (e.g., laboratory versus home) and the methodology (e.g., experimental design, naturalistic observation, parent report). Deictic gestures often first appear as open-handed reaching, reaching to be picked up, ritualized gestures to indicate refusal (e.g., pushing away), or consistent attention-getting body movements (e.g., leg and arm flailing) (Carpenter, Mastergeorge, & Coggins, 1983; Crais et al., 2004; Thal & Tobias, 1992). As noted by Iverson and Thal (1998), deictic gestures account for nearly 88% of the gesture repertoire in young children. Deictic gestures are often divided into contact and distal gestures (Bates, Camaioni, & Volterra, 1975). Contact gestures require contact between a child and object or caregiver, such as giving a toy or pushing away an adult's hand, and are considered "early" gestures. Distal gestures, in contrast, require no contact with the caregiver or object, such as pointing and waving, and are typically later appearing (10–12 months). One distinction that needs to be made, however, is that a few distal gestures (e.g., reaching toward objects, reaching to be picked up), in fact, defy the typical progression of contact gestures preceding distal gestures. One explanation, as noted by Crais et al. (2004), may be that although reaching is considered distal, it is also more contextually bound to the actions from which it emerges (e.g., grabbing, being lifted up).

The second major type of gestures, *representational* gestures, both establish reference and indicate a particular semantic content. They often appear around 12 months of age (Acredolo & Goodwyn, 1988; Bates et al., 1979) and typically after the emergence of a few deictic gestures (Crais et al., 2004). Using Iverson and Thal's (1998) categorization, representational gestures can be *object-related gestures* that signify some feature of the referent (e.g., cupped hand to mouth to represent "drinking"), referred to by some as "symbolic" gestures. They can also be culturally defined *conventional* gestures that are used socially (e.g., waving "bye," finger to lips for "quiet"), which have no specific object represented but do have specific semantic content. Most studies of gesture development have examined either deictic or representational object-related gestures. Although some researchers have chosen not to examine conventional gestures in their analyzed samples (Acredolo & Goodwyn, 1988; Goldin-Meadow & Morford, 1985), Iverson and Thal (1998) argue for their inclusion, so as not to underestimate the child's overall gesture repertoire. Carpenter et al. (1998) similarly suggest there is a need to study a greater variety of gestures than is examined in most studies. Two recent studies by Crais et al. (2004) and Iverson, Capirci, Longobardi, and Caselli (1999) have targeted both deictic and representational gestures (including some conventional gestures). Crais et al. (2004) followed 12 typically developing children from 6 to 24 months of age using a parent report methodology with monthly researcher observations and videotaping in the home. They were able to identify the earliest, and the progression of, emergence of a variety of gestures. Iverson and colleagues (Iverson et al., 1999) videotaped 12 Italian mother-child dyads when the children were 16 and 20 months old. As highlighted throughout this chapter, examples from studies of both deictic and representational gestures are utilized in support of an interactionist perspective.

INTERACTIONIST GENERALIZATION 1: OLD FORMS EXPRESS NEW MEANINGS

It has been well documented that representational gestures emerge within familiar games and routines that parents and other caregivers utilize to engage children (Acredolo & Goodwyn, 1988; Caselli, 1990; Goodwyn & Acredolo, 1993; Iverson & Thal, 1998; Werner & Kaplan, 1963). Games and routines such as "Itsy Bitsy Spider" or even exaggerated "blowing" on hot food contain many interactive, joint attention opportunities for the child to observe and produce representational gestures. These gestures are then extracted from their ritualized routines and extended to novel instances and in novel contexts (Werner & Kaplan, 1963). For example, Caselli's (1990) young son first "danced" to music in a social routine, whereas later he used it to request turning on the radio. In Crais et al. (2004), one child who initially used the "sh" gesture (index finger to lips) as part of the imitative routine during the song "Wheels on the Bus" later used it to request that verse in the song, and even later to signal for everyone to be quiet during naptime. Another child who initially shook her head "no" to indicate she wasn't supposed to do something (e.g., put her shoes on the couch, turn her sippy cup upside down) later used the same gesture to refuse unwanted objects. As suggested by Werner and Kaplan (1963), this "decontextualization" may serve as a rehearsal for the same phenomenon employed later with words. Similarly, Goodwyn, Acredelo, and Brown (2000) utilize the term *context flexible* to define when a child generalizes the gesture to a new context. Some studies of representational gestures in fact have used context flexibility as one of the criteria for evidence that a gesture was exhibited (Goodwyn et al., 2000). For example, Goodwyn and colleagues trained parents to model representational gestures to their 11-month-old infants, and only those gestures exhibited by the children in a new context were considered as acquired.

In terms of deictic gestures, Crais et al. (2004) provide multiple examples of the use of particular "forms" to express certain "functions" and the later use of the same forms to represent "new functions." Their data documented the mean emergence of giving objects to "comment" at 9.33 months, whereas giving objects to "request action" (e.g., open a jar, fix a toy) emerged later at a mean of 11.91 months. Similarly, all 12 children in their sample pointed to request objects (10.64 months) and to comment (10.75 months) before pointing to request actions (13.58 months) or request information (14.42 months). In addition, Crais et al. noted many examples of children using old forms in new contexts to represent the same function (e.g., pointing to get toys, drinks, books).

INTERACTIONIST GENERALIZATION 2: NEW FORMS EXPRESS "OLD" MEANING

Chapman's (2000) second generalization regarding "new forms" is especially relevant for the examination of gesture development. Bruner (1977) suggested the behavioral basis for referential skills occurs initially through eye gaze and motor movements. With experience the child gains more efficient means (or forms), such as gestures and words. As noted by Chapman (2000), these "new forms" when exhibited reflect the content that already exists in the child's repertoire, previously expressed by "old forms." There are numerous examples within the area of gesture development where this generalization is apparent. For instance, one child in the Crais et al. (2004) study initially pointed to signal wanting to go outside, whereas later he brought his mother her shoes to indicate the same desire. Another child refused certain foods first by turning her head away, whereas later she used a repeated spitting gesture with much, as her mother described, "fanfare" even on sight of the despised foods.

Another example of the second generalization within deictic gestures is the relative emergence of contact gestures before distal ones (except for the exceptions noted previously). This overall pattern supports Werner and Kaplan's (1963) "distancing hypothesis" in noting that children's first gestures emerge through actions on objects in interaction with others and only later is there a distance between person and object. Relevant examples could include the child who early in development seeks to gain access to objects by grabbing the adult's hand holding the object, whereas later in development pointing may be used for the same purpose. The move from contact to distal gestures also reflects the shift in ability from dealing with objects as "ego-bound things-of-action" to "ego-distant objects-of-contemplation" (Werner & Kaplan, 1963). As McLean, McLean, Brady, and Etter (1991) suggested, the transition from contact to distal gestures may be related to the symbol acquisition process, and children or adults who use *only* contact gestures may be manifesting a pervasive symbolic deficit. The question then becomes one focused on whether the lack of (or delay in) distal gestures may signal a concurrent lack or delay of language. Certainly in observing children on the autism spectrum, there are examples of children who use primarily contact gestures with little to no pointing or other distal gestures (Lord & Pickles, 1996). This population by definition is one with language and social deficits.

The transition from the use of gestures (with or without vocalizations) to a predominant use of words is another strong example of the second generalization. This transition occurs for both deictic and representational gestures. There are numerous links between gesture development and the emergence of language. Indeed, Bates and Dick (2002) describe language and gesture as "close family." Early in development, infants primarily use vocalizations and gestures to communicate. Between 8 and 12 months, gestural and gestural/vocal combinations predominate, and approximately half of deictic gestures exhibited between 8 and 11 months are accompanied by vocalizations (Carpenter et al., 1983). With increasing age, the use of gestures or vocalizations alone decreases as gesture–vocalization combinations increase until a point when they predominate at 15 months (Carpenter et al., 1988; Wetherby, Cain, Yonclas, & Walker, 1988). Thus, even as children enter into the one-word stage, gestures (with or without vocalizations) continue to play a prominent role.

The transition from gestural labels to verbal labels also provides support for the second generalization. As the data of Crais and colleagues (Crais et al., 2004) and that of others indicate, both deictic gestures and some representational gestures precede the emergence of naming. In this study, common early representational gestures included waving "bye bye," "dancing" to music, and "hugging" objects. Indeed, Bates and colleagues (Bates & Dick, 2002; Shore, Bates, Bretherton, Beeghly, & O'Connell, 1990) argue that before the use of words to name, children produce "recognitory" actions associated with objects (e.g., cup to lip, phone to ear). They suggest these early recognitory gestures serve as "gestural names" in the same manner as early verbal naming. The evidence they use to support this position comes from the fact that recognitory gestures and verbal naming emerge around the same time, they are positively correlated, gestures and first words share similar content or meaning, and recognitory gestures are brief and stylized in their form, as are first words (Bates & Dick, 2002). Others (Acredelo & Goodwyn, 1985, 1988; Iverson, Capirci, & Caselli, 1994; Namy & Waxman, 1998) suggest these early symbolic gestures are also used for requesting objects (e.g., Caselli's son who used "dancing" for requesting the turning on of the radio).

By 16 months, infants use both words and representational gestures interchangeably to name objects. However, by 20 months they have almost stopped using representational gestures as names for objects or object categories in favor of the use of words (Iverson et al., 1994; Namy, Acredolo, & Goodwyn, 2000). As noted by Namy and Waxman (1998), the use of words begins to diverge from the use of representational gestures as words take on "privileged status" in the infant's repertoire. Iverson et al. (1994) have also documented the decline in the spontaneous use of representational gestures over time with gestures becoming more supplementary in function. Acredolo and Goodwyn (1988) noted that most representational/symbolic gestures are used in the first half of the second year of life and continue only until a comparable word develops. A parallel decline in *comprehension* of representational gestures also appears at this time (Namy & Waxman, 1998), suggesting developmental changes in the use of gestures as object names as a result of "a shifting conceptualization of the relative function of words and gestures" (Namy et al., 2000, p. 65). Later in development, gestures and words again emerge in a parallel nature as seen when gesture–word and/or gesture–gesture combinations accompany or precede word combinations (Iverson & Goldin-Meadow, 1998). As word combinations become more prevalent, however, gesture–word and gesture–gesture combinations decline—another example of Chapman's second generalization.

In sum, the examples from gesture development provide strong support for Chapman's (2000) two important generalizations, yet what impact do these generalizations have on language learning? Chapman suggested from the interactionist perspective that the generalizations may provide advice to parents so that if they respond to their child's communicative attempts, the correct form will eventually develop. And more particularly, she noted that the acquisition of some forms should lead to development in other areas.

THE IMPORTANCE OF CAREGIVER INPUT

The following subsections focus on Chapman's (2000) arguments relative to parental input to young language learners and the effect this input has on gesture development.

Mothers' and Children's Use of Gesture

Iverson et al. (1999) noted that mothers' gesture use could be characterized as "gestural motherese" when compared to adults' use of gestures when talking with other adults. Not only do mothers use fewer gestures overall, but they also tend to use a larger number of conceptually simple and concrete gestures that are redundant with and reinforcing of the message conveyed in speech. Iverson and colleagues' study with 12 Italian mother–child dyads documented that only 15% of the mother's conversational acts at both 16 and 20 months were or included gestures, similar to what has been reported in American mothers (Bekken, 1989; Shatz, 1982). The children by comparison used or included gestures in 42% of their acts at 16 months and in 27% at 20 months. In addition, the mothers' gestures were primarily redundant or reinforcing of the verbal message, in contrast to gesture use in adult–adult interaction that is primarily complementary or supplementary to the verbal message (McNeill, 1992). Iverson et al. (1999) suggest that one possible reason that mothers use redundant gestures is to accommodate the needs of their young child. They cite the results of gesture comprehension studies in young children as evidence for this view. For example, although children under 2 years can comprehend pointing and other deictic gestures, they have much more difficulty with representational gestures, even when these same gestures are within their productive repertoire (Morford & Goldin-Meadow, 1992; Petitto, 1988).

Iverson et al. (1999) present convincing evidence of the direct link between maternal use of gestures and the child's use. Their study reported that for 16-month-old children, the mother's total gesture production significantly correlated with the child's total gesture production. Maternal verbal production was also correlated with the child's gesture production, vocabulary size, and total verbal production. In addition, maternal pointing was significantly correlated with the child's vocabulary size. Namy et al. (2000) also documented that the number of gestures used by the parents was highly correlated with the number of gestures used by their 15-month-old children.

The fact that children's learning of both gestural and verbal communication appears to be guided by parental input highlights the effect that social context and parental structure of the environment may have on symbol acquisition (Namy et al., 2000). This view reflects Bruner's (1966) and Vygotsky's (1962) early theories of development whereby the social setting provides the primary source of learning early in life. Yet what part does nature play in this development? The variable development of both deictic and representational gestures in young children serves as a prime example of the mutual influence of nature and nurture reflected in Chapman's (2000) interactionist model. For example, although there appears to be good agreement across a number of studies as to the mean age of acquisition of the most commonly studied deictic gestures (i.e., reach, show, give, point), a good deal of individual variability across children has been reported. In addition, a recent study by Crais et al. (2004) indicated earlier emergence for deictic gestures than had been previously reported in the literature (Carpenter et al., 1983, 1998; Masur, 1983). Reasons for these results may include methodological differences between the studies. For example, the Crais et al. (2004) children were seen at home versus in a lab, gestures were first documented by parents and validated by researchers, and the elicitors of the gestures were parents rather than researchers. Thus "social context" appeared to be an important factor in the age of emergence across a variety of deictic gestures. This finding could also be viewed as providing at least modest support for Werner and Kaplan's (1963) theory of decontextualization in that the children in Crais and colleagues' (2004) study were using gestures in familiar contexts, whereas many studies have elicited gestures in "new" contexts and therefore gestures may not be "decontextualized" until a later time. Previous studies (Coggins, Olswang, & Guthrie, 1987; Wetherby et al., 1988) have shown variations in the frequency and type of communicative acts exhibited by young children due to familiarity of the examiner and the degree of structure in the setting. Thus, gesture use is very likely affected by context, from a broader social setting context as well as direct parental input.

Further evidence of the influence caregivers may have on their children's gesture use comes from examining representational gestures. Crais et al. (2004) noted a good deal of individual variability in the emergence of representational gestures, and Goodwyn et al. (2000) reported a range of forms of representational gesture types used between 10 and 24 months. In Crais and colleagues' (Crais et al., 2004) longitudinal study, parents were asked over an 18-month period to indicate on a series of forms when and in what context each of a large number of deictic and representational gestures emerged. All the deictic gestures listed were exhibited by the children in at least some context, whereas some representational gestures were never exhibited. Parents who reported playing frequently with their children in pretend ways (e.g., pretending to sleep, smacking lips to signal eating) had children who also used these gestures. For the children who never used particular representational gestures, their parents reported that they themselves did not use the gestures. For example, one family noted that they never used the forefinger to the lips to signal "Sh" in any context (e.g., asking for quiet, pretending a baby doll was sleeping) as they did not want to give their child the impression that they did not want him to talk. Indeed, Zinober and Martlew (1985) argued that when compared to deictic gestures, representational gestures are more dependent on modeling by caregivers.

If caregiver gesture use is critical to child gesture use, then we would expect to see decreases in caregiver gestures as child gesture use decreases between 16 and 20 months. Although Iverson et al. (1999) saw no differences in amount of maternal gesture use between 16 and 20 months, Hodapp, Goldfield, and Boyatzis (1984) documented a decrease over time in parental use of gestural scaffolding in parent–child routines such as peek-a-boo. In fact, Namy et al. (2000) suggest that as children's verbal comprehension and language proficiency increase, parents may decrease their use of gestural naming. Thus, there is some evidence (at least in gestural and verbal naming) that changes in parental input may help account for the child's parallel shift over time toward decreases in gesture use as word use increases. Further, given that using words is typically the fastest way to get one's needs met, the child's shift toward the predominant use of words may also simply represent parental shaping of the child's output (although probably unintentionally) through enhanced responsiveness to the most easily interpreted communication. This is an assumption naturally associated with the interactionist perspective (Chapman, 2000) in which child and maternal output are reciprocally linked and the child's changing use of gestures is both a reflection of the child's inherent growth and the responsivity of the environment.

Purpose of Parental Use of Gestures

How then do caregivers view the purpose of gestures when used to communicate with their child? In general, the type of gestures used by the caregiver depends on the purpose or function of the gesture. Specifically, deictic gestures are directed toward getting the child's attention for declarative (joint attention) purposes, such as when showing, giving, or pointing to objects or actions that may be of interest to the child. In addition, deictic gestures are used to get the child to do something (instrumental/behavior regulation function) such as to give up an object in response to the adult's reach or to avoid doing something (e.g., putting sticky fingers on mom's suit). When looking at the informational role played by the gesture in respect to speech, these gestures are often "complementary" to the verbal communication and thus the gesture acts as an "aid" to getting the adult's message across to the child. Some deictic gestures may also serve to disambiguate the verbal communication, such as when pointing to a specific toy and saying "Not that one, this one" (Iverson et al., 1999). They can also serve to "add" information to the verbal message, such as when the gesture indicates a referent and the verbal component describes an attribute of the referent (e.g., pointing to a dog and saying "dirty").

Representational gestures in contrast are focused primarily on adding information to the communication and on getting and/or keeping the child's attention for social purposes. Common examples are those observed by Acredolo and Goodwyn (1988) such as "sniffing" a picture of a flower or flapping the arms to signify "birdie." These gestures have more of a "teaching" function as they add detail to the child's knowledge about objects and events. They may also have a social function when caregivers use this type of gesture to get or keep the child's interest in a book or the interaction itself. Examples could include a parent pretending to "eat" an apple from a page in a book or playing social games with the child, such as "Peekaboo."

What then of caregivers' intentional versus unintentional use of gestures? There are clearly some gestures that specifically are used to elicit the child's imitation, and the caregiver's clear goal is to get the child to produce the gesture spontaneously. Examples include what some would call "conventional" or "culturally determined" gestures (Iverson et al., 1999; Iverson & Thal, 1998), such as waving "bye bye" or shaking the head for "Yes" or "No." Caregivers may work very hard to elicit these types of gestures from their young children. Representational gestures may include both intentional and unintentional gestures used by caregivers to add information (or as noted to keep the social exchange going). Blowing on hot food or sniffing a real flower could be viewed as unintentional, whereas "dancing" by moving arms and body to music or producing "high fives" could be viewed as part of caregivers' efforts to encourage the child's imitation. Deictic gestures, in contrast, are not typically viewed by parents as ones used to encourage the child to imitate the adult. In the study by Crais et al. (2004), parents verbally (and their children by performance) clearly distinguished between deictic gestures and the broad class of representational gestures. As noted, all the children exhibited the targeted deictic gestures, whereas several children failed to exhibit one or more of the representational gestures. Thus, it is possible that parents in this study were subtly aware of the different functions of different types of gestures, using only the representational gestures that they valued and the deictic gestures more unintentionally in the natural course of interaction.

The Role of Gesture Imitation

Gestural imitation is viewed as part of the learning process, but why and when do young children imitate gestures? As indicated by the work of Shore et al. (1990) in examining the comprehension of recognitory gestures by young children, both gesture imitation and gesture comprehension exhibit a U-shaped relationship. In this study of gestural comprehension, children were not required to imitate the gesture produced by the examiner (e.g., combing hair with no comb), but only to indicate the item associated with the gesture (i.e., the comb). The results indicated that neither the "high" nor "low" gesture comprehenders used spontaneous imitation, but all the children who used imitation fell in the middle range on the comprehension task. As noted by Bates and Dick (2002), this finding supports Kagan's (1981) early argument regarding the function of imitation wherein children imitate those actions and sounds that are just beyond their current level of understanding. They further suggested that the relationship between gestural imitation and gesture comprehension is dependent on the child's level of development within each domain. This finding can be likened to Chapman's (1978) early description of the comprehension strategy "do what others do," when a child imitates someone else's action when unsure of the verbal message. Can this finding also be linked with anecdotal reports from parents that toddlers later lose interest in (and show limited imitation of) early infant games that they used to play (and imitate) readily? And if parental input and imitation play important roles in gesture use, can this knowledge be utilized by parents and professionals to facilitate gesture development?

Parental Impact on the Rate of Gesture Learning

From two studies by Goodwyn and colleagues (Acredolo & Goodwyn, 1990; Goodwyn et al., 2000) comes evidence that parents can impact the rate at which their children learn representational gestures. In these two studies, parents were trained to use representational gestures along with words (e.g., flapping arms while saying "birdie"). The children used more representational gestures than reported in the normative literature, and used approximately four times as many as had been reported in the authors' previous studies where no training had taken place. Thus, it appears that parents can facilitate the development of representational gestures through conscious modeling.

Given the findings of parental impact, some might argue that the Crais et al. (2004) results of earlier emergence of common deictic gestures may have been caused by parental awareness of the gestures targeted (i.e., parents received a checklist every 2 months of gestures that may emerge during that interval). However, as argued by Crais and colleagues, to speed up emergence of the gestures so uniformly, many of the parents would have had to either "teach" the gestures to their children and/or increase their feedback as the children used the targeted gestures. Although the parents very likely were more aware of gestures, the facts that there was a large number of gestures documented in the study and that earlier emergence was seen across many gestures make it unlikely that the parents could have been so successful. In addition, although the mean ages of emergence across the children were earlier than other studies, there was also a good bit of variability in individual children. Thus, the question remains of whether rate of acquisition of deictic gestures can be enhanced in children whose parents are either made aware of potential gestures or are trained to model these types of gestures. Because Crais and colleagues did not study the same representational gestures as did Goodwyn and colleagues (Acredolo & Goodwyn, 1990; Goodwyn et al., 2000), it is impossible to make comparisons across studies. Therefore, it is not clear whether just having awareness of possibly emerging representational gestures may make a difference in parents' use and thereby children's use of these gesture types. This leads us to the discussion of the relationship of gesture use and later language development.

GESTURE USE AND LATER LANGUAGE DEVELOPMENT IN TYPICALLY DEVELOPING CHILDREN

The interactionist perspective argues that development of some forms leads to development in other areas and that large individual differences across children should be expected (Chapman, 2000). By this account, the speed of acquisition of some subsystems may slow or facilitate the acquisition of other systems that build on them as a result of what the child brings to the learning arena as well as what the environment contributes.

Associations Between Gesture Use and Later Language

Further support for the interactionist perspective can be seen in the positive relationship that gesture development has on later language learning. This relationship is evident in the representational gesture training study by Goodwyn et al. (2000). Goodwyn and colleagues documented a positive correlation between representational gestures and verbal development, and further, increases in representational gestures at 19 months predicted an increase in verbal vocabulary at 19 and 24 months. Iverson et al. (1999) also present data to support the predictability of earlier maternal gesture use on later gesture and language use. They found positive correlations between maternal gesture use at 16 months and later amounts of both child gestures and verbalizations at 20 months. Thus, the degree to which mothers gestured with their children at younger ages had an impact on both gesture and verbal productions by the child at a later age.

Regarding the reasons for the positive correlations between early gesture use and later language skills, Goodwyn et al. (2000) highlighted several possibilities. In their representational gesture training study, not only did the children increase their use of gestures, but increases in both social interaction and parental attention to language development occurred. Specifically, children whose parents were trained to model gestures had higher receptive and expressive language as well as syntactic levels, when compared to children whose parents did not receive training or children whose parents received training only in labeling words. The fact that the "label only" children did not experience the same effect indicates that it was the gesture training that produced the significant enhancement in later language scores. Goodwyn et al. suggest this effect may be explained by the fact that representational gestures are typically learned at earlier ages than the accompanying words (Goodwyn & Acredelo, 1993), and therefore infants who have more representational gestures may more easily gain attention and feedback from parents. Thus, a young child with 10 representational gestures may elicit twice as many caregiver responses as a child with half as many gestures. Because representational gestures (and other gestures as well) when produced by parents are often accompanied by words (Iverson et al., 1999), the parent also may have more opportunities for labeling when the child produces this type of gesture. In addition, when caregivers are trained to model gestures to their child, they may also be more likely to respond to and reinforce the child's use of those (or perhaps any) gestures and therefore increase their opportunity to provide language input (Goodwyn et al., 2000). Caregiver responsivity and amount of caregiver input have clearly been associated with the rate of language acquisition (Huttenlocher, Haight, Bryk, Seltzer, & Lyons, 1991).

Goodwyn et al. (2000) also suggest that increasing the child's gesture repertoire could contribute to the child's ability to direct the "topic," thereby increasing the likelihood that the adult will comment on objects/actions that are of interest to the child rather than adult-generated ones. The ability to focus topics becomes particularly important given the work that has shown that parental use of names for objects on which the child is already focusing is a positive predictor of later vocabulary size (Tomasello & Farrar, 1986). Finally, as suggested by Goodwyn et al. (2000), the child is using representational gesturing as a type of scaffolding through which concepts can be explored and perhaps shaped/corrected. When a child has a symbol for something, not only can the child "comment" on it, ask questions about it (along with facial expressions), or request it, but the child can also gain increasing information about it through these interactions. Think of the child who "flaps" her arms to represent a duck after previously having done so for a bird. When the child's caregiver says "Oh, that's not a bird, it's a duck" or perhaps "It does have wings but it lives in the water," the child's database of information that binds objects/actions together as well as distinguishing them from one another is enriched. In sum, gesture use in both parents and children is a strong predictor of later language use and thus the early use of gestures can be an indicator of later typical development in a related domain.

Dissociations Between Gesture Use and Language Skills

Despite the fact that gesture production and word production have been shown to be correlated significantly, there are times when they are not. In addition, although there is a strong link between word comprehension and word production, the relationship is also variable. Three factors that appear to have an impact on both sets of relationships are the group versus the individual nature of the data, the child's developmental level, and the context of evaluation or use. For example, word comprehension and production are highly correlated when considered at a group level; however, there is considerable dissociation between the two when looking at individual children (Bates & Dick, 2002). For example, Fenson, Dale, Reznick, and Bates (1994) observed a number of children with receptive vocabularies over 200 words who produced no words productively. Similarly, across studies of gesture production, group means often represent a wide range of variation across children. In the larger data set from which the Crais et al. (2004) data were taken, the children who had the largest number of early gestures were not necessarily the first to use words. Indeed, one of the children who produced the most deictic and representational gestures at 12 months produced no words at all.

As noted by Bates and Dick (2002), with early correlations between the emergence of gestures and words, it is natural to assume that gesture production continues to be highly correlated with word production. Clearly, the association between word production and gestural naming is strong between 12 and 18 months, but disassociation occurs when verbal language takes over (Bates & Dick, 2002). Iverson et al. (1994) noted that 16-month-olds use both words and representational gestures to name objects, but by 20 months they have almost stopped using gestures and rely more heavily on words. As they suggest, word and symbol learning diverge as words take on "privileged status" in the infant repertoire. Word comprehension and word production, however, seem to have a reverse relationship in that early in development they are less well correlated, whereas later they become more closely associated. Paul (1996) uses the Fenson et al. (1993) data on vocabulary acquisition to illustrate the large standard deviations in word production seen at early ages. For example, although the mean vocabulary size at 18 months is over 100 words, the standard deviation is 111 (102% of the mean as noted by Paul). By the age of 24 months, average vocabulary size is over 300 words with a standard deviation of 175 (58% of the mean). Thus, as production vocabulary increases, the standard deviation decreases.

Indeed, as shown in several studies in older toddlers (Bretherton & Bates, 1984; Thal & Bates, 1988; Thal & Tobias, 1992), gesture production and *word comprehension* prove to be more closely linked than word comprehension and word production. Thus the relationship between gesture production and word production as well as the link between word comprehension and word production change over time.

In addition, despite the fact that maternal gesture use and child gesture use at 16 months is highly correlated, the relationship at 20 months (although still positive) is not significant (Iverson et al., 1999). In Iverson and colleagues' study, mean gesture production (tokens not types of gestures) in the children increased between 16 and 20 months (although not significantly), whereas gesture use compared proportionally to use of verbalizations decreased. This decrease was caused by a significant increase in word production between 16 and 20 months. For mothers, however, both gesture use and word use were almost identical when compared across the two time periods. Therefore, developmental level also appears to affect the relationship between maternal and child gesture use, especially with increases in the child's word production skills.

In terms of context, both gesture production and word comprehension are well correlated with word production; however, this effect is most evident when elicited under experimental conditions with little or no contextual support (Bates & Dick, 2002). As defined by Bates and Dick, "context" refers to the presence or absence of the object and the familiarity of the gesture modeled. There is also a strong link between word comprehension and gesture production, although the linkage is strongest when both are assessed in highly supportive contexts. These contexts typically include naturalistic observation and parental report. Within these contexts, both word comprehension and gesture production are dissociated from word production. Bates and Dick (2002) argue that these apparent disassociations are not influenced by domain (language or gesture) or the contrast between production and comprehension, but reflect the presence or absence of contextual support. In sum, individual children break away from the group trends, and developmental level and context both play a role in the relationships among communicative processes. Thus taken together, these results could be accounted for from the interactionist perspective (Chapman, 2000) in viewing each child and his or her surrounding context as a transactional unit in which each influences the other.

GESTURE USE AS A PREDICTOR FOR IDENTIFYING CHILDREN WITH COMMUNICATION DEFICITS

Increasingly, delayed and/or limited use of gestures is being correlated with deficits in later language learning. For example, children who are significantly delayed in both gestural and word naming often exhibit delays in language at later stages of development (Thal, Bates, Goodman, & Jahn-Samilo, 1997). For children with atypical development, Bates and Dick (2002) argue that word production does not typically emerge until the child has begun to produce recognitory gestures (even though both may be delayed). This developmental trend has been demonstrated in children with Down syndrome and Williams syndrome (Singer Harris, Bellugi, Bates, Jones, & Rossen, 1997) and in children with autism (Happé & Frith, 1996). Moreover, negative correlations between gestural and verbal naming are seen at later stages, and therefore persistence in gestural naming in some children beyond 18 months may indicate language delays (Bates & Dick, 2002).

As suggested by Thal and Tobias (1994), late talkers who appear to have adequate word comprehension and gesture production appear to be "late bloomers" and typically "catch up" in the next 1–2 years. Children who show delays in both word comprehension and gesture production, however, continue to show delays over time and may later be identified as language impaired. Thus, both the amount of gesture use and the relationship to word comprehension are predictive of later group membership for late talkers.

Further, the emergence of deictic gestures, culturally defined gestures (e.g., waving "bye"), and word comprehension are significantly correlated and all are predictive of later expressive language delays. These developmental processes are closely linked with cognitive and imitative growth suggesting not only the likelihood of shared underlying neural causes (Bates, Thal, & Janowsky, 1992), but also the possibility of interactive effects. Strong concurrent relationships between joint attention gestures and language have been demonstrated in both children with typical development and those with autism (Mundy, Sigman, & Kasari, 1994). In addition, the presence or absence of other gesture types (e.g., head nodding or shaking) has been strongly linked with expressive language levels in children with autism, language impairments, and mental impairments (Lord & Pickles, 1996). Moreover, the finding that word comprehension and gesture production are significantly delayed in children with mental retardation (Singer Harris et al., 1997), children with autism (Happé & Frith, 1996), and a portion of late talkers (Thal & Bates, 1988; Thal & Tobias, 1994) further indicates the importance of examining gesture use and its relationship to other areas of development.

In addition, the varied profiles of gesture use in children with diverse communication disorders (e.g., autism, Down syndrome, Williams syndrome, mental retardation) argue for different cognitive and neurological processes underlying communication development in these children (Mundy & Willoughby, 1998). Potential genetic contributions suggest differing manifestations of gesture development and use in these groups. For example, children with autism have been reported to use imperative (i.e., instrumental, behavior regulation) gestures more commonly with few or no declarative gestures (McEvoy, Rogers, & Pennington, 1993; Mundy et al., 1994), whereas children with Down syndrome have more difficulty using imperatives, yet use social interaction and joint attention acts more readily (Mundy, Kasari, Sigman, & Ruskin, 1995). However, Sigman, Mundy, Sherman, and Ungerer (1986) reported less frequent use of imperative gestures in preschool children with autism compared to typically developing children, but noted that the differences were less than the differences in joint attention use. A recent unpublished study by Watson, Baranek, Crais, Downing, and Popovich (2003), through retrospective video analysis, also indicated different profiles of gesture use in 15- to 18-month-old children later diagnosed with autism and those with typical development. Their findings, however, revealed that although the two groups had smaller differences between the frequency of use of social interaction gestures (e.g., social games, conventional gestures) there were much larger differences between the use of both behavior regulation and joint attention gestures. Thus, are there developmental differences in the gesture profiles of children later diagnosed with autism when examining them at younger (i.e., infancy) versus older (i.e., preschool) ages? To support this supposition, DiLavore and Lord's (1995) longitudinal study indicated that the differences between children with autism and those with other developmental problems in instrumental gestures had disappeared at age 3, whereas the differences in joint attention persisted.

Finally, the interactionist perspective (Chapman, 2000) would suggest that specific language and conceptual understanding of events of interest give weight and cue value to particular aspects of meaning and form. As suggested by Chapman from the work of Dale et al. (1998) examining late talkers and their twins, genetic influences play a strong role in child language disorders, whereas environmental factors play a strong role in language learning within normal variations. This does not mean, however, that for each group the alternate factor (i.e., environment in children with language disorders, genetics in typical language development) does not have an influence, just that the influence may not be the primary factor. The work exploring gesture development in children with diverse communicative disorders may help enlighten the field as to the influence of genetic components and their interactions with the surrounding environment.

IMPLICATIONS FOR FUTURE RESEARCH

It is clear that a growing body of research supports the increased focus on gesture development and use and its concurrent and predictive relationships with other developmental domains. Not only is gesture development a critical skill in overall communicative ability, it is also very likely a pivotal skill through which other communication behaviors are gained. As suggested by many, although the focus on a small number of gestures (e.g., show, give, reach, point) has helped move the field toward greater understanding of gesture development and its relation to other domains, there is a need to expand the types of gestures examined. The majority of gesture work has been on deictic gestures, with much less attention to other gesture forms. Thus, little is known about the relationship between deictic and other types of gestures and the predictability of these gesture types and other domains. Further, the interplay between gesture type and communicative function has been explored in children with typical development and increasingly with children with various types of communication deficits. The finding that a similar pattern of gesture use can be seen in children from a common disability grouping may provide insight into the underlying processes surrounding the disability. In addition, patterns of gesture use may also help identify children in need of early intervention and pinpoint potential targets for intervention. It is unclear, however, how stable these patterns are across groups and what factors might lead to individual variation. Recent work revealing differences across communicative functions between early and later gesture use across groups of children signals the need to continue to pursue longitudinal study of gesture use in infants and toddlers with differing disabilities. In addition, the factors that mediate gesture development across children (individually and by disability group) and how these factors can be used to enhance the development of gestures remain a mystery. Although there have been great strides in the knowledge base related to gesture development, much of the research has highlighted further questions to be answered.

REFERENCES

Acredolo, L., & Goodwyn, S. (1985). Symbolic gesturing in language development: A case study. *Human Development, 28,* 40–49.

Acredolo, L., & Goodwyn, S. (1988). Symbolic gesturing in normal infants. *Child Development, 59,* 450–466.

Acredelo, L., & Goodwyn, S. (1990). Sign language in babies: The significance of symbolic gesturing for understanding language development. In R. Vasta (Ed.), *Annals of child development* (Vol. 7, pp. 1–42). London: Jessica Kingsley.

Bates, E. (1976). *Language and context.* New York: Academic Press.

Bates, E., Benigni, L., Bretherton, I., Camaioni, L., & Volterra, V. (1979). *The emergence of symbols: Cognition and communication in infancy.* New York: Academic Press.

Bates, E., Camaioni, L., & Volterra, V. (1975). The acquisition of performatives prior to speech. *Merrill-Palmer Quarterly, 21,* 205–226.

Bates, E., & Dick, F. (2002). Language, gesture, and the developing brain. *Developmental Psychobiology, 40,* 293–310.

Bates, E., & Goodman, J. (1997). On the inseparability of grammar and the lexicon: Evidence from acquisition, aphasia, and real-time processing. *Language and Cognitive Processes, 12,* 507–584.

Bates, E., Thal, D., & Janowsky, J. (1992). Early language development and its neural correlates. In E. Sidney, J. Segalowitz, E. Rapin, et al. (Eds.), *Handbook of Neuropsychology* (Vol. 7, pp. 69–110). Amsterdam: Elsevier.

Bekken, K. (1989). *Is there motherese in gesture?* Unpublished doctoral dissertation, University of Chicago, Chicago.

Bretherton, I., & Bates, E. (1984). The development of representation from 10–28 months: Differential stability of language and symbolic play. In R. Emde & R. Hammon (Eds.), *Continuities and discontinuities in development* (pp. 229–259). New York: Plenum Press.

Bruner, J. (1966). On cognitive growth. In J. Brunner, R. Oliver, & P. Greenfield (Eds.), *Studies in cognitive growth* (pp. 1–20). New York: Wiley.

Bruner, J. (1977). Early social interaction and language acquisition. In H. Schaffer (Ed.), *Studies in mother–infant interaction* (pp. 271–289). New York: Academic Press.

Bruner, J. (1983). *Child's talk: Learning to use language.* New York: Norton.

Carpenter, R. L., Mastergeorge, A. M., & Coggins, T. E. (1983). The acquisition of communicative intentions in infants eight to fifteen months of age. *Language and Speech, 26,* 101–116.

Carpenter, M. , Nagell, K., & Tomasello, M. (1998). Social cognition, joint attention, and communicative competence from 9 to 15 months of age. *Monographs of the Society for Research in Child Development, 63*(4, Serial No. 255).

Caselli, M. (1990). Communicative gestures and first words. In V. Volterra & C. Erting (Eds.), *From gesture to language in hearing and deaf children* (pp. 56–67). New York: Springer-Verlag.

Chapman, R. (1978). Comprehension strategies in children. In J. Kavanaugh & P. Strange (Eds.), *Language and speech in the laboratory, school, and clinic* (pp. 308–327). Cambridge, MA: MIT Press.

Chapman, R. (2000). Children's language learning: An interactionist perspective. *Journal of Child Psychology and Psychiatry, 41*(1), 33–54.

Chapman, R., Streim, N., Crais, E., Salmon, D., Strand, E., & Negri, N. (1992). Child talk: Assumptions of a developmental process model for early language learning. In R. Chapman (Ed.), *Processes in language acquisition and disorders* (pp. 3–19). St. Louis, MO: Mosby-Year Book.

Coggins, T., Olswang, L., & Guthrie, J. (1987). Assessing communicative intents in young children: Low structured observation or elicitation tasks? *Journal of Speech and Hearing Disorders, 52,* 44–49.

Crais, E., Douglas, D., & Campbell, C. (2004). The interaction of gesture development and intentionality. *Journal of Speech, Language, and Hearing Research, 47,* 678–694.

Dale, P., Simonoff, E., Bishop, D., Eley, T., Oliver, B., Price, T., Purcell, S., Stevenson, J., & Plomin, R. (1998). Genetic influences on language delay in two-year-old children. *Nature Neuroscience, 1,* 324–328.

DiLavore, P., & Lord, C. (1995, April). *Do you see what I see? Requesting and joint attention in young autistic children.* Paper presented at the Conference for the Society of Research in Child Development, Indianapolis, IN.

Fenson, L., Dale, P., Reznick, S., Thal, D., Bates, E., Hartung, J., Pethick, S., & Reilly, J. (1993). *The MacArthur Communicative Development Inventories: User's guide and technical manual.* San Diego, CA: Singular.

Fenson, L., Dale, P., Reznick, S., Bates, E., Thal, D., & Pethick, S. (1994). Variability in early communicative development. *Monographs of the Society for Research on Child Development, 59*(Serial No. 242).

Goldin-Meadow, S., & Morford, M. (1985). Gesture in early child language: Studies of hearing and deaf children. *Merrill-Palmer Quarterly, 31,* 146–176.

Goodwyn, S., & Acredolo, L. (1993). Symbolic gesture versus word: Is there a modality advantage for the onset of symbol use? *Child Development, 64,* 688–701.

Goodwyn, S., Acredelo, L., & Brown, C. (2000). Impact of symbolic gesturing on early language development. *Journal of Nonverbal Behavior, 24*(2), 81–103.

Happé, F., & Frith, U. (1996). The neuropsychology of autism. *Brain, 119,* 1377–1400.

Hodapp, R., Goldfield, E., & Boyatzis, C. (1984). The use and effectiveness of maternal scaffolding in mother–infant games. *Child Development, 55,* 772–781.

Huttenlocher, J., Haight, W., Bryk, A., Seltzer, M., & Lyons, T. (1991). Early vocabulary growth: Relation to language input and gender. *Developmental Psychology, 27,* 236–248.

Iverson, J., Caprici, O., & Caselli, M. (1994). From communication to language in two modalities. *Cognitive Development, 9,* 23–43.

Iverson, J. M., Capirci, O., Longobardi, E., & Caselli, M. C. (1999). Gesturing in mother–child interactions. *Cognitive Development, 14,* 57–75.

Iverson, J., & Goldin-Meadow, S. (Eds.). (1998). *New directions for child development, No. 79. The nature and functions of gestures in children's communication.* San Francisco: Jossey-Bass.

Iverson, J., & Thal, D. (1998). Communicative transitions: There's more to the hand than meets the eye. In A. Wetherby, S. Warren, & J. Reichle (Eds.), *Transitions in prelinguistic communication* (pp. 59–86). Baltimore: Paul Brookes.

Kagan, J. (1981). *The second year*. Cambridge, MA: Harvard University Press.

Lord, C., & Pickles, A. (1996). Language level and nonverbal social-communicative behaviors in autistic and language-delayed children. *Journal of American Academy of Child and Adolescent Psychiatry, 35*(11), 1542–1550.

Masur, E. F. (1983). Gestural development, dual-directional signaling, and the transition to words. *Journal of Psycholinguistic Research, 12*, 93–109.

McEvoy, R., Rogers, S., & Pennington, R. (1993). Executive function and social communication deficits in young autistic children. *Journal of Child Psychology and Psychiatry, 34*, 563–578.

McLean, J., McLean, L., Brady, N., & Etter, R. (1991). Communication profiles of two types of gesture using nonverbal persons with severe to profound mental retardation. *Journal of Speech and Hearing Research, 34*, 294–308.

McNeill, D. (1992). *Hand and mind: What gesture reveals about thought*. Chicago: University of Chicago Press.

Miller, J., Chapman, R., Branston, M., & Reichle, J. (1980). Language comprehension in sensorimotor stages V and VI. *Journal of Speech and Hearing Research, 23*, 284–311.

Morford, M., & Goldin-Meadow, S. (1992). Comprehension and production of gesture in combination with speech in one-word speakers. *Journal of Child Language, 19*, 550–580.

Mundy, P., Kasari, C., Sigman, M., & Ruskin, E. (1995). Nonverbal communication and early language acquisition in children with Down syndrome or normal development. *Journal of Speech and Hearing Research, 38*, 157–167.

Mundy, P., Sigman, M., & Kasari, C. (1994). Joint attention, developmental level, and symptom presentation in young children with autism. *Development and Psychopathology, 6*, 389–401.

Mundy, P., & Willoughby, J. (1998). Nonverbal communication, affect, and social-emotional development. In A. Wetherby, S. Warren, & J. Reichle (Eds.), *Transitions in prelinguistic communication* (pp. 111–133). Baltimore: Paul Brookes.

Namy, L., Acredolo, L., & Goodwyn, S. (2000). Verbal labels and gestural routines in parental communication with young children. *Journal of Nonverbal Behavior, 24*(2), 63–79.

Namy, L., & Waxman, S. (1998). Words and gestures: Infants' interpretations of different forms of symbolic reference. *Child Development, 69*, 295–308.

Paul, R. (1996). Clinical implications of the natural history of slow expressive language development. *American Journal of Speech-Language Pathology, 5*, 5–21.

Petitto, A. (1988). "Language" in the prelinguistic child. In F. Kessel (Ed.), *The development of language and language research: Essays in honor of Roger Brown* (pp. 187–221). Hillsdale, NJ: Lawrence Erlbaum Associates.

Piaget, J. (1970). *Genetic epistemology* (Trans. E. Duckworth). New York: Columbia University Press.

Shatz, M. (1982). On mechanisms of language acquisition: Can features of the communicative environment account for development? In E. Wanner & L. Gleitman

(Eds.), *Language acquisition: The state of the art* (pp. 102–127). New York: Cambridge University Press.

Shore, C., Bates, E., Bretherton, I., Beeghly, M., & O'Connell, B. (1990). Vocal and gestural symbols: Similarities and differences from 13 to 28 months. In V. Volterra & C. Etting (Eds.), *From gesture to language in hearing and deaf children* (pp. 79–91). New York: Springer.

Sigman, M., Mundy, P., Sherman, T., & Ungerer, J. (1986). Social interactions of autistic, mentally retarded and normal children and their caregivers. *Journal of Child Psychology and Psychiatry, 27*(5), 647–656.

Singer Harris, N., Bellugi, U., Bates, E., Jones, W., & Rossen, M. (1997). Contrasting profiles of language development in children with Williams and Down syndromes. *Developmental Neuropsychology, 13*, 345–370.

Thal, D., & Bates, E. (1988). Language and gesture in late talkers *Journal of Speech and Hearing Research, 31*, 115–123.

Thal, D., Bates, E., Goodman, J., & Jahn-Samilo, J. (1997). Continuity of language abilities: An exploratory study of late- and early-talking toddlers. *Developmental Neuropsychology, 13*, 239–273.

Thal, D., & Tobias, S. (1992). Communicative gestures in children with delayed onset of oral expressive vocabulary. *Journal of Speech and Hearing Research, 35*, 1281–1289.

Thal, D., & Tobias, S. (1994). Relationships between language and gesture in normally developing and late-talking toddlers. *Journal of Speech and Hearing Research, 37*, 147–170.

Tomasello, M., & Farrar, J. (1986). Joint attention and early language. *Child Development, 57*, 1454–1463.

Vygotsky, L. (1962). *Thought and language*. Cambridge, England: Cambridge University Press.

Vygotsky, L. (1987). *The collected works of L. S. Vygotsky: Vol. 1. Problems of general psychology*. New York: Plenum Press.

Watson, L., Baranek, G., Crais, E., Downing, K., & Popovich, A. (2003, March). *Stability and change in symptoms of autism in infancy*. Paper presented at the Gatlinburg Conference on Theory and Research in Intellectual Development. Annapolis, MD.

Werner, H., & Kaplan, B. (1963). *Symbol formation*. New York: Wiley.

Wetherby, A., Cain, D. H., Yonclas, D. G., & Walker, V. G. (1988). Analysis of intentional communication of normal children from the prelinguistic to the multiword stage. *Journal of Speech and Hearing Research, 31*, 240–252.

Zinober, B., & Martlew, M. (1985). Developmental changes in four types of gesture in relation to acts and vocalizations from ten to twenty-one months. *British Journal of Developmental Psychology, 3*, 293–306.

6

Dissociations in the Development of Early Communication in Autism Spectrum Disorders

Rhea Paul[1,2]
Katarzyna Chawarska[2]
Ami Klin[2]
Fred Volkmar[2]
[1]Southern Connecticut State University
[2]Yale Child Study Center

Robin Chapman's work has encouraged us to examine the ways in which language acquisition interacts with other aspects of development. As a teacher and mentor of researchers in language disorders, one of her most important contributions is her insistence on seeing language development within the context of the child's social and emotional world. This orientation is especially relevant to work with children whose disabilities create social and emotional contexts that can differ from those of other children. In this chapter we discuss the case of language acquisition in autism spectrum disorders (ASD). We outline the course of early communicative development in children with ASD, and describe the language profiles of a group of children with ASD followed in our laboratory from the age of 18 months into the preschool period. This discussion outlines some of the ways in which communicative development diverges from typical patterns. We then speculate about how some of these divergences happen and what they might mean, both for understanding language development and disorders, and more specifically for understanding and ameliorating the severe communicative deficits seen in autism spectrum disorders.

Autism is a developmental disability with a neurobiological basis that is characterized by a triad of symptoms including difficulties in social interaction, difficulties in communication, and a pattern of restricted, repetitive, and stereotyped interests and activities (APA, 1994). It can be expressed with a range of severity; thus, conditions of this sort are commonly referred to as *autism spectrum disorders* (ASD). As a core symptom of ASD, communication is impaired in all children with these syndromes—even in the one condition (Asperger's syndrome) described subsequently in which some aspects of early language development are preserved. Some children are slow to begin talking or may not learn to talk at all; others may learn to produce words and sentences but have difficulty using them effectively to accomplish social interactive goals. Autism is primarily a disorder of communication, with secondary effects on the development of language. As such, impairments emerge prior to the point at which children normally begin speaking.

OVERVIEW OF EARLY DEVELOPMENT IN ASD

Infancy

Many parents of children with ASD report that these babies were very quiet and didn't babble, that they sometimes seemed deaf and did not respond to voices or their name, that they did not spend much time looking at faces, tried less frequently to attract others' attention, and were less eager to engage in early social games, such as "patty-cake," that involve smiling at others and vocalizing (see Volkmar, Charwarska, & Klin, 2005, for review). Although data like these are mainly retrospective and may be biased by knowledge that the child did turn out to have ASD, they suggest that deficits in communication and social interaction exist prior to the onset of language in this syndrome.

The Second Year of Life

Between 12 and 24 months of age, children who were later diagnosed with ASD have been found to be less responsive and to pay less attention to people in their environment and to show a lower frequency of looking at objects shown to them by others (Chawarska & Volkmar, 2005). They may begin to produce some communication, but their acts are usually for the purpose of getting others to do or not do things (regulatory acts), rather than for the purpose of sharing and social interaction that characterizes the majority of communicative acts of typical toddlers (Mundy, Sigman, & Kasari, 1994; Wetherby, 1986; Wetherby et al., 2004). Even when they do communicate, their rates are lower and they are less likely to engage people visually or to direct their acts to the communication partners with gaze (Chawarska & Volkmar, 2005; Mundy & Burnette, 2005). They also tend to use unusual gestures, such as pushing an adult's hand toward a desired object, rather than pointing or showing in a more conventional way (Stone, Ousley, Yoder, Hogan, & Hepburn, 1997).

Parents of children with ASD often report that the second year of life was the time they became seriously concerned about their affected child's development. These toddlers continue to show reduced attention to voices (Lord, 1995; Osterling & Dawson, 1994), but parents' most pressing concerns in the child's second year are typically around speech, either because the child failed to begin saying words, or because he or she learned a few words and never went farther, or lost the early words acquired. About 20% of children who end up on the autism spectrum are reported to experience a regression in skills, usually loss of the ability to say words, during their second year (Hoshino et al., 1987; Kobayashi & Murata, 1998; Kurita, 1985; Rogers & DiLalla, 1990; Tuchman & Rapin, 1997). Some children with ASD do not develop the ability to speak beyond a few single words (Tager-Flusberg, Paul, & Lord, 2005), and the issue is more one of developmental stagnation than regression (Siperstein & Volkmar, 2004). Our data, for example, suggest that 40% of 18- to 36-month-olds with ASD had no functional speech (compared to 10–15% of children from large, epidemiological samples; Beitchman et al., 1989; Rescorla, 1989), although a year later, when the children were between 3 and 4 years of age, this proportion dropped to 22% in our data.

Preschool Language Development

Even children with ASD who do speak are often very slow to acquire words and word combinations, and speak very little until late in the preschool years (LeCouteur, Bailey, Rutter, & Gottesman, 1989, August). Delays in language acquisition in the preschool period, of course, are not specific to ASD (Cantwell, Baker, & Mattison, 1980). In fact, delayed language development is the most common presenting problem for preschool children referred for special educational or psychiatric evaluations (Rosetti, 2001). Moreover, a small portion of children with ASD do not show any delays in language development or can even be precocious in their acquisition of words and sentences. In our data, 10% of children with ASD between the ages of 18 and 36 months had language scores within the normal range on a standardized test; 1 child (out of 51 children seen) scored in the superior range. These children may turn out to have Asperger's syndrome, a variant of ASD in which children show normal cognitive and language development, but significant difficulties in social uses of language and social interaction (Klin & Volkmar, 1997). The existence of this syndrome suggests that, even though abnormalities in communication are a core feature of pervasive developmental disorders, and slow language acquisition is common in this syndrome, early deficits in the formal aspects of language are not universal. In addition, Tager-Flusberg and Joseph (2003) and Roberts, Rice, and Tager-Flusberg (2004) have presented some evidence to suggest that language acquisition in ASD is variable, and that there may be subgroups of individuals within the autism spectrum who have language profiles that resemble those seen in children with specific language impairment.

PATTERNS OF COMMUNICATION SPECIFIC TO ASD

Although communication deficits have been identified in children with ASD from Kanner's (1943) initial description of the syndrome, Tager-Flusberg (1981) was the first to outline a basic pattern in the communication of children with this syndrome. This initial description consisted of relative preservation of the formal aspects of language (syntax, morphology, phonology), with deficits in the areas of semantics and pragmatics. Advancing research, in which Tager-Flusberg continues to play a major role, has modified this view somewhat. Current descriptions suggest that most areas of semantics, too, are more or less appropriate for mental age. For example, studies have shown that verbal children with ASD use semantic groupings (e.g., *bird, boat, food*) in typical ways to categorize and to retrieve words (Boucher, 1988; Tager-Flusberg, 1985; Minshew & Goldstein, 1993). Children with autism have been shown to use real-world probabilities to assist them in responding to complex sentences forms, as typical children do (Naito & Kikuo, 2004; Paul, Fisher, & Cohen, 1988). Kjelgaard and Tager-Flusberg (2001) report some difficulties in the use of higher order and abstract semantic skills, particularly the ability to use and understand words for affective and mental states. Basic word knowledge, however, appears to be more or less developmentally appropriate. The current consensus description of language acquisition in children with ASD who speak holds basic form and content of language to be comparable to mental age (Tager-Flusberg, 1994), with some exceptions in the area of words that reflect knowledge of others' affects and internal states. Syntactic development, too, appears to be similar to that seen in other developmental disorders (Tager-Flusberg et al., 1990). It is also now thought there may be subgroups of speakers with ASD who show additional delays in the production of obligatory tense markers (a "delay within a delay"), similar to the pattern seen in children with SLI. However, the most significant deficits for all children with ASD are concentrated in the area of pragmatic uses of language. Tager-Flusberg (1994) described this pattern as a "dissociation of form and function" in the language acquisition of children with ASD.

There are, in addition, some special features of language form and content that often appear when children with ASD begin to talk. One feature that is sometimes noted is *pronoun reversal* (Fay, 1969), usually in the form of substituting *you* for *I* (e.g., "Pick you up!"). Although this was originally thought to represent a failure of ego development, Fay (1971) pointed out that, rather than actually reversing pronouns, children with ASD were *failing* to reverse them; preserving the pronoun used in speaking to them when speaking themselves (Adult: "Do you want me to pick you up?" Child: "Pick you up!"). Tager-Flusberg (1994) found that many young children with ASD went through a stage of reversing pronouns, although as they got older the more linguistically advanced children stopped making these errors. Pronoun reversal is now seen as an instance of another feature of early language in ASD, *echolalia.*

Echolalia is the repetition, with similar intonation, of words or phrases that someone else has said. When children with ASD echo, they can use their echoes for a variety of communicative purposes (Prizant & Duchan, 1981). Shapiro (1977) and Carr, Schreibman, and Lovaas (1975) found that children with ASD were most likely to echo questions and commands that they did not understand or for which they did not know the appropriate response. Although echolalia is one of the most classic symptoms of ASD (Kanner, 1946), not all children with ASD echo, nor is echoing seen only in ASD. It also occurs in blind children, in children with other language impairments, in older people with dementia, and in some normally developing children at early stages of communication (Yule & Rutter, 1987). For all children, including those with ASD, echolalia declines over the course of development. It appears to function primarily to help children maintain communication with others, especially when they have limited ability to express their own intentions through spontaneous language. As expressive ability grows, echoing decreases. However, Tager-Flusberg et al. (1990) showed that imitated speech is neither longer nor more grammatically complex than spontaneous production, in children with ASD or in those with Down syndrome (DS) or typical development (TD).

Another area of special difficulty for children with ASD who speak is the use of *prosody.* Prosody includes features such as vocal quality, intonation, and stress patterns, which are frequently noted to be unusual in individuals with ASD spectrum disorders (Rutter, Mawhood, & Howlin, 1992). Ricks and Wing (1976) carried out one of the first studies in this area, looking at parents' identification of the meaning of the prelinguistic vocalizations of young children with ASD. They found that parents of children with ASD were unable to understand the preverbal vocalizations of other children with ASD, even though they could understand their own child's messages. In contrast, parents of typically developing children could understand vocalizations of typical children who were not their own, as well as those of their own child. Sheinkopf and his colleagues conducted a detailed examination of the vocal behavior of young preverbal children with ASD and a group of comparison children with developmental delays (Sheinkopf, Mundy, Oller, & Steffens, 2000). They reported that children with ASD showed significant impairments in vocal quality. In addition to their odd intonation, vocalizations of children with ASD were less likely to be paired with other nonverbal communication, such as shifts in gaze or gesture or changes in facial expression, than they were for the other children (Hellreigel, Tao, DiLavore, & Lord, 1995). These findings suggest that the source of the difference between the vocalizations of the young children with ASD and those of other young, nonverbal children was in both social intent and in a more basic aspect of the form of the vocalization. However, there are few data available regarding the phonological characteristics of language in very young children with ASD.

In children with ASD who speak, intonation or "tone of voice" differences are also often reported. The most frequently cited tone is monotony, but Fay and Schuler (1980) also describe a subset of autistic individuals who used an exaggerated singsong rather than flat pattern. Goldfarb, Braunstein, and Lorge (1956) and Pronovost, Wakstein, and Wakstein (1966) found unusually high pitch levels in speakers with ASD. Other voice disorders, such as hoarseness, harshness, and hypernasality, have also been reported, as well as poor control of volume, with unexplained fluctuations (Pronovost et al., 1966). Fay (1969) reported frequent whispering among children who echo.

By far, of course, the greatest difficulties in the language of speakers with ASD are in the area of language use. Unlike typically developing agemates, who are expanding and elaborating their forms and functions of communication during the preschool period, children with ASD show less frequent and less varied communicative functions in spontaneous speech, although their responses to highly structured situations may be similar to those of control groups (Landry & Loveland, 1989; Mermelstein, 1983; Wetherby & Prutting, 1984). Preschool children with ASD rarely use language for comments, showing off, acknowledging the listener, initiating social interaction, or requesting information. The speech acts that are missing or rarely used in the conversations of children with ASD all have in common an emphasis on social rather than regulatory uses of language (Wetherby, 1986). Moreover, unlike other children with language disorders, of whom, generally, it can be said that the more they talk, the more typical they become, the opposite is true for children with ASD (Tager-Flusberg et al., 2005). That is, the pragmatic deficits seen in verbal children with this syndrome result in increasing perceptions of oddity the more they say. Obsessive, perseverative topics may confuse or alienate peers. Repeated, stereotyped questions can try listeners' patience. Failure to listen and respond contingently to others' remarks often results in peers giving up on trying to converse with these children. Many of the pragmatic deficits seen in speakers with autism are thought to be related to their difficulties with "theory of mind"—that is, the ability to understand what others have in mind, what they know and want to know from conversation (Tager-Flusberg, 2000).

As we've said, some children with ASD do not develop useable spoken language. For these nonspeakers with ASD, again, problems go beyond not talking, to include difficulty in attending to and understanding language, in initiating communication to share attention and emotion, in using normal vocal quality even in preverbal vocalization, in directing communication to others with gaze, and in using conventional gestures to get messages across (Tager-Flusberg et al., 2005). Efforts to provide nonspeaking children with ASD with alternative forms of communication, such as Sign language or pictures, afford some help in increasing the child's ability to express wants and needs, but they rarely result in fluent and fully functional use of the alternative system, as is seen, for example, in the use of Sign by children who are deaf. However, very little is known about communication development in nonspeaking children with ASD, because very little research has focused on this population.

In the next section, we present a set of longitudinal data regarding a cohort of toddlers suspected of ASD in their second year and followed to preschool age. We discuss their profiles of communicative development, to begin to trace the trajectory of their language growth. We then speculate on what the observed patterns mean for understanding language development in autism and for thinking about its remediation.

DATA FROM THE YALE DEVELOPMENTAL DISABILITIES CLINIC

The Studies to Advance Autism Research and Treatment (STAART) clinical research program at the Yale Child Study Center has for the past 3 years been involved in a longitudinal investigation of the development of toddlers (16–37 months of age) who exhibit symptoms of ASD. As part of this study, we have provided in-depth evaluation in language, cognitive, motor, social, and adaptive areas for these children, and have followed them to preschool age. To date, over 100 children have been seen before their third birthday. The data to be reported here concern the 51 children who have been seen for both an initial visit before age 3 and a follow-up evaluation at least 1 year later, when they are at least 3 years of age.

Subjects

Subjects aged 16 to 37 months at their first visit were referred to the Developmental Disabilities Clinic due to behavioral and developmental concerns. The sample was predominantly Caucasian (94%), with African Americans and Asians constituting 4% and 2% of the sample, respectively.

Procedures, Visit 1

Detailed pre-, peri-, and postnatal history as well as evaluations and treatment history were collected according to a structured protocol. Assessment procedures used in this evaluation are listed here.

Clinical Diagnosis

The majority of these toddlers had not received an "official" diagnosis at the time of the assessment. As a result of their evaluation at our center, a best estimate clinical diagnosis was assigned by the members of the clinical team participating in the assessment. In rare cases of disagreement, the discrepancies were reexamined and consensus diagnosis was given. The diagnosis took into account direct observation, testing, and parent interview data, as well as review of medical and developmental history, and was based on the *DSM–IV* criteria modified for children under the age of 3 (see Stone et al., 1997, and Chawarska & Volkmar, 2005) with emphasis on the absence of early emerging dyadic and triadic interaction skills and limited nonverbal communication skills, with a lesser emphasis on the presence of stereotypic behaviors. All subjects reported on here received a diagnosis of ASD (either autism or pervasive developmental disorder—not otherwise specified) by means of this process at their first visit and maintained a diagnosis within the autism spectrum at their follow-up visit a year later.

Standardized Measures

Autism Diagnostic Observation Scale-G (ADOS; Lord et al., 2000). All toddlers were tested with Module 1 of the ADOS, a set of semistructured play probes designed for pre-verbal individuals and those using single words or simple phrases with fewer than three meaningful components. Spontaneous social and communicative behavioral responses are coded on a 0 to 3 scale, ranging from no evidence of abnormality to the highest severity of an abnormality. Based on selected items in the Communication and

Socialization domains, the ADOS provides two sets of cutoff points for *DSM–IV* based diagnostic classification: one for autism and one for pervasive developmental disorders—not otherwise specified (PDD-NOS). Children whose scores fall below the cutoff are classified as non-ASD. Detailed discussion of the findings from ADOS analyses are presented elsewhere (Chawarska, Klin, Paul, & Volkmar, 2005).

The Mullen Scales of Early Learning (Mullen, 1995). The Mullen consists of five scales assessing development from birth to 68 months: Visual Reception (VR) (visual discrimination and visual-spatial memory), Receptive Language (RL) (auditory comprehension and auditory memory), Expressive Language (EL) (spontaneous language production and verbal concept formation), Fine Motor (FM) (visual-motor ability and motor planning), and Gross Motor (GM) (gross motor control and mobility) domains. The Mullen yields standard *T*-scores in all five domains ($M = 50$, $SD = 10$) and age-equivalent scores.

The MacArthur-Bates Communicative Development Inventory (CDI; Fenson et al., 2003). For this test the infant version, "Words and Gestures," was also collected at visit 1 from each family. The CDI is a parent checklist that asks parents to check off words their child says and/or understands, and also asks about early gesture use and play behavior. This measure has well-established reliability and validity for indexing early language development (Dale, 1991).

The Communication and Symbolic Behavior Scales–Developmental Profile (CSBS–DP) Behavior Observation (Wetherby & Prizant, 2003). The CSBS–DP was used to provide a norm-referenced assessment of communication, social interaction, and play. The CSBS–DP presents the child with a series of "temptations" to communicate for requests, joint attention, and social interaction functions. It provides scales for the use of gestures and vocal and speech behaviors and also includes probes for lexical comprehension and symbolic and construction play.

The Vineland Adaptive Behavior Scales Survey Form (Sparrow, Balla, & Cicchetti, 1984). This is a nationally standardized semistructured caretaker interview instrument that assesses day-to-day adaptive functioning and was administered to primary caregivers by research assistants extensively trained in Vineland interview and scoring procedures. The Vineland consists of four domains: Communication, Daily Living, Socialization, and Motor. The Communication Domain is subdivided in Expressive and Receptive Language. Several studies have confirmed that the Vineland can be used to document delays in adaptive development in individuals with autism (Carter et al., 1998; Jacobson & Ackerman, 1990; Liss et al., 2001;

Loveland & Kelley, 1991; Rodriguez, Morgan, & Gefken, 1991; Schatz & Hamdan-Allen, 1995). Gillham, Carter, Volkmar, and Sparrow (2000) reported that autism could be differentiated from any nonautistic developmental disorder (DD) by means of scores on the Socialization and Daily Living scales of the Vineland.

Nonstandard Measures

Two additional measures were collected at the children's first visit: data on auditory preferences for speech stimuli in a preferential head-turn task, and an assessment of phonological production, based on transcription of a speech sample collected during the CSBS procedure.

Auditory Preferences. Subjects' listening preferences for speech versus nonspeech stimuli were tested in an auditory preference paradigm. Figure 6.1 provides a schematic of the auditory preference laboratory setup. Subjects were seated on a parent's lap between the two speakers, 4 feet from each. Two sets of stimuli were presented, one of a series of 15-s segments of a recording of a mother using natural child-directed speech (CDS) during free play with her toddler (with the child's responses and other extraneous sounds electronically removed), and the other the same segments electronically rotated so as to have the same acoustic properties as the first but to be unintelligible as speech (Scott, Blank, Rosen, & Wise, 2000).

A trial began with a light flashed directly in front of the child, calling the subject's attention to midline. When the child oriented to the center, the central light went out and the light above one speaker began to flash. If the child turned his or her head to the right or left in the direction of the light, the light stopped flashing and the speech or rotated speech segment was

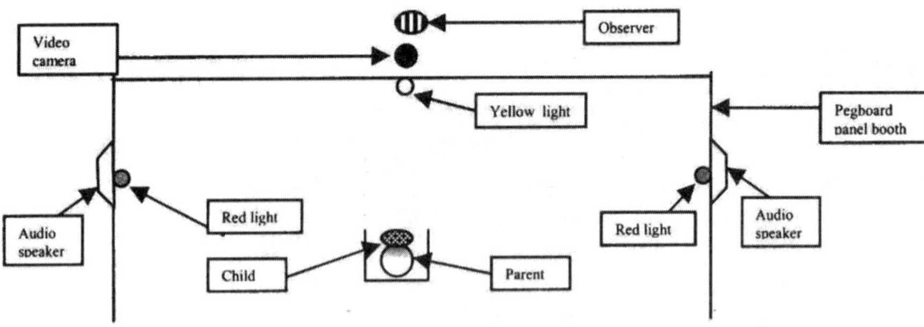

FIG. 6.1. Auditory preference laboratory (following Nelson et al., 1995).

played. The stimulus continued until the child turned away for at least 2 s, or until the entire trial was completed (about 15 s). Then the center light flashed to bring the child's attention back to midline and the next trial was begun. During the four pretest training trials, one presentation of each type of stimulus (speech or nonspeech) was given at each of the two locations (left/right sides). During all trials, the side light was extinguished as soon as the child looked toward that side, and only the sound continued throughout the head-turn. Test stimuli within each set were presented in individualized random order, controlled by the computer software.

A single observer sat behind the center panel, observing through a small porthole. The observer operated the response button box, connected to the computer, which controlled stimulus presentation and registered response timing. The observer signaled with one button when the child's attention was centered at the beginning of a trial, and then with another button when the child turned at least 30° in the direction of a stimulus location, as indicated to the observer by the side of the flashing light. An additional button was pressed when the infant changed from this orientation. On test trials, these observer responses initiated one of the flashing side lights, began an auditory stimulus, and terminated the sound and light when 2 s passed without any orientation to stimulus.

To guard against observer bias, the observer was blind to the stimulus and location order, which are both determined by the computer program. Both observer and parent wore tight-fitting earphones through which recordings of instrumental music were played loud enough to mask the stimuli being presented.

Phonological Production. To gather data on phonological production abilities of children in the sample, the CSBS assessment was videotaped and a timed, and a 15-min segment of each CSBS video was analyzed. The first 50 utterances produced during the 15-min CSBS segment were transcribed using broad phonemic transcription. Any additional utterances produced by the toddler were tallied, but not transcribed; if fewer than 50 utterances were present in the 15-min segment, all utterances produced were transcribed. These transcriptions were then analyzed for:

- *Percent utterances containing consonants:* Each utterance produced, whether meaningful or babbled, was scored as to whether it contained any consonant sound production. For each toddler, the number of utterances containing consonants was divided by the total number of utterances in the communication sample to derive a percentage of utterances containing consonants.

- *Inventory of consonant types produced:* The first appearance of each consonant type was tallied; voicing differences were not counted when tallying different consonant types (Shriberg & Kwiatkowski, 1982) (see Table 7.6).
- *Number of different consonant types:* the number of consonant types produced by each toddler was counted (see Table 6.5).
- *Percent consonants correct:* The percentage of consonants correctly produced (PCC) relative to the adult target word was computed for speaking toddlers (who produced 10 or more word or word approximations) using methods from Shriberg and Kwiatkowski (1982).

Procedures, Visit 2

The Vineland, Mullen, and ADOS were repeated at visit 2, which occurred at least 1 year following the first visit, when children were at least 36 months of age. At visit 2, the Reynell Developmental Language Scale, a direct assessment that contains both a receptive and expressive scale, was also administered as a standardized measure of language development.

Results

Descriptive Profiles: Visit 1. Table 6.1 presents data on performance at visit 1 on our assessment measures for these 51 children. There it can be seen, first, that on average, these toddlers with ASD scored below their chronological age on measures of both verbal and nonverbal function. Expressed as a developmental quotient (DQ; derived by dividing chronological age by nonverbal age-equivalent), the average nonverbal score for the group as a whole is 76.2, at the low end of the normal range. However, the measures of language, one direct (Mullen) and two using parent report (Vineland, CDI), uniformly show more significant delays in language than in nonverbal function.

Descriptive Profiles at Visit 1: Speakers and Nonspeakers. Because children with ASD who speak can show a quite different range of ability than those who do not, we divided our cohort into two groups: those with and those without functional speech. For this purpose, we define functional speech as the production of more than 10 words by parent report on the CDI after 18 months of age. Thirty-one of the 51 subjects (60.8%) were reported by parents to use more than 10 words on the CDI. Eighteen of the remaining 20 subjects who had no functional speech were over 18 months of age. Because it might be premature to expect functional speech from children under 18 months of age, only these 18 children's data will be considered. Table 6.2 shows the same descriptive profile as Table 6.1, with

TABLE 6.1
Average Scores on Assessment Measures

	Mean	*SD*	*Range*
Age (months)	28.1	5.0	16–37
Mullen Non-verbal Age-Equivalent (months)	21.4	7.4	13–69
Mullen Expressive Language Age-Equivalent (months)	15.0	7.3	5–46
Mullen Receptive Language Age-Equivalent (months)	12.5	7.8	4–51
Vineland Expressive Language Age-Equivalent (months)	13.1	6.0	10–35
Vineland Receptive Language Age-Equivalent (months)	15.1	6.2	10–35
CDI Words Produced and Age-equivalents (months)	62.8 (16 months)	87.1	0–395
CDI Words Understood and Age-Equivalents (months)	154.4 (15 months)	96.7	2–395

TABLE 6.2
Average Scores on Assessment Measures
for Subjects With and Without Speech

	Subjects With Functional Speech (n = 31)			*Subjects Without Functional Speech over 18 Months of Age (n = 18)*		
	Mean	*SD*	*Range*	*Mean*	*SD*	*Range*
Age (months)	28.8	4.4	20–37	27.6	5.0	18–35
Mullen Non-verbal Age-Equivalent (months)	23.5	9.2	14–69	19.1	3.5	13–26
Mullen Expressive Language Age-Equivalent (months)	19.0	6.8	8–46	9.5	3.5	5–15
Mullen Receptive Language Age-Equivalent (months)	14.7	8.5	6–51	8.33	3.6	4–19
Vineland Expressive Language Age-Equivalent (months)	15.6	5.4	6–35	8.8	2.9	1–12
Vineland Receptive Language Age-Equivalent (months)	16.8	6.0	8–31	12.7	4.5	1–189.6
CDI Words Produced (and Age-Equivalents, months)	101.5 (18 months)	93.2	11–395	3.2 (11 months)	3.4	0–10
CDI Words Understood (and Age-Equivalents, months)	200.9 (18 months)	87.0	30–395	90.9 (13 months)	57.4	13–220

subjects divided into 2 groups: those with more than 10-word expressive vocabularies, and those without functional speech who were over 18 months of age at their first visit. Student's *t*-tests revealed no significant differences between the two groups in terms of age ($t = 0.87$; $p < .39$) or nonverbal mental age on the Mullen ($t = 1.94$; $p < .06$), although the latter difference approached significance.

Looking at the data this way, we see that "speakers" and "nonspeakers" reveal a pattern of communicative performance, as measured both by direct assessment (Mullen) and parent report (Vineland, CDI), that is markedly depressed relative to nonverbal performance (although, of course, scores for the nonspeakers are more depressed than for speakers). For both groups, though, the pattern of communicative deficit is similar: Comprehension skills are not far in excess of production, as they often are for "late-talking" children (Paul, 1991; Thal, 1991); in fact, on direct testing with the Mullen, scores on comprehension are lower than production for both groups.

Data from the Communication and Symbolic Behavior Scales (CSBS; Wetherby & Prizant, 2003) can also be considered with regard to this observation. Although the CSBS does not yield age-equivalent scores, we can examine the scaled score data from this measure for patterns of communication in this population. Scaled scores on the CSBS have a mean of 10 and a standard deviation of 3, so that scores between 7 and 13 fall within normal limits (Wetherby & Prizant, 2003). These data are presented in Table 6.3. Student's *t*-tests reveal that on the scale that measures social behaviors (which includes use of gaze, gestures, and rate of communication) and on the one assessing receptive language (the ability to identify simple objects, familiar persons, and body parts when named) the speaking and nonspeaking groups do not differ significantly ($t = 1.43$, $p < .16$; and $t = 1.25$, $p < .21$, respectively). However, on the scale that measures speech (production of sounds, words, and word combinations), the speakers do score significantly higher than nonspeakers ($t = 3.26$; $p < .002$). This, of course should not be surprising, because the two groups were differentiated on the basis of speech production.

TABLE 6.3
CSBS Scale Scores for Speaking and Nonspeaking Subjects

	Subjects With Functional Speech (n = 31)	*Subjects Without Functional Speech (n = 18)*
	Mean (and SD) Scale Score	*Mean (and SD) Scale Score*
Social	5.1 (2.3)	4.3 (1.6)
Speech	9.3 (3.6)	6.4 (2.6)
Understanding	5.7 (4.2)	4.6 (1.9)

However, it is noteworthy that the nonspeakers are not significantly less likely to display social behaviors or to understand words than the speakers. This is not because the two groups show similarly high levels performance; instead, they are similarly low. For the both groups, social behaviors and receptive language scores are below the normal range, with scale scores of 4–5. For both groups, also, one-way analysis of variance (ANOVA) reveals that speech scores are significantly higher than scores in the other two domains: For the speaking group ($F = 13.37$; $p < .0001$), speech scores are within normal limits; for the nonspeaking group ($F = 2.37$; $p < .02$) speech scores approach the normal range at 6.4.

Descriptive Profiles: Visit 2. To examine growth in communicative ability in this cohort, Table 6.4 presents data on assessment measures collected at the subjects' second visit, at least 1 year following their first visit, when they were at least 36 months of age. At this point, children who had no speech at age 2 now score significantly lower on Mullen Visual Reception than those who spoke at the early age ($t = 2.59$; $p < .006$). Speakers had developmental

TABLE 6.4
Average Scores on Assessment Measures: Visit 2

	Subjects with Functional Speech at Visit 1			*Subjects Without Functional Speech at Visit 1*		
	Mean	*SD*	*Range*	*Mean*	*SD*	*Range*
Age (months)	49.2	6.8	42–55	48.3	3.7	36–59
Mullen Nonverbal Age-Equivalent (months)	44.0	11.5	25–60	34.4	11.6	20–60
Mullen Expressive Language Age-Equivalent (months)	42.2	10.5	20–63	27.3	15.5	8–70
Mullen Receptive Language Age-Equivalent (months)	44.4	12.7	22–69	27.7	14.7	7–65
Vineland Expressive Language Age-Equivalent (months)	40.8	16.0	20–78	22.8	10.2	8–50
Vineland Receptive Language Age-Equivalent (months)	39.5	17.3	12–96	26.2	12.8	12–48
Reynell Expressive Language Age-Equivalent (months)	41.2	12.2	24–64	30.7	11.9	18–61
Reynell Receptive Language Age-Equivalent (months)	40.1	13.1	22–72	28.1	11.6	13–57

quotients of 89 on average for Visual Reception; those without speech at age 2 had average developmental quotients of 71 for Visual Reception.

The two groups also differed significantly on all language measures at this age; however, there were no significant differences within the groups in terms of expressive versus receptive scores on any of the measures. Children showed similar scores across measures, whether direct (Mullen, Reynell) or parent report measures (Vineland). Children who had some speech at age 2 now showed developmental quotients for expressive and receptive language in the range of 80–85. These scores do not represent a significant gap relative to nonverbal scores on the Mullen. Thus, for children who began speaking in their second year, nonverbal and verbal skills appear more or less on par at preschool age. Those without speech at age 2 showed developmental quotients ranging from 56–64 on language measures, somewhat lower than their nonverbal levels.

Seven of the 18 children who had no functional speech at 18–35 months continued to score below 18 months on the Vineland Expressive scale at preschool age. In other words, 61% of children who were not speaking at age 2 had some speech by preschool age, and of all 51 children seen at age 2, 78% had some speech at 3–4 years.

Developmental Profiles: Summary

These data add to our understanding of the nature and course of language development in ASD. They reveal, first, that at 18–36 months of age, children with ASD show significant delays in language relative to nonverbal development, but this gap is only significant for those children who have not yet developed verbal language. For both children who do and children who do not use some speech in the second year, sound production appears somewhat ahead of social communication and understanding of language. And although parents of children with ASD, like other parents, tend to attribute comprehension to their children on parent report measures (as evidenced by higher receptive scores on parent report than on direct measures of comprehension), formal testing for both speakers and nonspeakers shows an aberrant pattern of better expressive than receptive performance.

A year later, a majority of the children who did not speak at age 2 are reported by parents to show some functional language, and average age-equivalent scores for this group generally exceed 24 months in expressive language measures both directly and by parent report. For the group who spoke during their second year, the rate of growth in language skills appears to be keeping pace with chronological age; during the average 20 months between assessments, average age equivalent scores on both direct testing (Mullen) and parent report (Vineland) increased at least 20 months in language areas. For the same period of time in the group who did not speak at 2, average age equivalent score increases were not quite as large, but averaged 18 months for formal testing and 14 months for parent report measures. Interestingly, receptive language skills in formal test contexts appear to have closed the gap seen earlier with expressive skills; receptive and expressive scores are similar on all measures at preschool age for both the group that spoke at 2 and the group that did not.

UNDERSTANDING LANGUAGE DEVELOPMENT IN ASD IN THE CONTEXT OF CURRENT MODELS OF LANGUAGE IMPAIRMENT

This thumbnail sketch of early communication development in ASD and brief presentation of data from our cohort bring us to the issue being raised in this chapter: How can we characterize the development of communication in ASD? How can we understand it in the context of what we know about typical development and the patterns seen in other disorders? And what might this understanding suggest about how best to address the serious impairments in communication seen in these children?

One concept to consider in addressing these questions is that suggested by Tager-Flusberg (1994): dissociations in development. One of the central observations about communication in autism concerns this notion. Unlike typical communicative development, in which a seamless tapestry of skills appears to be woven by the forces of biological predispositions and supportive environmental interactions in which the child actively and joyfully participates (Bloom, 1997; Chapman, 1992), in ASD we see "loose threads," developmental strands that fail to assume find their rightful place in the overall tapestry. But evidence emerging from the study of other disorders of language development suggests that dissociations are not unique to ASD.

Contemporary theorists in language disorders discuss the fact that there are selective impairments in language development in a variety of syndromes, such as Williams syndrome (WS), specific language impairment (SLI), and fragile X syndrome (fraX), to name a few. These "impairments within impairments" result in uneven profiles and "fractionations" of skills that are usually integrated in typical development. Thomas and Karmiloff-Smith (2005) discuss some examples. They cite WS, in which they report finding fewer errors made in syntax than morphology and that syntactic complexity is generally lower than receptive vocabulary would predict. Numerous other examples can be drawn from detailed studies of the language skill of children with SLI (e.g., Rice, 2004; Rice, Warren, & Betz, 2005), fraX (Fowler, 1998), and others. The consensus emerging from these investigations is that it is necessary to define fine-grained differences in specific components (e.g., syntax) and subcomponents (e.g., regular vs. irregular verb formation) of the language system relative to overall developmental level when describing development in populations with disorders. So, in this view, we would observe, for example, in Williams syndrome, that there are aspects of language that are MA-appropriate (vocabulary), aspects that are below MA expectations (syntactic complexity), and aspects that appear to be dissociated from others within a specific component (more errors in morphological than syntactic forms at the same developmental level). Recent investigations of language form reveal widespread fractionations within domains in a variety of disordered populations.

The important question becomes, then, how do these dissociations in development arise? Thomas and Karmiloff-Smith (2005), Locke (1994), Pinker (2001), and Rice (2004) have addressed this issue. In various ways, what these theorists have proposed is that the development of language, like other aspects of phylogeny, is the result of an unfolding complex of processes; it consists of a series of interdependent events, the disruption of any of which influences subsequent processes and pathways.

Locke (1994), for example, discussed the speculation that timing mechanisms might be involved in syntactic delays in late talkers. He speculated that the slowed acquisition of the first 50 productive vocabulary words in this group may lead to a failure to trigger, at the appropriate developmental time, the mechanism designed to reorganize these first-learned words into a grammar. Without the input of those first 50 words at the critical time, when other systems are developing in parallel, the grammatical system may fail to be activated so that later syntactic development must create less efficient compensatory mechanisms rather than making use of the biologically designed system that would have come online at 18 months, given appropriate lexical input.

Thomas and Karmiloff-Smith (2005) suggest mechanisms in addition to developmental mistiming by which a language-learning system can be perturbed. These include absent or atypical perceptual or computational biases, such as failure of early orienting systems that attract infants to faces and voices, resulting in a dearth of the requisite input on which developing systems build; anomalies in the emergence of specialized neural circuits due to abnormal pruning or competition; and changes in interaction among brain regions that force the system to develop compensatory mechanisms rather than employing optimal, biologically predetermined pathways for language acquisition. The point to be made is that although there may be a species-universal course of language acquisition that is mediated by a range of genetic events, neural structures, and interactive processes, disruptions in any component of the substrate for this acquisition can lead to a range of missed crucial opportunities. These disruptions can include failures to orient to, process, and store necessary data from the environment, or to achieve time-sensitive milestones that trigger subsequent neural or genetic events. These failures, in turn, can perturb the establishment of connections among neural areas that need to communicate in order for language acquisition to proceed optimally, or to compensatory processes that lead to less efficient mechanisms for accomplishing language decoding and encoding. One way to think about developing an understanding of communication development and disorders in ASD, then, would be to examine the dissociations specific to this syndrome.

DISSOCIATIONS IN EARLY COMMUNICATIVE DEVELOPMENT IN ASD

To attempt to provide some of the same fine-grained analysis of dissociation in strands of development of communication in ASD, similar to that emerging in the literature for other disorders, we discuss two aspects of dissociation revealed in our data on the early communication of our cohort of young children with ASD: dissociation between expressive and receptive language development, and dissociation between lexical and phonological production.

Expressive Versus Receptive Language

On both direct assessments of language in our study (Mullen and CSBS), toddlers with ASD score higher on measures of speech than on measures of understanding language. Bruinsma, Koegel, and Koegel (2004) also found that comprehension skills are depressed relative to production in the second year of life.

Although the parent report measures do not corroborate this observation, we should bear in mind, as Chapman taught us many years ago (1978), that parents characteristically overestimate their children's understanding of language. Data reported on the development of the CDI also suggest that parents are less reliable reporters regarding their children's language comprehension than their production (Dale, 1991). Moreover, studies of language comprehension in children with ASD suggest that these children, like their typical peers, make use of the same strategies that lead parents to this overestimation (Naito & Kikuo, 2004; Paul et al., 1988). Thus the direct assessment of language comprehension in toddlers, which reveals a decrement relative to production in both the speaking and nonspeaking groups, may represent more valid data.

These data would appear to suggest that, at least during the second year of life, toddlers with ASD demonstrate developmental levels of speech production that are in advance of their developmental level of language comprehension, with speech skills at near-normal to mildly delayed levels, on average, and receptive skills moderately to severely affected. A pattern such as our speaking group displays, with age-appropriate use of speech but significantly delayed receptive abilities, represents a profile not common to other kinds of language disorders. How can children learn to speak without understanding the language spoken to them?

To try to answer this question, we must first understand more fully the pattern displayed by this cohort. Although scores on measures of expressive language appear to be close to age level, the tasks involved in scoring at age level at this point in development are somewhat limited. On the Mullen, they involve single-word naming of objects and pictures; on the CSBS, they involve spontaneous labeling of concrete objects in the environment and the production of a range of consonant sounds and syllable shapes. Neither of these skills requires that the language produced be truly communicative in nature (children can label objects without using the label for any particular communication function). Moreover, these behaviors can be emitted on the child's own schedule, when each notices an object, and not necessarily in response to an adult's communicative bid. Receptive language items, on the other hand, require the child to focus on an adult utterance, leave off whatever was being attended to beforehand, match the content of the adult stimulus to objects in the environment, and indicate to the adult which object matches the stimulus. Both Chapman (1974) and Reznick, Corley, and Robinson (1999) suggested that differing task demands of measures of expressive and receptive language during this developmental period can help to explain differences in findings on expressive and receptive language tasks. It may be that the sequence of perceptions and actions necessary to demonstrate receptive language ability represents particular difficulty for children with ASD.

Our data from the auditory preference study help us to understand why receptive language might be particularly difficult for young children with ASD. Results of analysis of variance (ANOVA) of the time spent listening to natural child-directed speech (CDS) versus electronically rotated speech in the experimental paradigm are shown in Table 6.5. There it can be seen that children with ASD showed significantly less attention to the CDS than did children with TD. This finding reinforces earlier obser-

TABLE 6.5
Results of ANOVA for Auditory Preference Study

	Main Effect: Diagnosis[a]	*Main Effect: Natural Speech*[a]	*Interaction: Diagnosis × Natural Speech*[a]
Natural Speech/ Rotated Speech	F[1, 39] = 5.2; p = .028	F[1,39] = 22.9; p = .0001	F[1, 39] = 6.3; p = .017

[a]Significant at $p < .05$.

vations, such as Klin's (1992), that child-directed speech is less preferred by children with ASD than it is by agemates, and extends this finding to an earlier developmental level, at a point in development at which auditory attention to child-directed speech is thought to be highly facilitative of language development (Snow, 1999). Children with ASD not only listened less to both CDS and rotated speech stimuli, however. They also showed a less pronounced preference for the CDS, as indicated by a significant Diagnosis × CDS interaction effect. Nonetheless, it is important to note that there was a preference for natural CDS in the ASD group; it was simply weaker than the TD preference. This finding suggests that orienting functions that normally direct attention to relevant stimuli in the environment may be less consistent for toddlers with ASD.

These observations may help to explain the patterns seen in our data, in which toddlers with ASD consistently score more poorly on receptive than expressive testing, but this gap declines over time, so that by preschool age, receptive and expressive skills are comparable. If there is a reduced preference for CDS during the second year, when it probably serves its most important language-teaching function, we would expect to see slower development in receptive skills. However, because the preference was present, although inconsistent, it would not be surprising if those early receptive skills were acquired in time, although on a slowed schedule. Still, this inconsistent orienting preference would result in toddlers with ASD spending less time listening to child-directed speech in their environment, and could result in reduced input to language learning mechanisms within the developing brain at critical time periods. These mechanisms, then, would have more impoverished data on which to operate in their biologically timed processes. Even when adequate input is acquired, and basic lexical comprehension developing, certain crucial sensitive periods may be missed, leading to cascading effects in subsequent developmental trajectories.

Lexical and Phonological Development

A second set of dissociations can be seen in the patterns of lexical and phonological development in our cohort. In typical development, words and sounds are closely connected in acquisition (Stoel-Gammon, 1998). Children with large repertoires of consonants tend to have large expressive vocabularies, and vice versa. We investigated the phonological production of the toddlers in this cohort to examine the relationships between their production of sounds and words in order to determine whether this typical connection is maintained in ASD. We have already discussed the fact that speech sound production in our cohort tended to be a relative strength, in terms of scores on the CSBS. However, lexical development, as measured by the CDI does not reflect this strength. Speaking toddlers with ASD scored within the normal range for speech sound production on the CSBS, but at the 8th percentile on the CDI Expressive Vocabulary measure (Fenson et al., 2003); nonspeaking toddlers scored just over one standard deviation below the mean for production of speech sounds (at the 10–15th percentile) but at the first percentile for lexical development (Fenson et al., 1993). Clearly, the speech sound capacities of these children are not being placed in the service of lexical production.

Table 6.6 presents the percentage of subjects using each consonant in English at least once during their CSBS communication sample. There it can be seen that there is nothing atypical about the order of acquisition of consonants in this cohort. Consonants typically seen early in development (Shriberg, 1993) are used by most children in the cohort (this table combines speakers and nonspeakers; consonants were inventoried regardless of their

TABLE 6.6
Consonants Produced by Toddlers with ASD

High-Frequency Consonants	*Percentage of Subjects Who Produced Consonant at least Once*
m	83
k/g	80
t/d	80
p/b	77
h	67
w	70
/j/	57
Low-Frequency Consonants	*Percentage of Subjects Who Produced Consonant at Least Once*
s/z	40
h	36
f/v	27
l	13
ʃ	7
θ/ð	3
tʃ	3
ʤ	3
ɳ, ʒ , r	0

TABLE 6.7
Phonological Behaviors or Toddlers With ASD, Compared to TD and SELD Agemates

	Toddlers With ASD	*Toddlers With TD (Carson, Klee, Carson, & Hime, 2003; Paul & Jennings, 1992)*	*Toddlers With SELD (Carson et al., 2003; Paul & Jennings, 1992; Thal, Oroz, & McCaw, 1995)*
Percentage of utterances containing consonants			
Speaking Ss	75	70	64
Nonspeaking Ss	58		34
Number of consonants in inventory	6.6 (3.0)	17.9 (2.4)	9.9 (5)
Percent of utterances containing a closed syllable (VC, CVC)	16 (15)	63 (97.6)	41 (16.1)

production in words or preverbal babble); consonants typically seen late in development are used by few. Table 6.7 presents data comparing phonological skills of our cohort of toddlers with ASD to those reported in the literature for children with typical language and those with slow expressive language development (SELD; defined as nonverbal skills in the average range and an expressive vocabulary size of less than 10 words at 18–23 months or less than 50 words at 24–36 months; Paul & Jennings, 1992; Rescorla, 1989).

This comparison shows, first, that our toddlers with ASD produced more syllables with consonants than their SELD peers. Speaking toddlers with ASD show similar rates of consonant production to those with TD; nonspeakers show rates similar to SELDs who speak and higher rates than nonspeaking SELD peers. Yet they produce significantly fewer consonant types than SELD peers ($t = 2.36$; $p < .02$). These observations suggest that toddlers with ASD are producing high levels of "favorite sounds," saying the same consonants over and over, with less consonant variety than either peers with TD or SELD. Moreover, the percentage of utterances containing a closed syllable was significantly lower for toddlers with ASD than for those with SELD ($t = 4.1$, $p < .01$), suggesting that consonants were not being incorporated into word-like syllable shapes. These data corroborate our observation based on the CSBS and CDI comparisons; that is, toddlers with

ASD would appear to be producing large numbers of "favorite sounds," but not to be marshaling these consonants in the service of producing words and word-like syllable shapes. This failure to "hook up" speech skills to the lexical system represents another area of dissociation between strands of communicative development in this population.

This failure to connect sound with meaning may be related to the high rates of echolalia seen in this population. Although these children often master the motoric aspects of speech, they may have acquired few meaningful purposes to which their speech can be put. Echoing what others say may serve as a compensatory mechanism, allowing the child to utilize speech skills in an interactive way, without having mastered the content of their forms. With increasing practice in the interactive opportunities provided by children's willingness to echo, the meaning of their productions may become increasingly clear. Like other children, those with ASD reduce their rate of echoing as they gradually attach meanings to the forms they can produce. But, too, changes in the timing of developmental events, as well as the compensatory mechanisms involved in using echoing as a form of communication, can have significant consequences for subsequent aspects of language development.

Dissociations in Development: Summary

To recap this discussion, then, young children with ASD show dissociations among aspects of communication that are usually linked in typical children. These include better performance on measures of naming than on responding appropriately to names for objects, and a lag in using the consonant sounds in their repertoire to produce word approximations. Each of these dissociations independently and in the aggregate can lead the child's development to diverge significantly from the normal path.

It would appear then that in ASD, as in other syndromes we've reviewed, dissociations within the development of language can be seen, and these dissociations both are affected by the basic deficits that characterize the syndrome and affect subsequent development. These dissociations are observed in other areas of development in children on the autism spectrum and are commonly evident during psychological testing (Burack, Iarocci, Flanagan, & Bowler, 2004; Burack & Volkmar, 1992; Klin, Saulnier, Tsatsanis, & Volkmar, 2005). In ASD, basic failures to orient to social signals such as voice, as evidenced by our listening preference data, are accompanied by other failures of social orientation, such as a reduced preference for faces over other visual stimuli (Klin, Jones, Schultz, Volkmar, & Cohen, 2002). Failure to integrate phonological skills in the service of lexical acquisition must also be seen in the context of reduced frequency of making joint reference (e.g., Mundy & Burnette, 2005), which provides the children with limited opportunities to link objects of shared interest with labels provided by adults with whom they interact. In typical development, for example, a baby may say /ba/ without intending a referent, but parents immediately direct their attention and share notice of an object to which that sound could apply ("Oh, you want the *ball!* Here it is. Here's the red *ball* for you!"). A little later in development, the child uses joint reference to direct attention to objects of interest, and parents happily share focus on the object and eagerly supply its name. If the child fails to engage in these joint attention activities, the myriad opportunities for linking names to things that occur in normal development will be vastly reduced, even as speech sound development proceeds on its neuromotoric schedule.

Thus, the language development of children with ASD seems to share with that of other disorders a general pattern of dissociations among the development of usually integrated communicative capacities. The particular deficits central to the syndrome, however—including reduced levels of orientation to visual and auditory social stimuli, and a reduced tendency to establish joint attention that may lead to limited opportunities to acquire referents to attach to emerging speech productions—would appear to result in the particular pattern of dissociations that characterizes language development in this syndrome. These observations suggest that perhaps whatever is necessary for language development is not specifically impaired in autism; rather, it is the impulse to share internal states, such as attention, and the dearth of contexts for learning created by failures of social orientation, including reduced preference for speech and faces, as well as reduced predilection for joint attention, that result in the delays seen in language acquisition in this population. For children with strong cognitive skills, compensatory mechanisms, such as echolalia, may be recruited to acquire language. For those with less cognitive power to bypass the obstacles inherent in their condition, language acquisition may be extremely protracted and may require intensive intervention. In either case, what seems clear is that the normal cascade of events that occurs in early development to enable language acquisition through the linkage of social, emotional, cognitive, and linguistic development is significantly perturbed by the deficits that characterize ASD. Understanding this process can cause us to consider how the particular dissociations seen in ASD might influence our thinking about its treatment.

CLINICAL IMPLICATIONS FOR ASD

Just as fine-grained analysis of the various strands of development leads to a more complex picture of development than merely looking for "delays," understanding this fine-grained picture of development leads us to consider in detail how best to ameliorate communication in this syndromes. In ASD, we see that basic failures in social orientation to both faces and voices can have an effect on the child's ability to take in the stimuli with which he is presented. This suggests that simply giving a child more of these normal inputs may not be adequate. For example, child-centered models of intervention, in which the adult follows the child's lead and provides CDS input to accompany the child's actions, may be less effective in this syndrome than it is in others, because in autism CDS appears to be less compelling during the language learning period than it is for typical children. Secondary reinforcers that reward the child for attending to inputs like CDS, which might not be intrinsically attractive, may be necessary. Similarly, knowing that children with ASD can, in general, produce the sounds of speech and that their delayed acquisition of words cannot, in most cases, be traced to speech sound deficits argues for more energy spent on helping children to move beyond "favorite sounds" in vocal play and on beginning direct training of the use of sounds in more word-like shapes and for more communicative functions. These activities might include providing rewards for vocal imitation. Several operant programs, such as that of Tsiouri and Greer (2003), have shown success in eliciting vocal and verbal production. A program adapting these methods in light of our findings on phonological development in ASD might first attempt to expand consonant production beyond the child's current repertoire, and eventually move toward rewarding closed over open syllables. At the same time, providing both operant and prompt-free (Mirenda & Santogrossi, 1985) activities in which the child's vocalizations were first treated "as if" they were words, linked to referents in the environment, tangibly rewarded, and ultimately shaped into more conventional production may help make the link between the child's existing phonological skills and lexical acquisition that the child is failing to make on his own.

Thus the implication of this discussion may be that we do need to learn in more detail where the dissociations in development occur for children with ASD (as well as for other children with communication impairments) and understand how these impact their ability to take advantage of input and instruction. Children with ASD are not only slower to learn to communicate but have fractionations in their development that not only retard its progress but reduce their access to important experiences that, in themselves, foster development and integration, and understanding this will have important implications for intervention programs. Research on this population that is aimed at identifying these unique disconnects and testing ways to link them up will be necessary to maximize the potential of these children for communication and interaction.

ACKNOWLEDGMENTS

Preparation of this chapter was supported by Research Grant P01-03008 funded by the National Institute of Mental Health (NIMH); by the STAART

Center grant U54 MH66494 funded by the National Institute on Deafness and Communication Disorders (NIDCD), the National Institute of Environmental Health Sciences (NIEHS), the National Institute of Child Health and Human Development (NICHD), and the National Institute of Neurological Disorders and Stroke (NINDS); by Research Grant RO1 DC07129 from the NIDCD; by a MidCareer Development grant to Dr. Paul, K24 HD045576 funded by NIDCD; as well as by the National Alliance for Autism Research. We also express our appreciation to Helen Tager-Flusberg and Catherine Lord for their contributions to this chapter.

REFERENCES

American Psychiatric Association. (1994). *Diagnostic and statistical manual of mental disorders* (4th ed.). Washington, DC: Author.

Beitchman, J. H., Hood, J., Rochon, J., Peterson, M., Mantini, T., & Majumdar, S. (1989). Empirical classification of speech/language impairment in children. I. Identification of speech/language categories. *Journal of the American Academy of Child and Adolescent Psychiatry, 28,* 112–117.

Bloom, L. (1997). Language acquisition in its developmental context. In W. Damon (Series Ed.) & D. Kuhn & R. Siegler (Vol. Eds.), *Handbook of child psychology: Vol. 2. Cognition, perception, and language* (pp. 119–132). New York: Wiley.

Boucher, J. (1988). Word fluency in high-functioning autistic children. *Journal of Autism and Developmental Disorders, 18,* 637–645.

Bruinsma, Y., Koegel, R., & Koegel, L. (2004). Joint attention and children with autism: A review of the literature. *Mental Retardation and Developmental Disabilities Research Reviews, 10,* 169–175.

Burack, J. A., Iarocci, G., Flanagan, T. D., & Bowler, D. M. (2004). On mosaics and melting pots: Conceptual considerations of comparison and matching strategies. *Journal of Autism and Developmental Disorders, 34*(1), 65–73.

Burack, J. A., & Volkmar, F. R. (1992). Development of low- and high-functioning autistic children. *Journal of Child Psychology & Psychiatry & Allied Disciplines, 33*(3), 607–616.

Cantwell, D. P., Baker, L., & Mattison, R. E. (1980). Psychiatric disorders in children with speech and language retardation. *Archives of General Psychiatry, 37,* 423–426.

Carr, E., Shriebman, L., & Lovaas, O. L. (1975). Control of echolalic speech in psychotic children. *Journal of Abnormal Child Psychology, 3,* 331–351.

Carson, C., Klee, T., Carson, D., & Hime, L. (2003). Phonological profiles of 2-year-olds with delayed language development: Predicting clinical outcomes at age 3. *American Journal of Speech-Language Pathology, 12,* 28–39.

Carter, A., Volkmar, F., Sparrow, S., Wang, J., Lord, C., Dawson, G., et al. (1998). The Vineland Adaptive Behavior Scales: Supplementary norms for individuals with autism. *Journal of Autism and Developmental Disorders, 28,* 287–302.

Chapman, R. (1974). Discussion summary: Developmental relationship between receptive and expressive language. In R. Schiefelbusch & L. Lloyd (Eds.), *Language perspectives: Acquisition, retardation, and intervention* (pp. 308–237). Baltimore: University Park Press.

Chapman, R. (1978). Comprehension strategies in children. In J. Kavanagh & W. Strange (Eds.), *Speech and language in the laboratory, school, and clinic* (pp. 308–327). Cambridge, MA: MIT Press.

Chapman, R. (1992). *Child talk: Processes in language acquisition and disorder*. Chicago: Mosby-Year Book.

Chawarska, K., Klin, A., Paul, R., & Volkmar, F. (2005). *Autism spectrum disorder in the second year: Stability and change in syndrome expression*. Manuscript submitted for publication.

Chawarska, K., & Volkmar, F. (2005). Autism in infancy and early childhood. In F. Volkmar, R. Paul, A. Klin, & D. J. Cohen (Eds.), *Handbook of autism and pervasive developmental disorders* (Vol. 1, 3rd ed., pp. 223–246). New York: Wiley.

Dale, P. (1991). The validity of a parent report instrument of vocabulary and syntax at 24 months. *Journal of Speech and Hearing Research, 34,* 565–571.

Fay, W. (1969). On the basis of autistic echolalia. *Journal of Communication Disorders, 2,* 38–47.

Fay, W. (1971). On normal and autistic pronouns. *Journal of Speech and Hearing Disorders, 36,* 242–249.

Fay, W., & Schuler, A. L. (1980). *Emerging language in autistic children*. Baltimore: University Park Press.

Fenson, L., Dale, P. S., Reznick, J. S., Thal, D., Bates, E., Hartung, J. P., & Reilly, J. (2003). *MacArthur Bates Communicative Development Inventories*. Baltimore: Paul H. Brookes.

Fowler, A. (1998). Language in mental retardation: Associations with and dissociations from general cognition. In J. Burack, R. Hopapp, & E. Zigler (Eds.), *Handbook of mental retardation and development* (pp. 209–333). Cambridge: Cambridge University Press.

Gillham, J., Carter, A., Volkmar, F., & Sparrow, S. (2000). Toward a developmental operational definition of autism. *Journal of Autism and Developmental Disorders, 30,* 269–278.

Goldfarb, W., Braunstein, P., & Lorge, I. (1956). A study of speech patterns in a group of schizophrenic children. *American Journal of Orthopsychiatry, 26,* 544–555.

Hellreigel, C., Tao, L., DiLavore, P., & Lord, C. (1995, April). *The effect of context on nonverbal social behaviors of very young autistic children*. Paper presented at the biannual meetings of the Society for Research in Child Development, Indianapolis, IN.

Hoshino, Y., Kaneko, M., Yashima, Y., Kumashiro, H., Volkmar, F. R., & Cohen, D. J. (1987). Clinical features of autistic children with setback course in their infancy. *Japanese Journal of Psychiatry and Neurology, 41,* 237–245.

Jacobson, J. W., & Ackerman, L. J. (1990). Differences in adaptive development among persons with autism and mental retardation. *Journal of Autism and Developmental Disorders, 20,* 205–219.

Kanner, L. (1943). Autistic disturbances of affective contact. *Nervous Child, 2,* 217–250.

Kanner, L. (1946). Irrelevant and metaphorical language. *American Journal of Psychiatry, 103,* 242–246.

Kjelgaard, M. E., & Tager-Flusberg, H. (2001). An investigation of language impairment in autism: Implications for genetic subgroups. *Language and Cognitive Processes, 16*, 287–308.

Klin, A. (1992). Listening preference in regard to speech: A possible characterization of the symptom of social withdrawal. *Journal of Autism and Developmental Disorders, 21*, 29–42.

Klin, A., Jones, W., Schultz, R., Volkmar, F., & Cohen, D. (2002). Visual fixation patterns during viewing of naturalistic social situations as predictors of social competence in individuals with autism. *Archives of General Psychiatry, 59*, 809–816.

Klin, A., Saulnier, C., Tsatsanis, K., & Volkmar, F. R. (2005). Clinical evaluation in autism spectrum disorders: Psychological assessment within a transdisciplinary framework. In F. R. Volkmar, R. Paul, A. Klin, & D. J. Cohen (Eds.), *Handbook of autism and pervasive developmental disorders* (3rd ed., pp. 772–798). New York: Wiley.

Klin, A., & Volkmar, F. (2005). Asperger's syndrome. In F. Volkmar, R. Paul, A. Klin, & D. Cohen (Eds.), *Handbook of autism and pervasive developmental disorders* (3rd ed., pp. 94–122). New York: Wiley.

Kobayashi, R., & Murata, T. (1998). Setback phenomenon in autism and long-term prognosis. *Actuarial Psychiatry Scandanavia, 98*, 296–303.

Kurita, H. (1985). Infantile autism with speech loss before the age of 30 months. *Journal of the American Academy of Child Psychiatry, 24*, 191–196.

Landry, S. H., & Loveland, K. A. (1989). The effect of social context on the functional communication skills of autistic children. *Journal of Autism and Developmental Disorders, 19*, 283–299.

LeCouteur, A., Bailey, A., Rutter, M., & Gottesman, I. (1989, August). *Epidemiologically based twin study of autism*. Paper presented at the First World Congress on Psychiatric Genetics, Churchill College, Cambridge, England.

Liss, M., Harel, B., Fein, D., Allen, D., Dunn, M., Feinstein, C., et al. (2001). Predictors and correlates of adaptive functioning in children with developmental disorders. *Journal of Autism and Developmental Disorders, 31*, 219–230.

Locke, J. (1994). Gradual emergence of developmental language disorders. *Journal of Speech and Hearing Research, 37*, 608–616.

Lord, C. (1995). Follow-up of two year-olds referred for possible autism. *Journal of Child Psychology and Psychiatry, 36*, 1365–1382.

Lord, C., Risi, S., Lambrecht, L., Cook, E., Leventhal, B., DiLavore, P., et al. (2000). The Autism Diagnostic Observation Schedule—Generic: A standard measure of social and communication deficits associated with the spectrum of autism. *Journal of Autism and Developmental Disorders, 30*, 205–223.

Loveland, K., & Kelley, M. (1991). Development of adaptive behavior in preschoolers with autism or Down syndrome. *American Journal of Mental Retardation, 96*, 13–20.

Mermelstein, R. (1983, October). *The relationship between syntactic and pragmatic development in autistic, retarded, and normal children*. Paper presented at the Eighth Annual Boston University Conference on Language Development, Boston.

Minshew, N. J., & Goldstein, G. (1993). Is autism an amnesic disorder? Evidence from the California Verbal Learning Test. *Neuropsychology, 7*, 209–216.

Mirenda, P., & Santogrossi, J. (1985). A prompt-free strategy to teach pictorial communication system use. *Augmentative and Alternative Communication, 1*, 143–150.

Mullen, E. (1995). *Mullen Scales of Early Learning* (AGS edition). Circle Pines, MN: American Guidance Service.

Mundy, P., & Burnette, C. (2005). Joint attention and neurodevelopmental models of autism. In F. Volkmar, R. Paul, A. Klin, & D. Cohen (Eds.), *Handbook of autism and pervasive developmental disorders* (Vol. 1, 3rd ed., pp. 650–682). New York: Wiley.

Mundy, P., Sigman, M., & Kasari, C. (1994). Joint attention, developmental level, and symptom presentation in autism. *Development & Psychopathology, 6,* 389–401.

Naito, M., & Kikuo, N. (2004). Autistic children's use of semantic common sense and theory of mind: A comparison with typical and mentally retarded children. *Journal of Autism and Developmental Disorders, 34,* 507–519.

Nelson, D., Jusczyk, P., Mandel, D., & Myers, J. (1995). The head-turn preference procedure for testing auditory perception. *Infant Behavior & Development, 18,* 111–116.

Osterling, J., & Dawson, G. (1994). Early recognition of children with autism: A study of first birthday home videotapes. *Journal of Autism and Developmental Disorders, 24,* 247–258.

Paul, R. (1991). Profiles of toddlers with slow expressive language development. *Topics in Language Disorders, 11*(4), 1–14.

Paul, R., Fisher, M., & Cohen, D. (1988). Comprehension strategies in children with autism and expressive language disorders. *Journal of Autism and Developmental Disorders, 18,* 669–679.

Paul, R., & Jennings, P. (1992). Phonological behavior in normal and late talking toddlers. *Journal of Speech and Hearing Research, 35,* 99–107.

Pinker, S. (2001). Talk of genetics and vice-versa. *Nature, 413,* 465–466.

Prizant, B., & Duchan, J. (1981). The functions of immediate echolalia in autistic children. *Journal of Speech and Hearing Disorders, 46,* 241–249.

Pronovost, W., Wakstein, M., & Wakstein, D. (1966). A longitudinal study of speech behavior and language comprehension in fourteen children diagnosed as atypical or autistic. *Exceptional Children, 33,* 19–26.

Rescorla, L. (1989). The Language Development Survey: A screening tool for delayed language in toddlers. *Journal of Speech and Hearing Disorders, 54,* 587–599.

Reznick, S., Corley, R., & Robinson, J. (1999). A longitudinal twin study of intelligence in the second year. *Monographs of the Society of Research in Child Development, 62*(1), Serial No. 249.

Rice, M. (2004). Growth models of developmental language disorders. In M. Rice & F. Warren (Eds.), *Developmental language disorders: From phenotypes to etiologies* (pp. 207–240). Mahwah, NJ: Lawrence Erlbaum Associates.

Rice, M., Warren, S., & Betz, S. (2005). Language symptoms of developmental language disorders: An overview of autism, Down syndrome, fragile X, specific language impairment, and Williams syndrome. *Applied Psycholinguistics, 26,* 7–27.

Ricks, D. M., & Wing, L. (1976). Language, communication and use of symbols. In L. Wing (Ed.), *Early childhood autism* (pp. 93–134). Oxford: Pergamon.

Roberts, J., Rice, M., & Tager-Flusberg, H. (2004). Tense marking in children with autism. *Applied Psycholinguistics, 25,* 429–448.

Rodriguez, J., Morgan, S., & Gefken, G. (1991). A comparative evaluation of adaptive behavior in children and adolescents with autism, Down syndrome, and normal development. *Journal of Autism and Developmental Disorders, 21,* 187–198.

Rogers, S. J., & DiLalla, D. L. (1990). Age of symptom onset in young children with pervasive developmental disorders. *Journal of the American Academy of Child & Adolescent Psychiatry, 29*, 863–872.

Rossetti, L. (2001). *Communication intervention: Birth to three* (2nd ed.). San Diego: Singular.

Rutter, M., Mawhood, L., & Howlin, P. (1992). Language delay and social development. In P. Fletcher & D. Hall (Eds.), *Specific speech and language disorders in children: Correlates, characteristics and outcomes* (pp. 63–78). London: Whurr Publishers.

Schatz, J., & Hamdan-Allen, G. (1995). Effects of age and IQ on adaptive behavior domains for children with autism. *Journal of Autism and Developmental Disorders, 25*, 51–60.

Scott, S. K., Blank, C. C., Rosen, S., & Wise, R. J. S. (2000). Identification of a pathway for intelligible speech. *Brain: A Journal of Neurology, 123*, 2400–2406.

Shapiro, T. (1977). The quest for a linguistic model to study the speech of autistic children: Studies of echoing. *Journal of the American Academy of Child Psychiatry, 16*, 608–619.

Sheinkopf, S., Mundy, P., Oller, K., & Steffens, M. (2000). Vocal atypicalities of preverbal autistic children. *Journal of Autism and Developmental Disorders, 30*, 345–354.

Shriberg, L. D. (1993). Four new speech and prosody-voice measures for genetics research and other studies in developmental phonological disorders. *Journal of Speech and Hearing Research, 36*, 105–140.

Shriberg, L. D., & Kwiatkowski, J. (1982). Phonological disorders III: A procedure for assessing severity of involvement. *Journal of Speech and Hearing Disorders, 47*, 256–270.

Siperstein, R., & Volkmar, F. R. (2004). Brief report: Parental reporting of regression in children with pervasive developmental disorders. *Journal of Autism & Developmental Disorders, 34*(6), 731–734.

Snow, C. (1999). Social perspectives on the emergence of language. In B. MacWhinney (Ed.), *The emergence of language* (pp. 257–276). Mahwah, NJ: Lawrence Erlbaum Associates.

Sparrow, S., Balla, D., & Cicchetti, D. V. (1984). *The Vineland Adaptive Behavior Scales* (Survey Form). Circle Pines, MN: American Guidance Service.

Stoel-Gammon, C. (1998). Sounds and words in early language acquisition: The relationship between lexical and phonological development. In R. Paul (Ed.), *Exploring the speech-language connection* (pp. 23–45). Baltimore: Paul H. Brookes.

Stone, W., Ousley, O., Yoder, P., Hogan, K., & Hepburn, S. (1997). Nonverbal communication in two- and three-year-old children with autism. *Journal of Autism & Developmental Disorders, 27*, 677–696.

Tager-Flusberg, H. (1981). On the nature of linguistic functioning in early infantile autism. *Journal of Autism and Developmental Disorders, 11*, 45–56.

Tager-Flusberg, H. (1985). The conceptual basis for referential word meaning in children with autism. *Child Development, 56*, 1167–1178.

Tager-Flusberg, H. (1994). Dissociations in form and function in the acquisition of language by autistic children. In H. Tager-Flusberg (Ed.), *Constraints on language acquisition: Studies of atypical children* (pp. 175–194). Hillsdale, NJ: Lawrence Erlbaum Associates.

Tager-Flusberg, H. (2000). Language and understanding minds: Connections in autism. In S. Baron-Cohen, H. Tager-Flusberg, & D. Cohen (Eds.), *Understanding other minds: Perspectives from autism and developmental cognitive neuroscience* (2nd ed., pp. 124–150). Oxford: Oxford University Press.

Tager-Flusberg, H., Calkins, S., Noin, I., Baumberger, T., Anderson, M., & Chadwick-Denis, A. (1990). A longitudinal study of language acquisition in autistic and Down syndrome children. *Journal of Autism and Developmental Disorders, 20,* 1–22.

Tager-Flusberg, H., & Joseph, R. M. (2003). Identifying neurocognitive phenotypes in autism. *Philosophical Transactions of the Royal Society, Series B, 358,* 303–314.

Tager-Flusberg, H., Paul, R., & Lord, C. (2005). Language and communication in autism. In F. Volkmar, R. Paul, A. Klin, & D. J. Cohen (Eds.), *Handbook of autism and pervasive developmental disorders* (Vol. 1, pp. 335–364). New York: Wiley.

Thal, D. (1991). Language and cognition in normal and late-talking toddlers. *Topics in Language Disorders, 11*(4), 33–42.

Thal, D. J., Oroz, M., & McCaw, V. (1995). Phonological and lexical development in normal and late-talking toddlers. *Applied Psycholinguistics, 16,* 407–424.

Thomas, M., & Karmiloff-Smith, A. (2005). Can developmental disorders reveal the component parts of the human language faculty? *Language Learning and Development, 1,* 65–92.

Tsiouri, I., & Greer, R. D. (2003). Inducing vocal verbal behavior in children with severe language delays through rapid motor imitation responding. *Journal of Behavioral Education, 12,* 185–206.

Tuchman, R. F., & Rapin, I. (1997). Regression in pervasive developmental disorders: Seizures and epileptiform electroencephalogram correlates. *Pediatrics, 99,* 560–566.

Volkmar, F., Chawarska, K., & Klin, A. (2005). Autism in infancy and early childhood. *Annual Review of Psychology, 56,* 315–336.

Wetherby, A. (1986). Ontogeny of communication functions in autism. *Journal of Autism and Developmental Disorders, 16,* 295–316.

Wetherby, A., & Prizant, B. (2003). *Communication and Symbolic Behavior Scales-Developmental Profile.* Baltimore: Paul H. Brookes.

Wetherby, A., & Prutting, C. A. (1984). Profiles of communicative and cognitive-social abilities in autistic children. *Journal of Speech and Hearing Research, 27,* 364–377.

Wetherby, A., Woods, J., Allen, L., Cleary, J., Dickinson, H., & Lord, C. (2004). Early indicators of autism spectrum disorders in the second year of life. *Journal of Autism & Developmental Disorders, 34,* 473–493.

Yule, W., & Rutter, M. (1987). *Language development and disorders.* London: MacKeith.

7

Language Learning and Use as Embedded Social Activities: Evidence From Autism and Fragile X Syndrome

Leonard Abbeduto
Andrea McDuffie
Waisman Center, University of Wisconsin–Madison

Nativist theories of language development (e.g., Chomsky, 1965; Fodor, 1983; Pinker, 1996) invariably include claims about the modularity of language. In these theories, language is conceptualized as a system of abstract, context-free rules, with different types of rules or rules governing different types of content comprising different "components" of language. Moreover, the rules within any one component are thought to be acquired and used with minimal input from other components, other modules of the mind, and, most definitely, domain-general learning mechanisms (Chomsky, 1975). Put more generally, there is something "special" about language that reflects its unique character and the unique character of the processes by which it is learned and used. And finally, this uniqueness is biologically based, arising from the innately given organization and structure of the human mind (Chomsky, 1988).

The nativist approach has been challenged on many grounds, and several alternative theoretical formulations have been proposed (for reviews, see Abbeduto & Chapman, 2005; Abbeduto, Evans, & Dolan, 2001). The Child Talk model proposed by Chapman and her colleagues (Chapman et al., 1992) embodies many of the themes of these alternative accounts. Chapman et al. argue that the nativist approach incorrectly characterizes the fundamental nature of the language learning process by assuming that its purpose is the mastery of a set of abstract, context-free rules. Instead, Chapman and her colleagues propose that children are acquiring knowledge about how to participate in the real-world social contexts and activities that populate their lives. Thus, the knowledge they acquire is procedural in nature and intrinsically tied to the social contexts and activities in which it is learned and used. Moreover, there is nothing special about language—at least not in the nativist sense; instead, language is thought to be only one of many cultural practices that must be learned in order to participate in the recurring social activities of one's life. In other words, children are learning how to do things in particular social contexts, and some of those things are verbal performances of one sort another.

The conceptualization of language learning that the Child Talk model embodies has proven very useful for investigating the language learning problems of children with neurodevelopmental disorders. In particular, the Child Talk model leads to the following predictions, among others:

1. Because the process of language learning depends heavily on the child's use of social-contextual information, differences in language learning and use across contexts should occur.
2. Because the process does not depend on language-specific mechanisms, it can be influenced by numerous dimensions of the child's behavioral phenotype, including auditory memory skills, attentional capabilities, knowledge of the social and physical worlds, and the presence of various forms of psychopathology (e.g., anxiety). Impairments or psychopathologies in the social realm should be especially deleterious in light of the need to process social-contextual information.

In this chapter, we briefly describe our own programs of research, each of which is focused on the language development of a particular neurodevelopmental disorder, namely, autism (McDuffie) and fragile X syndrome (Abbeduto). We highlight those results that address the predictions of the Child Talk model.

AUTISM

Autism is a neurodevelopmental disorder, probably present from birth, that is identified on the basis of a triad of behavioral characteristics (Lord & Bailey, 2002), including impairments in communication and social reciprocity and the presence of unusually repetitive or stereotyped behaviors and interests (APA, 1994). Autism and other pervasive developmental disorders represent a continuum of impairments. Children and adults with autism spectrum disorders can exhibit any combination of characteristic behaviors in any degree of severity. Recent epidemiological studies have reported overall prevalence rates for autism and pervasive developmental disorders of 20 cases per 10,000 (National Research Council, 2001). The recent increase in prevalence of autism from rates historically reported can be most likely attributed to more standardized diagnostic practices, greater public awareness, and a more inclusive definition of disorders on the autism spectrum (Volkmar, Lord, Bailey, Schultz, & Klin, 2004).

Behavioral Phenotype of Autism

The social and communicative impairments of very young children with autism are likely to manifest as an absence of typical behaviors rather than as the presence of unusual behaviors (Stone, 1997). During the preschool years, impairments that distinguish children with autism from children with other developmental delays include deficits in social communicative skills, such as directing attention and responsiveness to another's voice (Lord, 1995), looking at faces and showing objects (Osterling & Dawson, 1994; Stone, Ousley, Yoder, Hogan, & Hepburn, 1997), gaze monitoring (Charman, Baron-Cohen, Swettenham, Baird, Cox, & Drew, 2000), pretend play (Baird et al., 2000), and motor imitation (Rogers, Hepburn, Stackhouse, & Wehner, 2003; Stone, Ousley, & Littleford, 1997). Recently, it has been suggested that delays in the emergence of joint attention skills represent a pivotal or core deficit in the behavioral phenotype of children with autism spectrum disorders (Charman, 2003). Joint attention behaviors allow children to coordinate attention between a social partner and an object or event in the environment (Bakeman & Adamson, 1984). Because the acquisition of conventional behaviors, especially language, relies on the young child's ability to participate in such triadic interactions, it is likely that deficits in joint attention skills will have cumulative and adverse implications for subsequent development.

Language Development in Children with Autism

Most children with autism spectrum disorders have delays in language development relative to their nonverbal mental ages (Stevens et al., 2000;

Tager-Flusberg, 1988; Tager-Flusberg & Sullivan, 1998), and approximately half of young children with autism fail to acquire speech as their primary mode of communication (Prizant, 1996). It is not yet known why some children with autism learn to talk and others do not; however, research has shown that early language ability is positively related to long-term outcomes for children with autism (Gillberg, 1991; Howlin, Mahood, & Rutter, 2000; Liss et al., 2001) and that measures of verbal skills are the strongest longitudinal predictors of social adaptive functioning (Venter, Lord, & Schopler, 1992). Given the predictive relationship between early vocabulary and later use of multiword utterances in typically developing populations (Bates, Bretherton, & Snyder, 1988; Bates, Dale, & Thal, 1995; Bates & Goodman, 1999, 2001; Fenson et al., 1994), understanding the process of early word learning by children with autism is a first step toward the goal of increasing the proportion of these children who develop functional language skills.

Word Learning and Fast Mapping

Learning the conventional meanings of words provides an excellent example of how the ability to access both social cues from conversational partners and contextual cues from the environment are necessary for language learning, as predicted by the Child Talk model. The rapid, associative process by which label and object are paired to establish the earliest representation of a word in the child's lexicon was termed "fast mapping" in a classic study by Carey and Bartlett (1978). Many subsequent studies have employed this theoretical construct as an explanation for how typically developing children acquire new vocabulary words (Akhtar & Tomasello, 1996; Baldwin, 1991, 1993a, 1993b; Baldwin & Markman, 1996; Woodward, Markman, & Fitzsimmons, 1994).

The general paradigm for these kinds of word learning studies has been to provide exposure to a novel word–referent pairing in either an ostensive or nonostensive training context and then to assess whether the novel word has been learned. Common to these studies is the examination of how children respond to the speaker's attentional focus within a referential context. None of these studies, however, has actually demonstrated an empirical association between attention following, fast-mapping ability, and the number of words that children understand and produce.

Typically developing children, as a group, are likely to display high levels of responsiveness to adult social cues when learning new words. Thus, studies with typically developing participants have focused on measuring the outcome of the fast-mapping process (i.e., whether or not the novel word is learned) or determining the age at which fast mapping occurs under conditions in which fast mapping requires responsiveness to social and contextual cues. These studies, therefore, have not attempted to quantify attention following as a correlate or predictor of fast mapping. However, children with autism, especially those with mental ages under 20 months, have a core deficit in responding to the attentional directives of conversational partners (Leekam, Hunnisett, & Moore, 1998; Mundy, Sigman, & Kasari, 1994a). In fact, a deficit in attention following is one of the primary indicators for the early diagnosis of autism spectrum disorder (Baird et al., 2000; Baron-Cohen et al., 1996). The ability to follow adult nonverbal cues to objects or events in the environment should relate to the efficiency with which children with autism map verbal labels to appropriate referents (Baldwin, 1991, 1993a, 1993b).

Only one study in the literature has examined fast mapping in children with autism (Baron-Cohen, Baldwin, & Crowson, 1997). This study is suggestive of the way that fast mapping and the ability to access adult social cues within a referential context dissociate in this group of children. Baron-Cohen and colleagues used a modified version of the Baldwin (1993a) paradigm and demonstrated that children with autism made mapping errors because they incorrectly used their own direction of gaze as a strategy for making word–object associations, rather than following the speaker's gaze direction. In fact, only 29% of the participants with autism in the Baron-Cohen et al. study were able to correctly map verbal labels to object referents when the speaker's direction of gaze was discrepant from their own. In two language-matched comparison groups, over 70% of participants with developmental delay and almost 80% of typically developing toddlers were able to correctly complete the experimental task. When the speaker's direction of gaze coincided with their own, children with autism were able to make word–object associations as often as language-matched controls. It is important to note that children with autism did not *fail* to make word–object mappings in the discrepant labeling condition. They simply selected the toy that was their own focus of attention as the referent, rather than the toy indicated by the experimenter's attentional focus. Thus, we have evidence that the fast-mapping process is intact for school-aged children with autism, but that the ability to make appropriate mappings is impaired, presumably due to a deficit in attention following.

Fast Mapping in 2-Year-Olds With Autism

Participants with autism in the Baron-Cohen et al. (1997) study were between 7 and 12 years of age (mean CA = 9 years, 2 months). The goal of the research I (McDuffie) recently completed, in collaboration with Paul Yoder and Wendy Stone, was to replicate and extend the findings of Baron-Cohen et al. (1997) by investigating whether younger children with autism, at the earliest stages of word learning, also demonstrated the ability to form a rapid association between a verbal label and an object referent. We predicted that if a positive relationship between attention following and either vocabulary comprehension or production was demonstrated, it would be mediated by the ability to learn a rapid word–object mapping.

Measuring Attention Following in Young Children With Autism. Deficits in attention following are most evident in children with autism at the youngest developmental ages (Leekam et al., 1998; Mundy et al., 1994). Many studies of attention following employ a frequency metric or report the percentage of trials administered to which the child accurately responds to a single adult attention-directing cue to a distal target. The challenge of measuring attention following in a developmentally young group of children with autism, however, is the likelihood that many would score a zero, thereby reducing the utility of the attention-following measure. We reasoned that measuring attention-following under more scaffolded conditions might be necessary to obtain sufficient variability in performance to test the associations of interest. This measure differed from most commonly used measures of attention following because proximal rather than distal adult cues were used and child attention was continually redirected to the target and continuously measured.

Demonstrating a Mediating Relationship. Demonstrating that fast mapping mediated the relationship between attention following and vocabulary outcomes required that four conditions be met (Baron & Kenny, 1986; Holmbeck, 1997, as cited in Hoff, 2003): (a) The predictor variable must be significantly associated with the outcome (e.g., attention following must be predictively related to comprehension or production); (b) the predictor variable must be significantly associated with the hypothesized mediator (e.g., attention following must be predictively related to fast mapping); (c) the hypothesized mediator must be significantly associated with the outcome (e.g., fast mapping must be concurrently related to either comprehension or production); and (d) the strength of the relation between the predictor and the outcome must be reduced by removing the variance attributable to the mediator (e.g., the relationship between attention following and either comprehension or production must be rendered nonsignificant when variance attributable to fast mapping is included in the analysis).

Study Design, Participants, and Method. Our study (McDuffie, 2004) used a concurrent and longitudinal correlational design. Attention following was measured at the initial visit and fast mapping was measured at the follow-up 6 months later. In addition, comprehension and production of object nouns were measured at the follow-up with a standardized parent-report instrument (CDI; Fenson et al., 1994). Participants were 29 children diagnosed with autism spectrum disorders. At the initial visit, 83% of the participants were under 36 months of age and mean chronological age was 32 months. All children had a clinical diagnosis of autism or pervasive developmental disorder—not otherwise specified (PDD-NOS), based on *DSM–IV–TR* criteria (APA, 2000).

During the attention-following procedure, eight colorful, novel objects were individually presented to the participants. For each trial, the examiner attempted to get the child's attention and excitedly presented the novel object to the child. The examiner used proximal gestures, head turns, gaze shifts, and movement of the object to scaffold and redirect child attention, encouraging the child to manipulate and explore each object. After continuing attempts to redirect the child's attention to the object for approximately 30 s, the object was removed and the next object was presented.

For each pair of objects, presentation of one object was accompanied by 10 repetitions of a nonsense label embedded in child-directed, connected speech and presented in sentence-final position ("Look! I have a modi! You can see my modi! I like how you are playing with my modi! Wow, it's a great modi!"). Presentation of the other object was accompanied by child-directed, connected speech without labeling ("Look! See what I have? It's mine! And you can play too! You're looking at my favorite!"). The metric for attention following was a duration variable, the *average proportion of child visual attention* to each object.

The attention-following procedure was repeated at the follow-up visit and a test of novel word learning followed the presentation of each pair of objects (i.e., one labeled, one not labeled). During testing, the examiner told the child that they were going to play a game ("Guess what? We're going to find the modi! Ready?"). The examiner slowly and simultaneously presented both objects to the child while encouraging child to look at the previously labeled object ("Here comes the modi! Look at the modi! Where's the modi?"). The examiner did not allow the child to grasp either object until the child had clearly looked toward the labeled object, even if this object was not the first one toward which the child looked. The metric for fast mapping was the *average latency until first look at the labeled object* during each testing trial.

Results and Conclusions. Our results indicated that fast mapping at follow-up met all the criteria for mediating the relationship between attention following at Time 1 and both comprehension and production of object noun vocabulary at Time 2. By meeting the empirical criteria for detecting a mediated relationship, the study provided empirical support for the hypothesis that attention following facilitates vocabulary by enabling accurate fast mapping. Given continuous and proximal attention-directing cues, young children with autism were able to follow into the adult focus of attention. Children who did so most proficiently mapped nonsense words most accurately 6 months later. Finally, children who mapped most effectively had the largest concurrent comprehension and production vocabularies for object nouns. As theorized for typically developing children, these data support the notion that children with autism can use both attention following and fast mapping to add new words to their lexicon.

One of the secondary goals in this research was to determine whether our measure of fast mapping was related to measures of constructs with which fast mapping could be expected to covary. By demonstrating that *latency of first look to the target object* was predictively related to attention following at Time 1 and concurrently related to vocabulary size at Time 2, the results support the construct validity of this new measure of fast mapping (Cronbach & Meehl, 1955). Attention following and vocabulary are two constructs with which a metric of fast mapping would be expected to covary. Replication of the current study's findings would strengthen the basis for generalizing these results to other samples of children with autism.

In any event, the results support the predictions of the Child Talk model: Learning words depends on the ability to attend to social and contextual cues. More generally, the results reinforce the notion that understanding language learning problems requires understanding the nonlinguistic strengths and weakness that comprise the full phenotype of the disorder in question.

FRAGILE X SYNDROME

Fragile X syndrome is the leading inherited cause of mental retardation (Hagerman, 1999). It is the result of a mutation in a single gene (FMR1) located on the X chromosome at Xq27.3 (Brown, 2002). In the full mutation, there are more than 200 repetitions of a trinucleotide (i.e., CGG) sequence, compared to the 54 or fewer repeats found in the normal allele (Oostra, 1996). The expansion of the sequence leads to methylation, or a silencing of the gene, so that its protein (FMRP) is not produced (Oostra & Willemsen, 2003). FMRP is involved in experience-dependent maturation and functioning of neural synapses, ensuring that neural activation is organized and appropriately constrained (Greenough et al., 2001). As expected for an X-linked disorder, fragile X syndrome differentially affects the sexes. Thus, the prevalence of affected individuals is 1 in 4,000 males and 1 in 8,000 females (Crawford, Acuna, & Sherman, 2001). Males with the full mutation typically meet diagnostic criteria for mental retardation (Hagerman, 1999). Only about half of females with the full mutation have IQs in the range of mental retardation; the remainder have learning disabilities and/or social-affective challenges (Keysor & Mazzocco 2002).

Behavioral Phenotype of Fragile X Syndrome

There are several features of the behavioral phenotype of fragile X syndrome that according to the Child Talk model would be expected to negatively affect language learning and use and distinguish it from other neurodevelopmental disorders (Belser & Sudhalter, 1995; Cohen, 1995; Cornish, Sudhalter, & Turk, 2004; Murphy & Abbeduto, 2003). Although many cognitive skills are delayed in their development in fragile X syndrome, some that are especially important for language are exceptionally delayed (Mirrett, Roberts, & Price, 2003), including those involved in the processing of sequential information (Burack et al., 1999; Dykens, Hodapp, & Leckman, 1987), auditory short-term memory (Freund & Reiss, 1991), and the directing and sustaining of attention (Bregman, Leckman, & Ort, 1988; Dykens et al., 1987; Mazzocco, Pennington, & Hagerman, 1993). In contrast, there are cognitive skills that appear to be relatively strong, including the ability to process simultaneous information (Dykens et al., 1989), long-term memory ability (Freund & Reiss, 1991), and the ability to distinguish between the self's representations of the world and those of other people (Garner, Callias, & Turk, 1999). This profile of impairments differs from those of many other neurodevelopmental disorders (Dykens, Hodapp, & Finucane, 2000); for example, individuals with Down syndrome have greater challenges in auditory than visual short-term memory and in social cognition compared to mental age expectations, but no special challenge in sequential processing (Abbeduto, Pavetto, Kesin, Weissman, Karadottir, O'Brien, & Cawthon, 2001; Marcell & Weeks, 1988; Seung & Chapman, 2000; Zelazo, Burack, Benedetto, & Frye, 1996).

Fragile X syndrome is also characterized by high rates of psychopathology. The psychopathology includes hyperarousal (Wisbeck et al., 2000), hyperactivity (Baumgardner et al., 1995; Bregman et al., 1988; Dykens et al. 1989; Mazzocco et al., 1993), and social anxiety (Bregman, Leckman, & Ort, 1988; Mazzocco, Baumgardner, Freund, & Reiss, 1998). Autistic-like behaviors are also frequent in fragile X syndrome (Feinstein & Reiss, 2001), and are sufficient to warrant a comorbid diagnosis of autism in between 10% and 40% of affected individuals (Demark, Feldman, & Holden, 2003), although there is controversy as to whether the mechanisms underlying the symptoms of autism are different in individuals with and without fragile X syndrome (Bailey et al., 2004). In any event, the behaviors associated with these psychopathologies can lead the individual with fragile X syndrome to avoid or have difficulties with participation in social interaction and thus in language (Cornish et al., 2004; Murphy & Abbeduto,

2003). Similarly high rates of psychopathology are not seen in many other neurodevelopmental disorders (Dykens et al., 2000); for example, individuals with Down syndrome, as a group are quite sociable (Kasari, Mundy, Yirmiya, & Sigman, 1990; Kasari, Freeman, Mundy, & Sigman, 1995), although they may bring quite limited social-cognitive skills to their interactions with others (Abbeduto, Pavetto, Kesin, Weissman, Karadottir, O'Brien, & Cawthon, 2001).

Language Development in Fragile X Syndrome

In our research on language learning and use by individuals with fragile X syndrome, we have uncovered numerous examples of contextual influences on language and of predictive relationships between various nonlinguistic dimensions of the behavioral phenotype and language development. In the remainder of this section, we briefly describe these findings.

Contextual Influences on Language. It is well-documented that the nature of the interaction in which talk is embedded can have an effect on many dimensions of the talk produced by typically developing children (Dollaghan, Campbell, & Tomlin, 1990; Evans & Craig, 1992). We (Abbeduto et al., 2002) have found similar contextual influences on talk for samples of school-age children and adolescents with mental retardation that were heterogeneous with respect to etiology (Abbeduto, Benson, Short, & Dolish, 1995). In examining this issue for individuals with fragile X syndrome, we collected samples of talk from adolescents and young adults ($n = 18$) in two contexts: conversation with an adult examiner, and narration of a wordless picture book to an adult examiner. In each context, the adult followed a predetermined script for introducing and responding to talk to ensure standardization of materials and examiner behavior across individuals within each context (see Abbeduto et al., 1995, for a description of the procedures). Such standardization is necessary for interpreting differences in talk among individuals or between different groups of individuals.

The talk produced in each context was transcribed and segmented into C-units, which is a standard unit of analysis in analyzing the talk of older children (Abbeduto et al., 1995). A C-unit is defined as an independent clause and any modifiers, with the latter including words, phrases, and even dependent clauses (Loban, 1976). Several measures were computed to characterize the nature of the talk in the samples, including five measures that are relevant here: (a) the number of C-units attempted per minute; (b) the percentage of C-units that were fully intelligible (i.e., understandable) to the transcriber; (c) the percentage of C-units containing a maze (i.e., *um, er,* and other dysfluencies, or repetitions of all or part of a word); (d) the number of different word roots produced in a 50-C-unit sample; and (e) the mean length of C-units in morphemes. These measures provided a characterization of the participants' talkativeness, articulation, utterance planning, vocabulary, and syntax, respectively. Comparisons were made with age- and IQ-matched adolescents and young adults with Down syndrome.

Contextual influences were observed for four variables: C-units attempted per minute; number of different word roots; utterance planning; and MLU. On average, the youth in both groups were more talkative and produced a great diversity of lexical items in conversation than in narration, but produced more fluently planned and syntactically complex language in narration than in conversation. Most interesting, however, was the fact that there was a Diagnostic Group × Context interaction for MLU. This interaction reflected the fact that the youth with fragile X syndrome displayed higher MLUs than did the youth with Down syndrome, but only in narration.

Together, these findings demonstrate that context influences important dimensions of talk. Some contexts are better suited to illuminating the boundaries of some dimensions of language skill than are other contexts; for example, conversation "pulls" for verbosity and lexical diversity, whereas narration "pulls" for syntax. As a result, differences between various groups of language users on any particular dimension of language are most apt to be seen in those contexts that place the greatest demands on that dimension; for example, the syntactic deficits associated with Down syndrome relative to fragile X syndrome are highlighted in narration compared to conversation because the former requires higher-level syntactic skills.

In addition to comparisons between fragile X syndrome and other diagnostic groups, we have also found that context effects in expressive language performance are important for understanding individual differences among those with fragile X syndrome. In particular, Pavetto and Abbeduto (2002a) compared the performance of males and females with fragile X syndrome in conversation and narration on the variables of talkativeness, articulation, utterance planning, vocabulary, and syntax. The males ($n = 14$) and females ($n = 9$) were similar in age (with all being adolescents or young adults), but, as is typical for the syndrome, the females had higher IQs than did the males. It was found that females had higher MLUs than did males in both conversation and narration, with the latter context eliciting higher MLUs on average; however, there was also a Gender × Context interaction, such that the difference in MLU between females and males was greater in narration than in conversation. Again, narration elicited more complex syntactic forms and thus, group differences in the upper bounds of syntactic capabilities are more likely to emerge in narration than in conversation.

We (Pavetto & Abbeduto, 2002b) have also investigated contextual influences on the occurrence of topic perseveration (i.e., the excessive repetition of utterances focused on the same, narrowly defined topic), which is thought to distinguish fragile X syndrome from Down syndrome, autism, and other neurodevelopmental disorders (Belser & Sudhalter, 2001; Ferrier, Bashir, Meryash, Johnston, & Wolff, 1991; Sudhalter, Cohen, Silverman, & Wolf-Schein, 1990). In particular, it was found that adolescent and young adult males and females with fragile X syndrome ($n = 14$) were more likely to perseverate on a topic in conversation than in narration. It has been suggested that perseveration in this population is a reflection of social anxiety and hyperarousal (Belser & Sudhalter, 1995; Cohen, 1995; Cornish et al., 2004). A challenge for this hypothesis is to explain contextual differences in perseveration.

In summary, these studies clearly demonstrate that the context in which language is used plays a critical role in shaping linguistic performance. Moreover, these studies suggest that an adequate characterization of language development, and of group differences in that development, require assessments in multiple contexts, with the contexts selected so as to probe the boundaries of language skill. Contextual influences such as these are difficult to reconcile with the nativist account of language development, but they are to be expected (indeed, they are central) to the Child Talk account.

Language in Relation to Other Dimensions of the Behavioral Phenotype. In our research, we have examined concurrent relationships among various measures of language and other, nonlinguistic, dimensions of the fragile X syndrome phenotype. Although determining the direction of causation is impossible in such cases, these relationships provide data relevant to the contrasting claims of the Child Talk and nativist approaches (Abbeduto & Chapman, 2005). The data thus far suggest that there are intimate connections between many dimensions of language and various aspects of cognition and social cognition.

In a study of receptive language, we (Abbeduto et al., 2003) administered the Test for Auditory Comprehension of Language–Revised (TACL–R; Carrow-Woolfolk, 1985) to adolescent and young adult males and females with fragile X syndrome ($n = 19$). The TACL–R includes subtests measuring comprehension of words, grammatical morphemes, and phrase-, clause-, and sentence-level syntactic patterns. We also administered several nonverbal subtests from the Stanford-Binet, 4th edition (Thorndike, Hagen, & Sattler, 1986), so as to derive a measure of nonlinguistic cognitive maturity (i.e., nonverbal mental age). Among other things, it was found that nonverbal mental age was significantly correlated with all of the TACL–R subtests for the youth with fragile X syndrome (as well for mental age-matched comparison groups of adolescents and young adults with Down syndrome and typically developing children). These findings are consistent with notion that language learning entails the use of a wide variety of cognitive skills and knowledge.

Connections with nonlinguistic dimensions of the phenotype also have emerged for the more social aspects of language use. In one study, for example, we (Abbeduto, Murphy, Richmond, Amman, Beth, Weissman, Cawthon, Kim, & Karadottir, 2006) examined the referential talk of adolescents and young adults with fragile X syndrome ($n = 18$) as they described novel shapes to an adult partner in a non-face-to-face communication game. The youths with fragile X syndrome were found to be less consistent than mental age-matched comparison groups of youths with Down syndrome or typically developing young children as regards the descriptions they used for repeated references to any given shape. Exploratory analyses not reported by Abbeduto et al. suggest that the use of inconsistent references by the youths with fragile X syndrome was positively correlated with their problems in attention. One interpretation of this finding is that the inability to direct and sustain attention that characterizes so many with fragile X syndrome prevents them from creating or attending to a representation of the previous discourse when making decisions about their talk.

In a second study focused on the social aspects of language use, we (Abbeduto, Murphy, Giles, Bruno, & Karadottir, 2004) examined the extent to which adolescents and young adults with fragile X syndrome ($n = 19$) signaled their noncomprehension (e.g., by saying "Which one?") when they encounter referentially inadequate messages from others. We found that the youths with fragile X syndrome were less likely to signal noncomprehension than were their typically developing mental age matches. In addition, the extent to which youths with fragile X syndrome signaled noncomprehension was positively correlated with their ability to distinguish between their representations of the world and those of other people.

We have also found some evidence of a relationship between psychopathology and language in individuals with fragile X syndrome. In particular, Murphy et al. (2004) found, in a small-scale preliminary study, that comprehension of vocabulary, grammatical morphemes, and syntactic patterns, as measured by the TACL–R (or TACL–3), was more impaired in youths with fragile X syndrome who also met diagnostic criteria for autism ($n = 8$) than for age- and mental age-matched youths with fragile X syndrome but without autism ($n = 18$). Similar findings have been obtained by other investigators (e.g., Philofsky, Hepburn, Hayes, Hagerman, & Rogers, 2004). Such findings raise the possibility that the social impairments that are at the core of autism interfere with the development of language in youth with fragile X syndrome.

Together, these studies clearly demonstrate that understanding the language problems associated with fragile X syndrome requires reference to other, nonlinguistic, dimensions of the behavioral phenotype. Various cognitive and social-cognitive impairments as well as some forms of psychopathology are associated with differences in mastery of the formal and social aspects of language. Although determining the direction of causation from concurrent correlations is not possible, such correlations are consistent with the Child Talk model while posing a challenge to the nativist account.

CONCLUSION

The nativists assume that language learning is a modular process of mastering abstract, context-free rules. In contrast, the Child Talk model of Chapman and colleagues embeds language learning in the social contexts of children's lives. The Child Talk model views children as attempting to learn how to participate in those contexts and as drawing on all of their cognitive and social-cognitive capabilities (and weaknesses) in the process. We have tried to show in this chapter the ways in which the Child Talk model, and other alternatives to the nativist account (e.g., social-interactionist theory and emergentist theory; Abbeduto, Evans, & Dolan, 2001), offer a useful explanatory framework for two developmental disorders associated with serious language impairments, namely, autism and fragile X syndrome. Indeed, the results emerging for both disorders are difficult to reconcile with the nativist account, suggesting, as they do, contextual influences on language and intimate connections among language learning, language performance, and the child's attentional and social-cognitive capabilities. The implication for clinical practice of the Child Talk model and these empirical findings is that assessment and intervention must target more than language as defined by the nativist. Assessment and intervention, like language learning itself, must be embedded social activities.

ACKNOWLEDGMENTS

Preparation of this chapter was supported by National Institutes of Health (NIH) grants R01 HD24356, and P30 HD03352, T32 HD007489, by NIH grant R21 HD42437 awarded to Dr. Wendy Stone of Vanderbilt University, and by a doctoral scholarship from the Bamford-Lahey Children's Foundation awarded to A. McDuffie.

REFERENCES

Abbeduto, L., Benson, G., Short, K., & Dolish, J. (1995). Effects of sampling context on the expressive language of children and adolescents with mental retardation. *Mental Retardation*, 33(5), 279–288.

Abbeduto, L., & Chapman, R. S. (2005). Language development in Down syndrome and fragile X syndrome. In P. Fletcher & J. F. Miller (Eds.), *Trends in language acquisition research* (pp. 53–71). Philadelphia: John Benjamins.

Abbeduto, L., Evans, J., & Dolan, T. (2001). Theoretical perspectives on language and communication problems in mental retardation and developmental disabilities. *Mental Retardation and Developmental Disabilities Research Reviews, 7,* 45–55.

Abbeduto, L., Murphy, M. M., Cawthon, S. W., Richmond, E. K., Weissman, M. D., Karadottir, S., & O'Brien, A. (2003). Receptive language skills of adolescents and young adults with mental retardation: A comparison of Down syndrome and fragile X syndrome. *American Journal on Mental Retardation, 108,* 149–160.

Abbeduto, L., Murphy, M. M., Cawthon, S. C., Kesin, E., Weissman, M. D., & Karadottir, S. (2002, July). *Expressive language and contextual influences in fragile X syndrome.* Paper presented at the biennial international conference of the National Fragile X Foundation, Chicago.

Abbeduto, L., Murphy, M. M., Giles, N., Bruno, L., & Karadottir, S. (2004). *Understanding misunderstanding: Comparison of youths with Down syndrome or fragile X syndrome.* Manuscript in preparation.

Abbeduto, L., Murphy, M. M., Richmond, E. K., Amman, A., Beth, P., Weissman, M. D., Cawthon, S. W., Kim, J. S. & Karadottir, S. (2006). Collaboration in referential communication: Comparison of youths with Down syndrome or fragile X syndrome. *American Journal of Mental Retardation, 111,* 170–183.

Abbeduto, L., Pavetto, M., Kesin, E., Weissman, M. D., Karadottir, S., O'Brien, A., & Cawthon, S. (2001). The linguistic and cognitive profile of Down syndrome: Evidence from a comparison with fragile X syndrome. *Down Syndrome Research and Practice, 7,* 9–15.

Akhtar, N., & Tomasello, M. (1996). Twenty four month old children learn words for absent objects and actions. *British Journal of Developmental Psychology, 14,* 79–93.

American Psychiatric Association. (1994). *Diagnostic and statistical manual of mental disorders* (4th ed.). Washington, DC: Author.

Bailey, D. B., Roberts, J. E., Hooper, S. R., Hatton, D. D., Mirrett, P. L., Roberts, J. E., & Schaaf, J. M. (2004). Research on fragile X syndrome and autism: Implications for the study of genes, environments, and developmental language disorders. In M. Rice and S. F. Warren (Eds.), *Developmental language disorders: From phenotypes to etiologies* (pp. 121–150). Mahwah, NJ: Lawrence Erlbaum Associates.

Baird, G., Charman, T., Baron-Cohen, S., Cox, A., Swettenham, J., Wheelwright, S. & Drew. A. (2000). A screening instrument for autism at 18 months: A 6-year follow-up study. *Journal of the American Academy of Child & Adolescent Psychiatry, 39,* 694–702.

Bakeman, R., & Adamson, L. (1984). Coordinating attention to people and objects in mother–infant and peer–infant interaction. *Child Development, 55,* 1278–1289.

Baldwin, D. (1991). Infants' contribution to the achievement of joint reference. *Child Development, 62,* 875–890.

Baldwin, D. (1993a). Early referential understanding: Young children's ability to recognize referential acts for what they are. *Developmental Psychology, 29,* 1–12.

Baldwin, D. (1993b). Infant's ability to consult the speaker for clues to word reference. *Journal of Child Language, 2,* 395–418.

Baldwin, D., & Markman, E. (1996). Infants' reliance on a social criterion for establishing word-object relations. *Child Development, 67,* 3135–3153.

Baron, R., & Kenny, D. (1986). The moderator-mediator variable distinction in social psychological research: Conceptual, strategic, and statistical considerations. *Journal of Personal and Social Psychological Research, 51,* 1173–1182.

Baron-Cohen, S., Baldwin, D., & Crowson, M. (1997). Do children with autism use the speaker's direction of gaze strategy to crack the code of language? *Child Development, 68,* 48–57.

Baron-Cohen, S., Cox, A., Baird, G., Swettenham, J., Nightingale, N., Morgan, K., Drew, A., & Charman, T. (1996). Psychological markers in the detection of autism in infancy in a large population. *British Journal of Psychiatry, 168,* 158–163.

Bates, E., Bretherton, I., & Snyder, L. (1988). *From first words to grammar: Individual differences and dissociable mechanisms.* New York: Cambridge University Press.

Bates, E., Dale, P., & Thal, D. (1995). Individual differences and their implications for theories of language development. In P. Fletcher & B. MacWhinney (Eds.), *The handbook of child language* (pp. 96–151). Cambridge, MA: Blackwell.

Bates, E., & Goodman, J. (1999). On the emergence of grammar from the lexicon. In B. MacWhinney (Ed.), *The emergence of language* (pp. 29–79). Mahwah, NJ: Lawrence Erlbaum Associates.

Bates, E., & Goodman, J. (2001). On the inseparability of grammar and the lexicon: Evidence from acquisition. In E. Bates & M. Tomasello (Eds.), *Essential readings in developmental psychology* (pp. 134–162). Malden, MA: Blackwell.

Baumgardner, T., Reiss, A. L., Freund, L., et al. (1995). Specification of the neurobehavioral phenotype of males with fragile X syndrome. *Pediatrics, 95,* 744–752.

Belser, R. C., & Sudhalter, V. (1995). Arousal difficulties in males with fragile X syndrome: A preliminary report. *Developmental Brain Dysfunction, 8,* 270–279.

Belser, R. C., & Sudhalter, V. (2001). Conversational characteristics of children with fragile X syndrome: Repetitive speech. *American Journal on Mental Retardation, 106,* 28–38.

Bregman, J. D., Leckman, J. F., & Ort, S. I. (1988). Fragile X syndrome: Genetic predisposition to psychopathology. *Journal of Autism and Developmental Disorders, 18,* 343–354.

Brown, W. T. (2002). The molecular biology of the fragile X mutation. In R. J. Hagerman & P. J. Hagerman (Eds), *Fragile X syndrome: Diagnosis, treatment and research* (3rd ed., pp. 110–135). Baltimore: Johns Hopkins University Press.

Burack, J. A., Shulman, C., Katzir, E., Schaap, T., Brennan, J. M., Iarocci, G., Wilansky, P., & Amir, N. (1999). Cognitive and behavioural development of Israeli males with fragile X and Down Syndrome. *International Journal of Behavioral Development, 23,* 519–531.

Carrow-Woolfolk, E. (1985). *Test for Auditory Comprehension of Language-Revised.* Allen, TX: DLM Teaching Resources.

Carey, S., & Bartlett, E. (1978). Acquiring a single new word. *Papers and Reports on Child Language Development, 15,* 17–29.

Chapman, R. S., Streim, N., Crais, E., Salmon, D., Strand, E., & Negri, N. (1992). Child talk: Assumptions of a developmental process model for early language learning. In R. S. Chapman (Ed.), *Processes in language acquisition and disorders* (pp. 3–19). St. Louis, MO: Mosby.

Charman, T. (2003). Why is joint attention a pivotal skill in autism? *Philosophical Transactions of the Royal Society of London, 358,* 315–324.

Charman, T., Baron-Cohen, S., Swettenham, J., Baird, G., Cox, A., & Drew, A. (2000). Testing joint attention, imitation, and play as infancy precursors to language and theory of mind. *Cognitive Development, 15,* 481–498.

Chomsky, N. (1965). *Aspects of theory of syntax.* Cambridge, MA: MIT Press.

Chomsky, N. (1975). *Reflections on language.* New York: Pantheon.

Chomsky, N. (1988). *Language and problems of knowledge: The Managua lectures.* Cambridge, MA: MIT Press.

Cohen, I. L. (1995). A theoretical analysis of the role of hyperarousal in the learning and behavior of fragile X males. *Mental Retardation and Developmental Disabilities Research Reviews, 1,* 286–291.

Cornish, K., Sudhalter, V., & Turk, J. (2004). Attention and language in fragile X. *Mental Retardation and Developmental Disabilities Research Reviews, 10,* 11–16.

Crawford, D. C., Acuna, J. M., & Sherman, S. L. (2001). FMR1 and the fragile X syndrome: Human genome epidemiology review. *Genetics in Medicine, 3,* 359–371.

Cronbach, L., & Meehl, P. (1955). Construct validity in psychological tests. *Psychological Bulletin, 52,* 281–302.

Demark, J. L., Feldman, M. A., & Holden, J. J. A. (2003). Behavioral relationship between autism and fragile X syndrome. *American Journal of Medical Genetics, 108,* 314–326.

Dollaghan, C. A., Campbell, T. F., & Tomlin, R. (1990). Video narration as a language sampling context. *Journal of Speech and Hearing Research, 55,* 582–590.

Dykens, E. M., Hodapp, R. M., & Finucane, B. M. (2000). *Genetics and mental retardation syndromes: A new look at behavior and interventions.* Baltimore: Brookes.

Dykens, E. M., Hodapp, R. M., & Leckman, J. F. (1987). Strengths and weaknesses in the intellectual functioning of males with fragile X syndrome. *American Journal on Mental Deficiency, 92,* 234–236.

Dykens, E., Hodapp, R., Ort, S., & Finucane, B. (1989). The trajectory of cognitive development in males with fragile X syndrome. *Journal of the American Academy of Child and Adolescent Psychiatry, 28,* 422–426.

Evans, J. L., & Craig, H. K. (1992). Language sample collection and analysis: Interview compared to free play assessment contexts. *Journal of Speech and Hearing Research, 35,* 343–353.

Feinstein, C., & Reiss, A. L. (2001). Autism: The point of view from fragile X studies. *Journal of Autism and Developmental Disorders, 28,* 393–405.

Fenson, L., Dale, P., Reznick, J., Bates, E., Thal, D., & Pethick, S. (1994). Variability in early communicative development. *Monographs of the Society for Research in Child Development, 59*(5, Serial No. 242).

Ferrier, L. J., Bashir, A. S., Meryash, D. L., Johnston, J., & Wolff, P. (1991). Conversational skills of individuals with fragile-X syndrome: A comparison with autism and Down syndrome. *Developmental Medicine and Child Neurology, 33,* 776–788.

Fodor, J. A. (1983). *The modularity of mind.* Cambridge, MA: MIT Press.

Freund, L. S., & Reiss, A. L. (1991). Cognitive profiles associated with the fra(X) syndrome in males and females. *American Journal of Medical Genetics, 38,* 542–547.

Garner, C., Callias, M., & Turk, J. (1999). Executive function and theory of mind performance of boys with fragile-X syndrome. *Journal of Intellectual Disability Research, 43,* 466–474.

Gillberg, C. (1991). Outcome in autism and autistic-like conditions. *Journal of the American Academy of Child and Adolescent Psychiatry, 30,* 375–382.

Greenough, W. T., Klintsova, A. Y., Irwin, S. A., Galvez, R., Bates, K. E., & Weiler, I. J. (2001). Synaptic regulation of protein synthesis and the fragile X protein. *Proceedings of the National Academy of Sciences, USA, 98,* 7101–7106.

Hagerman, R. J. (Ed). (1999). *Neurodevelopmental disorders.* Oxford: Oxford University Press.

Hoff, E. (2003). The specificity of environmental influence: Socioeconomic status affects early vocabulary development via maternal speech. *Child Development, 74,* 1368–1378.

Howlin, P., Mahood, L., & Rutter M. (2000). Autism and developmental receptive language disorder—A follow-up comparison in early adult life: Social, behavioral, and psychiatric outcomes. *Journal of Child Psychology and Psychiatry, 41,* 561–578.

Kasari, C., Freeman, S., Mundy, P., & Sigman, M. (1995). Attention regulation by children with Down syndrome: Coordinated joint attention and social referencing looks. *American Journal on Mental Retardation, 100,* 128–136.

Kasari, C., Mundy, P., Yirmiya, N., & Sigman, M. (1990). Affect and attention in children with Down syndrome. *American Journal of Mental Retardation, 95,* 55–67.

Kasari, C., Sigman, M., Mundy, P., & Yirmiya, N. (1990). Affective sharing in the context of joint attention interactions of normal, autistic, and mentally retarded children. *Journal of Autism and Developmental Disorders, 20,* 87–100.

Keysor, C., & Mazzocco, M. (2002). A developmental approach to understanding fragile X syndrome in females. *Microscopy Research Technology, 57,* 179–186.

Leekam, S., Hunnisett, E., & Moore, C. (1998). Targets and cues: Gaze following in children with autism. *Journal of Child Psychology and Psychiatry, 39,* 951–962.

Liss, M., Harel, B., Fein, D., Allen, D., Dunn M., Feinstein, C., Morris, R., Waterhouse, L., & Rapin, I. (2001). Predictors and correlates of adaptive functioning in children with developmental disorders. *Journal of Autism and Developmental Disorders, 31,* 219–30.

Loban, W. (1976). *Language development: Kindergarten through grade twelve.* Res. Rep. No. 18. Urbana, IL: National Council of Teachers of English.

Lord, C., & Bailey, A. (2002). Autism spectrum disorders. In M. Rutter & E. Taylor (Eds.), *Child and adolescent psychiatry: Modern approaches* (4th ed., pp. 636–663). Oxford: Blackwell Scientific.

Lord, C. (1995). Follow-up of two year olds referred for possible autism. *Journal of Child Psychology and Psychiatry, 36,* 1365–1382.

Marcell, M. M., & Weeks, S. L. (1988). Short-term memory difficulties in Down's syndrome. *Journal of Mental Deficiency Research, 32,* 153–162.

Mazzocco, M. M., Baumgardner, T., Freund, L. S., & Reiss, A. L. (1998). Social functioning among girls with fragile X or Turner syndrome and their sisters. *Journal of Autism and Developmental Disorders, 28,* 509–517.

Mazzocco, M. M., Pennington, B., & Hagerman, R. J. (1993). The neurocognitive phenotype of female carriers of fragile X: Further evidence for specificity. *Journal of Development and Behavioral Pediatrics, 14,* 328–335.

McDuffie, A. (2004). *The relationship of four prelinguistic skills and rapid word-object mapping to vocabulary outcomes in young children with autism*. Unpublished doctoral dissertation, Vanderbilt University, Nashville, TN.

Mirrett, P. L., Roberts, J. E., & Price, J. (2003). Early intervention practices and communication intervention strategies for young males with fragile X syndrome. *Language, Speech, and Hearing Services in Schools, 34,* 320–331.

Mundy, P., Sigman, M., & Kasari, C. (1994). Joint attention, developmental level and symptom presentation in autism. *Development and Psychopathology, 6,* 389–401.

Murphy, M. M., & Abbeduto, L. (2003). Language and communication in fragile X syndrome. In L. Abbeduto (Ed.), *International Review of Research in Mental Retardation* (Vol. 27, pp. 83–113). New York: Academic Press.

Murphy, M. M., & Abbeduto, L. (in press). Indirect genetic effects and the early language development of children with genetic mental retardation syndromes: The role of joint attention. *Infants and Young Children.*

Murphy, M. M., Abbeduto, L., Giles, N., Bruno, L., Richmond, E. K., & Schroeder, S. (2004). *Cognitive, language, and social-cognitive skills of individuals with fragile X syndrome with and without autism*. Poster presented at the annual Gatlinburg Conference on Mental Retardation, San Diego, CA.

National Research Council. (2001). *Educating children with autism.* Washington, DC: National Academy Press.

Osterling, J., & Dawson, G. (1994). Early recognition of children with autism: A study of first birthday home videotapes. *Journal of Autism and Developmental Disorders, 24,* 247–257.

Oostra, B. A. (1996). FMR1 protein studies and animal models for fragile X syndrome. In R .J. Hagerman & A. C. Cronister (Eds.), *Fragile X syndrome: Diagnosis, treatment and research* (2nd ed., pp. 193–209). Baltimore: Johns Hopkins University Press.

Oostra, B. A., & Willemsen, R. (2003). A fragile balance: FMR1 expression levels. *Human Molecular Genetics 12: Review Issue, 2,* R249–R257.

Pavetto, M. M. & Abbeduto, L. (2002a, June). *Characteristics of expressive language among males and females with fragile X syndrome.* Poster session presented at the annual meeting of the Academy of Mental Retardation, Orlando, FL.

Pavetto, M. M., & Abbeduto, L. (2002b, June). *Gender differences in repetitive talk among adolescents with fragile X syndrome.* Paper presented at the 126th Annual Meeting of the American Association on Mental Retardation, San Diego.

Philofsky, A, Hepburn, S. L., Hayes, A., Hagerman, R., & Rogers, S. J. (2004). Linguistic and cognitive functioning and autism symptoms in young children with fragile X syndrome. *American Journal on Mental Retardation, 109,* 208–218.

Pinker, S. (1996). *The language instinct.* New York: Norton.

Prizant, B. (1996). Brief report: Communication, language, social, and emotional development. *Journal of Autism and Developmental Disorders, 26,* 173–178.

Rogers, S., Hepburn, S., Stackhouse, T., & Wehner, E. (2003). Imitation performance in toddlers with autism and those with other developmental disorders. *Journal of Child Psychology and Psychiatry, 44,* 763–781.

Seung, H.-K., & Chapman, R. S. (2000). Digit span in individuals with Down syndrome and typically developing children: Temporal aspects. *Journal of Speech, Language, and Hearing Research, 43,* 609–620.

Stevens, M., Fein, D., Dunn, M., Allen, D., Waterhouse, L., Feinstein, C., & Rapin, I. (2000). Subgroups of children with autism by cluster analysis: A longitudinal examination. *Journal of the American Academy of Child and Adolescent Psychiatry, 39,* 346–352.

Stone, W. (1997). Autism in infancy and early childhood. In D. Cohen & F. Volkmar (Eds.), *Handbook of autism and pervasive developmental disorders* (2nd ed., pp. 266–282). New York: Wiley.

Stone, W., Ousley, O., & Littleford, C. (1997). Motor imitation in young children with autism: What's the object? *Journal of Abnormal Child Psychology, 25,* 475–485.

Stone, W., Ousley, O., Yoder, P., Hogan, K., & Hepburn, S. (1997). Nonverbal communication in two and three year old children with autism. *Journal of Autism and Developmental Disorders, 27,* 677–695.

Sudhalter, V., Cohen, I. L., Silverman, W., & Wolf-Schein, E. G. (1990). Conversational analyses of males with fragile X, Down syndrome, and autism: Comparison of the emergence of deviant language. *American Journal on Mental Retardation, 94,* 431–441.

Tager-Flusberg, H. (1988). On the nature of a language acquisition disorder: The example of autism. In F. Kessel (Ed.), *The development of language and language researchers* (pp. 249–267). Hillsdale, NJ: Lawrence Erlbaum Associates.

Tager-Flusberg, H., & Sullivan, K. (1998). Early language development in children with mental retardation. In J. Burack, R. Hodapp, & E. Zigler (Eds.), *Handbook of mental retardation and development* (pp. 208–239). New York: Cambridge University Press.

Thorndike, R. L., Hagen, E. P., & Sattler, J. M. (1986). *Stanford-Binet Intelligence Scale* (4th ed.). Chicago: Riverside.

Venter, A., Lord, C., & Schopler, E. (1992). A follow-up study of high functioning autistic children. *Journal of Child Psychology and Psychiatry, 33,* 489–507.

Volkmar, F., Lord, C., Bailey, A., Schultz, R., & Klin, A. (2004). Autism and pervasive developmental disorders. *Journal of Child Psychology and Psychiatry, 45,* 135–170.

Wisbeck, J. M., Huffman, L. C., Freund, L., Gunnar, M., Davis, E. P., & Reiss, A. L. (2000). Cortisol and social stressors in children with fragile X: A pilot study. *Developmental and Behavioral Pediatrics, 21,* 279–282.

Woodward, A., Markman, E., & Fitzsimmons, C. (1994). Rapid word learning in 13–18 month olds. *Developmental Psychology, 30,* 553–566.

Zelazo, P. D., Burack, J. A., Benedetto, E., & Frye, D. (1996). Theory of mind and rule use in individuals with Down's syndrome: a test of the uniqueness and specificity claims. *Journal of Child Psychology and Psychiatry, 37,* 479–448.

8

Fragile X Syndrome: Memory Skills and the Emergence of Reading in Males

Mina C. Johnson-Glenberg
Waisman Center, University of Wisconsin–Madison

This chapter reports on a pattern of memory strengths and weaknesses observed in males with fragile X syndrome. In addition, some preliminary findings on the relationships between memory, sequencing skills, and word-level reading skills are explored against the framework of typically developing memory and reading skills. Both memory and reading are cognitive constructs that develop over time. They interact with one another and have large and important dynamic effects on all other cognitive processes. Memory and reading skills are considered emergent (see Abbeduto & Chapman, this volume) and are discussed throughout with this terminology.

Fragile X syndrome (FXS) is the most prevalent form of heritable mental retardation in the world. It affects approximately 1 in 4,000 males and 1 in 8,000 females (Hagerman, 1999). The mutation consists of an unstable expansion of CGG trinucleotide repeats on the 5′ untranslated region of the FMR1 gene (Oberle et al., 1991; Verkerk et al., 1991). There is much variability in the symptoms manifested at the cognitive, linguistic, and social levels of functioning. The mutation is X-linked and, on average, females are less affected. Females with FXS present a much wider range of cognitive deficits and psychological dysfunction (Mazzocco & Reiss, 1999); therefore this chapter focuses on affected males. The central question is, how do males with FXS compare in a fine-grained memory profile to nonverbal mental age-matched typically developing (TD) children? In order to ask a developmental and reading-related question, the males with FXS are also compared to an older TD group matched on word reading.

PROFILE OF COGNITION IN INDIVIDUALS WITH FXS

Individuals with FXS possess a profile of relative strengths and weaknesses. When assessing higher levels of cognitive functioning, it appears that males with FXS have difficulty integrating past experiences with present (Sobesky, Hull, & Hagerman, 1992) and with abstract reasoning (Freund & Reiss, 1991). They are resistant to environmental change (Reiss & Freund, 1992), and demonstrate a need for sameness. They often overreact to novelty (Scharfenaker et al., 1996). Males with FXS often demonstrate problems with self-regulatory behavior, hyperactivity, poor attention, and concentration. They also perform significantly worse on arithmetic measures when compared to the mean performance of children with Down syndrome and nonspecific retardation (Hodapp et al., 1992). In addition, males with FXS perform significantly worse on hand movement imitation (K-ABC, Kaufman Assessment Battery for Children; Hodapp et al., 1992). Regarding some of their relative strengths, those with FXS perform better than individuals with Down syndrome on several other *simultaneous* K-ABC measures—Magic Window (identifying a partially occluded object passing through a window) and significantly better on gestalt memory closure (identifying partially obscured line drawings) (Hodapp et al., 1992). These results have led researchers to put forth the theory that those with FXS have relatively stronger skills in simultaneous processing compared to other groups with mental retardation (MR). It may be useful to analyze these processing skills in reference to an established memory framework such as the working memory model proposed by Baddeley (1986).

MEMORY RESEARCH IN TYPICALLY DEVELOPING INDIVIDUALS AND INDIVIDUALS WITH MENTAL RETARDATION

It is possible to discuss memory using a developmental framework with TD individuals because decades of research of been done. FXS is a relatively recent diagnosis (compared to Down syndrome for example) that is still somewhat underdiagnosed; thus, there is not a large body of research on memory in FXS. Certainly there is not a clear picture of the development and the working memory subprocesses in this population. This chapter's cross-sectional data should add to the growing body of memory research.

In the typically developing population children ages one through 12 years demonstrate a linear increase in skill for digit, letter and word span measures (Dempster, 1981). Cowan (1997) highlights six developmental changes postulated to account for memory increases with age. These changes can occur in (a) knowledge, (b) processing strategies, (c) processing speed, (d) use of attention, (e) passive memory loss over time, and (f) memory storage capacity. All of these are correlated with age and brain growth (in particular myelination). Each process will be described briefly. Knowledge aids memory because it reduces the memory load by laying down schemata or permanent memory structures for incoming information to systematically adhere to. Processing strategies are extremely useful in aiding recall and increasing working memory. This is an area where individuals with MR show consistent differences when compared to TD groups. In particular, covert rehearsal of items often occurs spontaneously in TD children. Flavell, Beach, and Chinsky (1966) examined children's lip movements during delays on a word list recall. They also found that the subvocal rehearsal strategy was much more infrequent in younger children than in older, who remembered more. In addition, Naus et al. (1977) found that sixth-grade children rehearsed spontaneously, whereas third graders did not. Processing speed is also responsible for memory increases over age. As the myelin increases, information is transmitted faster throughout the brain. This suggests faster and more effective rehearsal, which would result in more items that can be maintained at the same time. These items could be refreshed in working memory before they are lost (Baddeley, 1986). Use of attention changes with age as well, and this can be demonstrated via incidental and intentional memory tasks. Maccoby and Hagen (1965) studied first-, third-, fifth-, and seventh-grade children. Recall on the intentional task increased with age. However, performance on the surprise or incidental recall task actually decreased with age. The older children were more adept at ignoring the distractors than the younger children. This finding is of interest because in this chapter we report on differences in incidental memory between FXS and TD groups.

Passive memory loss over time refers to how long original signal information can be maintained in working memory. Cowan (1997) examines experiments in the auditory domain that show differences between 6- to 7-year-olds, 10- to 12-year-olds, and adults. The adults outperformed the children. Finally, memory storage capacity may increase with age. Pascual-Leone (1970) conducted several experiments that discouraged rehearsal and found that the number of items recalled still increased with age.

Of course, as Cowan points out (1997), it would be difficult to separate larger capacity from enhanced processing associated with age.

Precise research on memory in individuals with MR has been hampered by a lack of etiological specificity. Over the decades, several theories of memory in individuals with MR have risen and fallen in prominence. Ellis (1963) was a proponent of the weak stimulus trace theory. This theory proposed that memory traces of those with MR were of weakened intensity and lesser duration than traces created by TD individuals (akin to the passive memory loss theory). In the late 1960s when strategy theories became influential (e.g., Atkinson & Shiffrin, 1968), researchers investigated rehearsal and processing strategies (Bellmont & Butterfield, 1977; Campione & Brown, 1977; Ellis, 1970). In the 1980s, researchers posited that memory deficits might be related to cognitive structural deficits (Winters & Semchuk, 1986). Before the advent of imagining technologies, the term *cognitive structures* (in this field at least) referred to "the organization of thinking and learning processes such as the logico-mathematical patterns that underlie human understanding, reasoning and information acquisition and use." (Weiss, Weisz, & Bromfield, 1986, p. 157). Over the years, all the factors that explain growth in memory in the TD population have been specifically postulated as the primary deficit(s) for those with MR, except for lack of attention, perhaps because some consider attention an overlying global deficit in most individuals with MR.

It has been difficult to come to a clear picture of some of the developmental cognitive differences between groups with MR and TD-match groups. In their thorough meta-analysis, Weiss et al. (1986) report that there is not a simple, favored outcome when comparing group performances on typically Piagetian tasks. Of the 24 studies analyzed 52% reported *no* significant group differences, and 45% reported a significant difference with TD mental age (MA) matches outperforming those with MR. In the end, Weiss et al. posit that those with MR may be deficient in more than one fundamental process, and that the differences seen across studies show that it might not be useful to try to describe cognition (or information processing) as a unitary process. This supports the arguments that many make against modularity—as defined by Fodor (1983) and refuted by the connectionists, such as Elman, et al. (1996), and now applied to MR populations (e.g., Abbeduto & Chapman, this volume; Karmiloff-Smith, Brown, Grice, & Paterson, 2003).

Munir, Cornish, and Wilding (2000) and Cornish et al. (2004) elegantly state the case for a developmental approach that does not view cognition as a highly modularized construct. Differences at the genetic and brain structure levels from conception onward affect growth and outcomes dynamically. This point of dynamicism in development and the emergence of relative strengths and weaknesses is now being explicitly advocated by researchers who study both TD and MR populations (Abbeduto, Evans, & Dolan, 2001; Chapman, 2000; Karmiloff-Smith & Thomas, 2002; Thelen, 1994). More research needs to be done with a longitudinal and developmental perspective for the MR populations to help solidify theories and guide remediation.

MEMORY AND READING

Memory and reading are dynamically intertwined. Increases in memory serve literacy, and increases in reading skill serve to enrich the knowledge base or schemata on which memory resides. Our lab is engaged in an ongoing study of prereading and reading skills in individuals with FXS. The decision was made to begin the research by gaining an understanding of memory subprocesses in males with FXS. In this chapter an effort is made to classify some of the memory and reading skill states of males with FXS and to compare those to states of matched TD children. The term *state* here means the value of the variables at a given moment in time (Abraham, Abraham, & Shaw, 1990); it does not imply "end state," wherein variable vector velocity would equal zero.

Before describing the memory matrix and the measures we would like to make the case for memory subprocesses to be viewed on a continuum. This is in response to the crisp boundaries that modularity would suggest, and the fact that many measures themselves do not tap pure processes. For example, many of the memory for geometric design tasks are categorized as nonverbal, but Howieson and Lezak (1995) warn that these items can be recalled using verbal rehearsal strategies as well. For ease of classification, the simplistic descriptors of verbal and nonverbal memory are used throughout the chapter, but with the understanding that these constructs are conceived of as existing on a continuum. That is, some measures are *more* verbal and some are *more* nonverbal than others. The memory measures are broken into a 2 × 2 × 2 matrix containing: mode—verbal versus nonverbal; time—immediate recall versus delayed recall; and processing—sequential versus simultaneous.

Memory: Verbal and Nonverbal

Baddeley's (1986) theory of working memory is a useful model for parsing memory. Baddeley posits that working memory is comprised of three elements. The first is a central executive (CE) in charge of planning, flexibility, and shuttling information. In addition, it has been proposed that the CE is in charge of more specific skills such as switching, updating and inhibition (Miyake et al., 2000). The CE system contains two slave systems, the phonological (or articulatory) loop and the visuo-spatial sketchpad. (Visuo-spatial tasks often map to the simultaneous processing tasks.)

One way of investigating differences between the FXS and TD groups is to ask how the slave systems differ. The prediction is that the FXS group should perform equally, or somewhat better, on the more simultaneous verbal tasks because they are older (have more world knowledge) and will not have to contend with the difficulties of sequencing. Abbeduto et al. (2003) found that the FXS group significantly out performed a Down syndrome (DS) match group on the TACL (Test for Auditory Comprehension of Language–Revised; Carrow-Woolfolk, 1985), which would be considered a verbal simultaneous task. In addition, Abbeduto et al. reported that the FXS group performed somewhat better than the TD mental age-match group. Hodapp et al. (1992) found that males with FXS were over half a year higher in their expressive vocabulary compared to the individuals with DS and to individuals with nonspecific MR, although these differences, too, were not statistically significant. Thus, there is some evidence that males with FXS possess relative verbal strengths. We are interested in the magnitude of these strengths, whether they remain after a recall delay, and how they compare with MA-match TD children.

Recall: Immediate and Delayed

Another important distinction in memory is that between working (short-term) and long-term memory. The guiding theory used by this article is that the two memory systems complement one another as learning systems. That is, new information passes through the prefrontal areas and the hippocampus (HC)[1] among other structures. The HC is designed to rapidly encode and retain novel input from the information stream. Neuroscientists agree that the HC plays an important role in learning and memory, but consensus has yet to be reached as to the exact role (Gluck & Myers, 2001). One prominent cognitive theory is that new information is then "slowly interleaved" with long-term memories that are stored neocortically (McClelland & Goddard, 1996; McClelland, McNaughton, & O'Reilly, 1995). Learning is the result of this complementary meshing of old and new information. By retesting individuals with FXS after longer delays, it is possible to assess how much of the new information has been retained, and to compare this performance to other relevant match groups.

An age-related increase in the volume of the HC has been found in individuals with FXS (Reiss, Lee, & Freund, 1994). This finding, coupled with the abnormal dendritic spine structures, observed both in humans and in

[1]Due to space constraints, the many other brain structures involved in learning are not described here.

FMRP knock-out mice (Irwin, Galvez, & Greenough, 2000), would predict dysfunctions in many processes associated with learning. We hypothesize that recall after a delay will be compromised in the FXS group regardless of whether the task is more verbal or more simultaneous.

Processing: Sequential and Simultaneous

This distinction came to prominence based primarily on findings by Hodapp et al. (1992) and Dykens, Hodapp, and Leckman (1987). Hodapp et al. (1992) assessed three groups composed of males with FXS, individuals with DS, and individuals with MR of nonspecific etiology. Sequential processing was assessed using three subtests from the K-ABC (Kaufman & Kaufman, 1983): hand movements, number recall, and word order. The FXS group performed significantly worse than the DS group on hand movements. Simultaneous processing was assessed with magic window (name an object that is being moved through a small window), face recognition, gestalt closure, triangles, matrix analogies, and spatial memory. Performance by the group with FXS was equivalent to that of the group with DS except on gestalt closure, where those with FXS performed significantly better. Using a within-group analysis on the K-ABC results, Dykens et al. (1987) reported that males with FXS performed significantly better in the simultaneous domain compared to the sequential.

In contrast, Munir et al. (2000) do not report a comparative strength of simultaneous processing on the classic spatial memory task from the K-ABC. Their FXS group performed significantly worse than the verbal mental age-matched group with DS, the TD verbal mental age-matched group, and the TD chronological age-matched group. However, the spatial memory task from the K-ABC may not represent a pure spatial, that is, simultaneous, task because the final stage of assessment involves serialization for recall. The participant must sequentially point to each empty grid cell, where an object had previously been located. Because so many sequential tasks are phonologically mediated using subvocal rehearsal strategies, one of the hypotheses of this study is that those with FXS will perform poorly across the board on sequential tasks, regardless of whether these tasks are deemed more verbal or nonverbal.

Table 8.1 demonstrates the memory framework. The plus signs indicate predicted relative strengths in the males with FXS. The final cell is empty because we did not have an appropriate nonverbal, delayed sequential test at the time of the study.

METHOD

There were two primary comparison groups in the following analyses, the males with FXS and the TD nonverbal mental age-matched children. A

TABLE 8.1
The Memory Framework: Predicted FXS Strengths Indicated by Plus Signs

Time and Mode	*Processing— More Simultaneous*	*Processing— More Sequential*
Verbal immediate	+	
Verbal delayed		
Nonverbal immediate	+	
Nonverbal delayed		

third group of reading-matched TD children was created to address certain developmental issues related to sequencing and reading skills. The TD reading-matched group is described later.

Participants

The two primary groups were individuals with FXS, age range 11;5 to 38;1 ($n = 15$), and typically developing individuals, age range 3;11 to 8;3 ($n = 22$). Data from four females with FXS were also gathered, but because their scores were significantly higher than the males their data are not included in these analyses. Participants with FXS were recruited through postings on the Internet at national FXS foundations, through advertisements in newsletters of regional organizations that focus on developmental disabilities, and via mailings to local genetics clinics and doctors who specialize in developmental disabilities. All participants with FXS either lived at home or in apartments with one or two other roommates with a developmental disability. TD children were recruited through a university-based birth registry. Parents of TD children indicated their children had no history of special education or hearing loss at the time of the study. English was the first language of all the participants.

The TD group was 55% male and contained one boy of Hispanic origin. The FXS group was 100% male and contained one Hispanic male and one African American male. FXS status was confirmed via certified doctor and geneticist reports. Four of the oldest participants (all over 28 years) were diagnosed through karyotype screening. These participants (and their parents) were not interested in subsequent DNA testing. Of the males with DNA testing, all were mosaic and CGG repeat size varied from 230 to 1200. None of the participants in the TD group were on medications. Eight of the 15 participants in the FXS group were currently on medications; these included Prozac, Zoloft, Adderall, Tenex, Risperadol, BuSpar, Ritalin, and Tegretol.

All participants were prescreened to know the most common colors and shapes. The number of participants in any task varied for several reasons; for example, the Continuous Performance Task (CPT) was added later to the test battery, there were occasional software failures, and for the Word Identification test many of the younger TD children could not read.

Testing Protocol

Participants were tested individually in a sound-attenuated room at a university research center. One or both parents or caregivers of all the FXS children, and of the majority of the TD children, viewed the session from an adjoining room through a two-way mirror. Software was administered with a Sony VIAO PCG-FX240 laptop; the software was written in E-Prime Beta and 1.0 versions. Measures were given in an invariant order. First the toy task was administered, then the Continuous Performance Attention task, then mental age and memory tests, then the Card Task, and finally the two surprise delay tasks.

For the Card Task data, two individuals' scores were gathered by another lab in the same building. Members of that lab were extensively trained in the protocol and demonstrated a high level of experimenter fidelity; in addition, experimenters followed a written script. All participants chose a prize and received a T-shirt after the study.

Materials

The tests conform to three categories: (a) grouping variables, (b) attention, and (c) memory.

Grouping

Mental Age. Mental age was assessed with two different measures. In an effort to reduce testing time, the Columbia Mental Maturity Scale (CMMS) was originally chosen to assess mental age. However, it became evident that many individuals with FXS exhibited a position bias, so its use was discontinued.[2] The test was administered to nine TD participants and three individuals with FXS when it was noticed that the last two FXS individuals were demonstrating a preference for choosing the item in the third position. Because this sort of test does not seem valid, nor reliable, for the

[2]The CMMS is based on the odd-one-out concept. Participants must pick which image does not belong on a long cardboard card (e.g., cup, magnifying glass, knife, glass, fork). When the experimenter noted the position bias (after a streak of five), it was brought to the participant's attention, "Remember, it is not always the third item." This did not appear to break the participant's perseveration or mental set.

FXS population, the decision was made to assess mental age with the Stanford-Binet (4th ed.) (Thorndike, Hagen, & Sattler, 1986) subtests of Bead Memory and Pattern Analysis. These subtests have been used extensively with individuals with developmental disabilities (Abbeduto et al., 2003; Miles & Chapman, 2002), and they scale properly for delayed populations. The CMMS scores called Maturity Index scores map to the Stanford-Binet's age-equivalents scores. The correlation of the CMMS with the first version of the Stanford-Binet is .67 for TD children, and .61 for children with MR (French & Worcester, 1956).

Bead Memory. The Stanford-Binet 4th ed. (Thorndike et al., 1986) was used. At the beginning level, participants view beads in the experimenter's hand for 2 s and then pick the same color and type on a picture card. At the next level, participants view a picture of various beads on a stick. The picture is removed after five seconds and the participants must build the bead sequence on a stick. No error feedback is given. The test is discontinued after three out of four items are incorrect.

Pattern Analysis. The Stanford-Binet 4th ed. (Thorndike et al., 1986) was used. At the beginning level, participants place geometric forms onto a board with cutout holes. At the next level, pattern blocks are used. Participants must first recreate the design the experimenter builds. Then participants must recreate the design from a picture in a test booklet. The last task is noticeably more difficult because the pictures do not include lines depicting block boundaries. No error feedback is given. The test is discontinued after three out of four items are incorrect. Performance is timed, and a time failure (usually longer than 45 s) is scored as a failure. Performance information for the grouping variables can be found in Table 8.2.

Word Identification. The Woodcock Reading Mastery Tests–Revised (Woodcock, 1998) were used. Participants read real words from an easel booklet until six consecutive errors were reached on a page. This test is used to match older typically developing individuals to the FXS group.

Attention

Continuous Performance Task (CPT). This experimenter-designed task is based primarily on Crosby's (1972) venerable CPT designed to be used with children with MR. It was necessary to create a new version for this study that would not be contingent on letter identification (as many of the younger TD children were nonreaders) and that would not last more than 15 min (as that might unduly fatigue our participants). We created our own computerized task composed of two parts. Part I measured simple

TABLE 8.2
Characteristics of FXS and MA-Matched Groups

	TD, M (SD)	*TD, Min: Max*	*FX, M (SD)*	*FX, Min: Max*	*t-Test*
n	22		15		
Chronological Age	5.39 (1.06)	3.92: 8.25	20.56 (8.74)	11.42: 38.08	$t_{(14.3)^a} = 6.69$, $p < .000$
Nonverbal mental age	5.73 (1.13)	3.45: 7.21	5.30 (1.26)	3.70: 7.88	$t_{(35)} = 1.09$, NS
N for CPT—Continuous Performance T	7		9[b]		
Attention—CPT D Prime I[c]	2.62 (1.07)	.28: 3.38	2.63 (1.45)	.71: 4.06	$t < 1.0$
Attention—CPT D Prime II[d]	1.91 (.89)	.90: 3.48	2.13 (.81)	.79: 3.40	$t < 1.0$

[a]Variance between groups differed significantly, degrees of freedom have been adjusted.
[b]Nonverbal mental age statistics were rerun for the CPT subsets, TD = 6.11 (.71); FXS = 5.04 (1.26), $t_{(14)} = 2.00$, $p = .065$.
[c]Simple attention task.
[d]Attention with inhibition.

attention and Part II measured impulsivity. In the instructions and practice before Part I, participants were asked to name the shapes and colors in the task (red square, blue triangle, green circle). They were then given nine practice items and instructed to hit the space bar every time a red square appeared. Immediate feedback was given. If less than two-thirds of the red squares were detected, the practice session was repeated. If participants still did not reach criterion, the CPT was not administered. Stimuli were present for 1000 ms, or until the space bar was hit. The interstimulus interval (ISI) was 400 ms, during which a fixation cross was presented. The duration of Part I was approximately 6 min with 176 items. Participants were also given 12 practice items before Part II. Part II assessed impulsivity, that is, attention with inhibition. The instructions were to hit the space bar when a red square was present, but *only* if it followed a blue triangle. Therefore, participants must inhibit the prepotent response to hit the space bar at every red square, and then they must monitor and recall for the presence of a preceding blue triangle. The duration of Part II was approximately eight minutes with 160 items. Scores were recorded as Hits (correct acceptances) and False Alarms (incorrect acceptances). Final scores are reported in the D prime statistic.[3] Table 8.2 lists the performance for the groups on the CPT. The groups performed equivalently on the simple attention task (Part I). Interestingly, the FXS group did better on the inhibition task than the TD mental age-match children, but not significantly so. Because the groups performed equivalently, it may be assumed that differences on the memory measures were not artifacts of more upstream cognitive functioning related to attention.

The memory measures were chosen to capitalize on the four distinctions at the ends of the memory processing continua described in the introduction: simultaneous versus sequential, and verbal versus nonverbal.

Memory Measures—More Simultaneous (Spatial)

Toy Recall. In an effort to assess simultaneous memory in an engaging manner that would lend itself to a delayed component, a classic spatial task used by Smith and Milner (1981) was slightly altered. When participants first entered the testing room they saw a table covered with 16 colorful, small toys. The toys appeared randomly placed over a 24 × 38 inch piece of tracing paper. Actually, the toys were placed over a specific number on a master sheet of paper. To ensure encoding, participants pointed to each item with a pen and named the item. The toys where then placed in a box, and participants were asked to immediately recall the toys. At the end of the entire testing session, participants were told there was a surprise task. They then performed a delayed recall of the toys (delay equal to approximately 2.5 h). Participants were then asked to replace the toys—on a fresh sheet of tracing paper. The instructions were, "Try to put these toys back in the place where you first saw them." The distance from original placement to participant's placement was later tallied.

Gestalt Closure. The K-ABC (Kaufman Assessment Battery for Children; Kaufman & Kaufman, 1983) was used. This test measures the participants ability to "fill in the gaps" in a partially completed inkblot drawing. Participants must name the image. The designers consider this a measure of holistic processing that is part of a greater dynamic organizing principle (Kaufman & Kaufman, 1983). The designers further claim that this test is a measure of "intellectual ability within the visual-vocal channel of communication and assesses the following ...: perceptual closure, perceptual inference, and conversion of abstract stimuli into concrete objects" (p. 42). It is our contention that for the younger children, the test is extremely depend-

---

[3]This is a measurement of the sensitivity of the participant to the stimuli. Essentially, low D prime scores demonstrate poor sensitivity (hitting the bar for every item would garner many Hits, in addition to many False Alarms). A perfect performance would result in a D prime approaching infinity.

ent on vocabulary skills. Indeed, the intercorrelation between Gestalt and the K-ABC Expressive Vocabulary is .47 (Kaufman & Kaufman, 1983) for preschool children. This is one of the highest intercorrelations seen between all the K-ABC subtests. Because Gestalt appears to tap into two processes that must occur in two steps, it is reported in two places: (a) immediate nonverbal (perceptual recognition), and (b) immediate verbal (for the second step, naming the recognized object).

Memory Measures—More Sequential

Card Task. This is an experimenter-designed measure. It is essentially a running *n*-back span test. The experimenter and the participant face a laptop. On the screen are three decks of cards; the bottom two decks are face down and belong respectively to the experimenter and the player. The upper deck placed in the middle of the screen represents the discard pile (see Fig. 8.1). The experimenter hits the space bar to control presentation of a card (i.e., to "flip up" a card) to the discard pile, and the participant hits any button on the mouse to flip up a card. These actions alternate. At quasi-random intervals, the experimenter hits a key that results in a picture of a hand covering up the discard pile. This is the cue to recall cards. Before cueing a recall the experimenter must wait until a set minimum number of cards have appeared and must also monitor that the participant's eyes have been on the screen throughout the sequence. The system does not allow the cards to be displayed at a rate faster than one per 2 s.

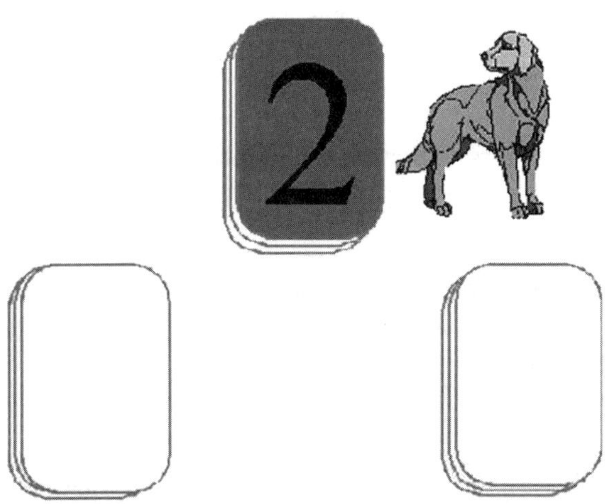

FIG. 8.1. Screen shot of Card Task color and number with distractor.

The participant is asked to recall the last card(s) viewed. The number of cards to be recalled varies by set. There are four sets of one, two, three, or, sometimes, four cards recalled in a sequence. Single cards that must be recalled after a sequence of intervening cards are called "onesies," two cards that must be recalled after a series of intervening cards are called "twosies," and so on. In each set there are four onesies, six twosies, three threesies—and if one threesie is recalled correctly, then three more threesies and two foursies are presented. Because none of the individuals with FXS got any of the foursies correct, those data are not reported here. In addition, there are two different blocks of difficulty, color only and color and number.

Before scoring begins, participants practice a onesie recall on the computer; then they practice a twosie recall with a real deck of cards. This is important because participants must understand the concept of recalling the card "on top" (the one closest to the hand) as the first card.[4] Participants practice with the real deck until they are correct. Participants then practice a twosie and a threesie on the computer. If they did not get a onesie correct, the game is sensitively terminated.

The Card Task contains two blocks. The first block is color only, consisting of red, green, yellow, and blue cards; the second block is color and number (col&num), consisting of the same four colors with the numerals 1, 2, 3, or 4 embedded in the middle of the colored card. Thus, there are 16 different cards in the second block and two pieces of information, or components, that must be recalled (e.g., "red three"). Participants practiced a onesie and a twosie on the computer before starting the task. In both blocks immediate feedback was given after every trial, and stickers or marbles were awarded for each correct trial. Participants seemed genuinely motivated throughout the task—and referred to it as the "game." Verbal encouragement was also given at approximately every third trial.

Card Task Distractors. Because incidental memory has been referred to as a potential relative strength in those with FXS, attractive distractors were displayed for 70 ms on the screen. Figure 8.1 shows a dog distractor. The hypothesis was that those with FXS may actually perform *better* when recalling the cards with distractors compared to the cards without distractors, and better when compared to the TD matched children. In the center of the color-only cards a small image of either a cow or a lion was displayed, and beside the col&num cards either a cat, whale, dog, or frog was displayed.

[4]In the piloted version, participants were allowed to recall either forward or backward, but that proved to be too confusing for both the participants and the experimenter. Therefore, participants were instructed to recall using the backward order strategy—which had been the most popular in the pilot sessions.

Distractor images were programmed to display in a random order at various intervals.[5]

The first time a distractor appeared on the screen the participant would often ask the experimenter what had just happened. The scripted reply was, "Sometimes those just show up." At the very end of the Card Task, participants were asked to recall all the distractor animals. Again, the hypothesis was that individuals with FXS would recall more of the incidental distractors than the TD matched children.

Verbal Auditory Learning (VAL). The Woodcock-Johnson III Tests of Cognitive Abilities (Woodcock, McGrew, & Mather, 2001) were used. Participants are first taught rebus symbols for words and then they read sentences written with the symbols. This test includes an immediate and delayed portion. At the end of the entire session, the delayed version is administered, approximately 1.5 h later. The symbols were not specifically retaught, although participants received immediate feedback on their performance (during both immediate and delayed versions).

Hand Movements. The K-ABC (Kaufman Assessment Battery for Children; Kaufman & Kaufman, 1983) was used. This test measures skill in imitating an experimenter's hand movements on a tabletop. The movements consist of a series of taps from a fist, flat palm, or side of the hand. This task is included because it has strong nonverbal components, although even the interpretive manual (Kaufman & Kaufman, 1983) admits that using mediating strategies, such as verbally labeling, would aid in performance. The purity of the measure may be further clouded by motor planning and execution issues.

RESULTS

As an overview, a comprehensive table that lists the memory measures in a two by four matrix is presented in Table 8.3. The group predicted to perform better is indicated.

Nonverbal Mental Age. The two groups were not significantly different; the scores included were based on either the CMMS or the mean of the Bead memory and Pattern analysis scores. See Table 8.1 for results.

---

[5]It was determined that there should be an approximate 50% chance of a distractor appearing in a given sequence. Thus, a 30% chance of seeing a distractor per card for onesies, a 16% per card chance for twosies, and an 11% chance per card for threesies were chosen. Stated another way, given the number of intervening cards per sequence, the chance of *not* having a distractor on a single card is .70 for onesies; thus the chance of *not* having a distractor on a two-card sequence would be (.7 × .7 or .49, for a three-card minimum threesie sequence it would be .84 × .84 × .84 or .59).

TABLE 8.3
Memory Tasks by Time, Mode, and Processing Type

Time and Mode	*Processing—More Simultaneous/Spatial*	*Predicted Favored Group*	*Processing—More Sequential*	*Predicted Favored Group*
Verbal Immediate	Toy Recall	FXS	Card Task (Twosies, Threesies—*reading TD match*)	TD
	Gestalt Mem. (vocab.)	FXS	Verbal Auditory Learning (VAL)	TD
Verbal Delayed	Card Task distractors	FXS (trend)	Verbal Auditory Learning (VAL—delay)	TD
	Toy Recall—delay			
Nonverbal Immediate	Gestalt Mem (recognition)	FXS	Hand movements	TD
Nonverbal Delayed	Toy Placement (delay)			

CPT Attention. Because there were no significant group differences, attention will be assumed to be similar for both groups. See Table 8.1 for results.

Memory—More Simultaneous/Spatial

Toy Recall. The TD group recalled on average 6.09 toys and the FXS group recalled on average 8.25 toys. This difference resulted in a statistical trend (two-tailed p value greater than .054 and less than .104) that favored the FXS group. See Table 8.4. There was no significant difference in the delayed toy recall.

Gestalt Closure. The TD group named on average 12.6 items and the FXS group named on average 18.07 items. The difference was statistically significant and the result favored the FXS group. Gestalt closure is listed twice in Tables 8.3 and 8.4 because it taps into both verbal (vocabulary) and nonverbal (perceptual recognition) aspects of immediate memory.

Naming Distractors From Card Task. Of the six animal distractors, on average the TD group recalled 28% and the FXS group recalled 39%; this difference resulted in a statistical trend favoring the FXS group. See Table 8.4.

TABLE 8.4
Results Comparing FXS and MA-Matched Groups With Effect Sizes and Favored Group (If Difference is a Trend or Better)

Measure	*TD, M (SD)*	*FX, M (SD)*	*t-Test*	*p*	*ES*	*Favored Group*
Verbal Immediate—Spatial						
Toy Recall I	6.09 (1.70)	8.25 (3.41)	$t_{(21)} = 1.89$	.07	.84	FX
Gestalt Mem. (vocab.)—raw	12.60 (3.86)	18.07 (3.35)	$t_{(21)} = 3.64$	.002	1.52	FX
Card Task—Onesies, %	57.88 (24.41)	56.67 (35.94)	$t < 1.0$			
Verbal Immediate—Sequential						
VAL—error count	32.60 (11.24)	50.71 (23.70)	$t_{(19.6)} = 2.23$	.04	1.04	TD
Card Task—Twosies, %	28.47 (22.24)	24.40 (22.35)	$t < 1.0$			
Card Task—Threesies, %	3.12 (8.54)	1.17 (4.38)	$t < 1.0$			
Verbal Delayed—Spatial						
Card Task Distractors						
Proportion recalled	.28 (.16)	.39 (.13)	$t_{(20)} = 1.71$	.10	.76	FX
Toy Recall II	4.63 (2.61)	5.92 (2.02)	$t_{(18)} = 1.25$		.56	
Verbal Delayed—Sequential						
VAL II—Delay-error count	28.67 (6.69)	49.43 (19.71)	$t_{(17.2)} = 3.63$	.002	.79	TD
Nonverbal Immed.—Spatial						
Gestalt Mem. (recog.)—raw	12.60 (3.86)	18.07 (3.35)	$t_{(21)} = 3.64$	.002	1.52	FX
Nonverbal Immed.—Sequential						
Hand Movements—raw	6.55 (2.46)	3.00 (2.16)	$t_{(22)} = 3.75$	.001	1.54	TD
Nonverbal Delayed—Spatial						
Toy Placement, mean cm	14.26 (4.47)	18.07 (7.85)	$t_{(22)} = 1.42$		.62	
Word Identification						
Raw Score	14.83 (23.24)	36.80 (23.16)	$t_{(18)} = 2.12$	.048	.95	FX
Age Equivalents	5.97 (1.51)	8.00 (1.34)	$t_{(18)} = 2.99$	.008		FX

Note. When variances are significantly unequal, the degrees of freedom are adjusted and contain a decimal place.

Memory—More sequential

Card Task. Results on the Card Task indicate that the two groups did not differ on percent correct in each set of the onesies, twosies, or threesies. Results for the onesies are listed in Table 8.4 under Verbal Immediate Spatial (rather than sequential, because participants were only recalling the very last item seen). The results for the twosies and threesies are listed in Table 9.4 under Verbal Immediate Sequential. Again, the FXS and MA matched groups performed equivalently when recalling cards.

Card Task—Recalling with Distractors. How did the distractors affect performance? The results were collapsed across sets; that is, onesie, twosie, and threesie performances have been aggregated. The blocks have been analyzed separately. For color only, the proportion correct of cards recalled when there was no distractor present was .48 (.14) for the TD group, and .37 (.19) for the FXS group. This difference resulted in a trend that favored the TD group; $F(1, 31) = 3.50$, $p = .07$. The proportion correct when a distractor was present on one of the cards recalled was .37 (.23) for the TD group and .44 (.37) for the FX group. This difference was not statistically significant. In addition, the group differences were not significant for the color and number performances. The overall pattern for color only (the simpler task) would lend some support to the hypothesis that when a distractor is present the FXS group would do somewhat better on the task than the TD group. That is, what is "distracting," incidental, and novel to a TD child may actually aid an individual with FXS in encoding an entire image and recalling it later.

Verbal-Auditory Learning (VAL), –Verbal–Sequential. The number of errors made on the VAL–Immediate recall was on average 32.60 for the TD group and 50.71 for the FXS group. Table 9.4 demonstrates that the TD performance was significantly better. For the delayed version of the VAL (given approximately 1.5 h later) the TD group extended their lead somewhat, making only 28.67 errors compared the FXS group's 49.43 errors. This difference significantly favored the TD group.

Hand Movements–Nonverbal–Sequential. The number correct of imitated hand movements was on average 6.55 for the TD group and 3.00 for the FXS group. This resulted in a statistically significant difference favoring the TD group. See Table 8.4.

Toy Placement–Nonverbal–Delayed–Spatial. When asked to replace the toys after an approximate 2-h delay, the TD group deviated 14.26 cm from the point of original placement (this represents the average for all 16 toys). The FXS group deviated 18.07 cm. The group difference was not statistically significant.

Reading and the Developmental Picture

In the first section the results are based on the differences between the FXS group and a TD group matched for nonverbal mental age. Those TD children had a chronological mean age of 5;5. In order to view a more developmental picture and ask how the FXS group will compare to a TD group that has increased in skill level and has attained the ability to sound out words, a second group of TD children was matched on real world reading. Word ID or real word reading is also of interest because it is one of the few variables on which the FXS group outperformed the younger TD matches. Further, we were interested in how the FXS group compared to a TD group that was matched on a more verbal measure, rather then a nonverbal measure. Because the recall of sequential items is often mediated via the phonological loop, the reading task was deemed appropriate. Because the focus of this chapter is on memory and sequencing skill, the Card Task was chosen as the dependent variable of interest for this section.

First, a review of reading for the TD population is offered, and then reading for the MR populations. Reading is very important for individuals with developmental delays, because reading can be a potent factor in increasing self-sufficiency and self-esteem. In addition, reading adds to the individual with MR's experience base a multitude of events that are outside of the present environment (Butler, 1979). Enhancing basic decoding (the ability to sound out or decipher print) skills would allow an individual many newfound and quality-of-life-enhancing opportunities, such as reading want ads, using a recipe, and finding the proper bus at the correct time.

Typically Developing Reading. In the simple view of reading, Gough and Tunmer (1986) portion reading into two distinct processes: decoding and linguistic comprehension skills. The latter are essentially all the higher level processing skills that occur after decoding. In the decoding realm, three letter-sound capabilities must be present for fluency: (a) knowledge of letter shapes, (b) knowledge of the grapheme (letter) to phoneme (sound) correspondences, and (c) phonemic segmentation skills (Adams, 1990; Ehri, 1998). In addition, some functional level of assembly, which includes both memory storage and processing, must be present. Assembly is the ability to sequence the sounds together and the Card Task is an appropriate estimate of these grosser level assembly skills.

Linnea Ehri (1991, 1994, 1995) describes four developmental phases that represent the sequence of learning to read in the typically developing population. These phases are:

1. The prealphabetic phase, in which memories for words are formed using visual cues in the words (e.g., two tall sticks are in the middle of *yellow*). Children here are typically 4 to 5.5 years old.
2. The partial alphabetic phase, in which partial cues are formed between graphemes and phonemes. In this phase salient positions are overimportant; often only the first and last letters may be used to

sound out the word. Readers lack full knowledge of the grapheme/phoneme mappings in this phase, particularly regarding vowels. Children here are typically 6 to 7 years old.

3. The full alphabetic phase, in which readers remember how to read sight words by forming a complete set of mappings between all graphemes and phonemes in the word. Reading is not yet fast and fluent. Children here are typically 7 to 8 years old.
4. Finally, the consolidated alphabetic phase, in which readers possess the ability to retain the full alphabetic phase in memory without much processing. Mastery here allows for an expanding print lexicon because letter patterns that recur across different words become consolidated or unitized. Consolidation means readers can now decode using flexible multiletter units. Children here are typically 8.5 and older.

Mastery of Phase 1 relies primarily on visuo-spatial memory skills. To achieve mastery in Phase 2 requires somewhat stable grapheme/phoneme correspondences, and rudimentary sequencing or assembly skills. To achieve mastery in Phase 3, a reader must possess stable enough correspondences and assembly skills to sound out nonwords. To achieve mastery at Phase 4, a reader must possess distinct and automatic letter/sound correspondences, as well as felicitous assembly skills, with adult-like levels of flexibility that are evident under cognitive load.

Our lab is interested in assessing how males with FXS progress through these phases. Are there particular sticking points in the progression? If so, where? This research will be important for guiding remediation. Ehri's research suggests that after the minimal baseline skills needed for the rote naming of whole words in Phase 1 has been attained, two subprocesses must be functioning for transition to Phase 2. These subprocesses involve phonological skills and assembly. In this section, we present data on phonological skills via the reading of nonwords and assembly via the Card Task.

Reading in Individuals With MR. Individuals with MR read well below their own mental ages (Katims, 2000; Singh & Singh, 1986). It has only been very recently that those with MR have been seriously and systematically instructed in learning how to read (Katims, 2000). Much of the instruction (until the mid 1990s) relied on isolated mastery of linear subskills which did not engage the students in connected, more authentic texts (Katims, 1996). Conners (2003) cautions that reading acquisition depends on instruction and exposure, and metions that there have been great advances in instruction and educational services for individuals with MR in the past 15 years. Many students with MR now have access to reading instruction and they are learning to read (Byrne, MacDonald, & Buckley, 2002). These individuals continue to make progress in reading throughout adolescence and young adulthood (Moni & Jobling, 2000).

We are interested in etiologically specific profiles. Even recently researchers (Conners et al., 2001) have analyzed samples of children with MR together without specifying etiology. We realize it is difficult to find large numbers, but attempts should be made even with smaller numbers. Indeed, the environment appears to be changing, Boudreau (2002) analyzed how early literacy skills (e.g., letter naming, rhyming, blending, etc.) in children and adolescents with DS compare with those found in MA-matched TD children. Roberts et al. (2005) report on individuals with FXS ages 4–13 using the Woodcock Johnson Psychoeducational Battery. At 8 years of age, they report an average W score on letter word recognition of 394 (TD average = 500), and an age slope of .77.

Unfortunately, there is not a clear picture of the reading subprocesses profile for those with FXS. This chapter represents an attempt to analyze some of the subprocesses involved in reading (memory, attention, sequencing, and nonwords reading skills) as they relate to reading real words. In addition, because assembly is an import skill in reading and is necessary for more emergent downstream functions, we present data on the Card Task for two groups.

Participants. The same FXS group was used for the following analyses and seven of the TD participants were retained. Six new TD participants were recruited. The TD group was created to match on reading skill as measured by the Word Identification subtest of the Woodcock Reading Mastery Tests–Revised (Woodcock, 1998). This resulted in a somewhat older TD group, mean age 7;6. The new TD reading match group is over 2 years older than the previous TD nonverbal mental age match group.

Measures. The Word Identification subtest of the Woodcock Reading Mastery Tests–Revised (Woodcock, 1998) was used to create the reading-match group. Participants read real words. In addition, performance on the Word Attack subtest of the Woodcock Reading Mastery Tests–Revised (Woodcock, 1998) is reported. In Word Attack participants read nonwords from an easel page until six consecutive errors. Analyses were also run on the Continuous Performance Task measuring attention. The descriptive statistics, *t*-tests, and effect sizes for the new, older group are listed in Table 8.5.

Card Task With Word ID Reading Match. Because there were significant differences in these group comparisons, the Card Task sets have been bro-

TABLE 8.5
Descriptives, *t*-Tests, and ES for the Reading (WordID) Match and FXS Groups

	TD	*FX*	*t-Test*	*ES*
n	13	15		
Chronological Age	7.60 (2.08)	20.56[a] (9.23)	$t_{(15.7)} = 5.04$, $p < .000$	2.29
Word ID raw	41.15 (33.84)	39.13 (22.36)	< 1.0	0.07
Word ID age equivalent	8.08 (2.63)	7.99 (1.30)	< 1.0	
Word Attack raw	16.38[a] (14.90)	5.23 (8.99)	$t_{(19.1)} = 2.35$, $p = .03$	0.93
Word Attack age equivalent	8.67[a] (3.43)	6.45 (1.57)	$t_{(16.3)} = 2.14$, $p = .04$	0.91
Nonverbal Mental Age	8.71[a] (3.94)	5.19 (1.33)	$t_{(14.3)} = 3.06$, $p = .008$	1.33
Attention-CPT D Prime 1	3.82[a] (0.86)	2.63 (1.45)	$t_{(13.3)} = 2.03$, $p = .06$	1.03
Attention-CPT D Prime 2	3.40[a] (1.37)	2.13 (0.81)	$t_{(9.2)} = 2.16$, $p = .06$	1.17

[a]Favored group.

ken down into their subcomponents. That is, for color and number there may have only been six trials for the twosies, but there were 24 components to be recalled when counting both color and number on each card as a component. Table 8.6 lists the results.

In the color-only block the TD reading-match group consistently and significantly outperformed the FXS group. In the color and number (col&num) block the component analyses revealed trends or significant differences between the groups. From twosies onward this task was very difficult for both populations, and only four of the FXS participants made it onto the threesie col&num set. These results support the contention that males with FXS may be able to perform sequential memory tasks similar to nonverbal mental age-matched TD children around 5 years of age, but when compared with reading-matched TD children around 7 years of age, males with FXS perform significantly worse. Performance on the color-only cards is actually *negatively* correlated with chronological age for the males with FXS (although this is not statistically significant; correlational coefficients range from –.09 to –.19). For the TD group only twosies was significantly correlated with chronological age; this was in the positive direction ($r = .48$, $p = .05$).

TABLE 8.6
Percent Correct and t-Tests on Card Task With WordID Match Group

Card Task	*WordID–TD*	*FX*	*t-Test*	*p*	*n*
Color only					On avg. TD = 13 FX = 15
Onesies (4 trials)	82.69 (21.37)	50.00 (36.59)	$t_{(26)} = 2.83$	.009	
Twosies (6 trials)	51.15 (24.69)	22.20 (23.06)	$t_{(26)} = 3.21$	.004	
Twosies—components, max. 12	66.69 (18.88)	45.07 (20.72)	$t_{(26)} = 2.87$	.008	
Threesies (3 or 6 trials)	18.75 (26.05)	1.17 (4.38)	$t_{(11.5)} = 2.31$	.040	
Threesies—components, max. 9 or 18	45.25 (25.11)	25.58 (21.69)	$t_{(22)} = 2.05$	.052	
Color and number					
Onesies (4 trials)	64.58 (34.47)	44.64 (32.79)	$t_{(24)} = 1.51$		
Onesie—components, max. 8	78.25 (24.55)	57.85 (31.37)	$t_{(22)} = 1.77$	.090	
Twosies (6 trials)	23.67 (35.07)	6.46 (10.85)	$t_{(12.9)} = 1.63$		
Twosies—components, max. 24	58.42 (23.88)	33.77 (18.39)	$t_{(22)} = 2.83$	.010	
Threesies (3 or 6 trials)	5.00 (11.19)	.00 (.00)	$t_{(12)} = 1.41$		TD = 10 FX = 4
Threesies—components, max.18 or 36	48.60 (18.05)	29.75 (14.45)	$t_{(12)} = 1.85$	.089	TD = 10

DISCUSSION

Simultaneous/Spatial Processing

The results here indicate that males with FXS demonstrate some relative strengths compared to TD MA-matched children. In the simultaneous verbal processing realm, males with FXS demonstrate impressive effect sizes ranging from .76 to 1.52 when performance is compared to the TD MA-matched group on both immediate (toy recall and gestalt memory) and moderately delayed recalls (recall of the Card Task distractors). Table 8.3 supplies a succinct summary of the memory tasks and favored groups. The tasks favoring the FXS group have simultaneous and spatial processing in common, and are not contingent on sequencing skills or long term delays. Additionally, they are not contingent on learning, where this term refers to the integrating of new information into a longer term store area (like the neocortex).

One of these tasks, gestalt memory, has a history of favoring FXS groups (Hodapp et al., 1992), but this outcome may be more reflective of world knowledge/vocabulary skills than actual processing differences. It is difficult to say with any authority because gestalt memory taps two distinct cognitive components: perceptual recognition and object naming at the lexical level.

Card Task Distractors

Regarding the trend favoring the FXS group in recalling card task distractors, results on this task are particularly interesting because delayed tasks were predicted to be difficult across the board for the FXS group. However, this recall task has two elements in it that need to be explicated. First, the delay in this task was very short compared to the other delay tasks (minutes vs. almost two hours). There may be a few-minutes-wide window in which information is considered "immediate," and after that access to and recall of the information fall off dramatically.[6] Second, there is some evidence that individuals with FXS are very attuned to incidental information, that is, information that does not serve the task's end goal. Munir et al. (2000) speculate that males with FXS may demonstrate lower scores when information to be recalled is "meaningless." One might predict that attending to the animal distractors would not aid an individual in the end goal of the task (i.e., recalling cards); however, the distractors might still be *meaningful* to the males with FXS, but in a very different manner than for the TD-matched group.

The animal distractors are new (novel and odd) and attractive (colorful). One of the functions of the hippocampus is to mark information as being novel (Gluck & Myers, 2001). Assessing and tagging incoming information as new, or as information that has not been codified before in a certain context, is valuable for learning and survival. Because the HC is larger in males with FXS (Reiss et al., 1994) and torturous dendritic spines have been observed in various parts of the brain—including cerebral cortex and visual and temporal cortices (Irwin et al., 2001)—we can assume there are differences in processes associated with these regions. Furthermore, Ivanco and Greenough (2000) investigated mossy fiber sprouting from the HC (the CA3 region) in FMRP knockout and wild-type mice. They discovered ex-

[6]Ericsson and Kitsch (1996) have proposed a "long-term working memory" that operates just such a manner, they explore its use primarily in text comprehension.

cess sprouting of the fibers in the knockout mice. One theory is that there is insufficient pruning in the brains of those with FXS. We hypothesize that inappropriate attention to incidental information may be one of the consequences of poor pruning.

One conjecture regarding the recall of distractors by the males with FXS in this study is that although the males with FXS recalled more distractors, suggesting they may have been more attuned to them, the distractors may also have aided the FXS group in recalling the paired cards. In the color-only condition, the FXS group demonstrated an ES of .23 compared to the TD children on recall of cards that were paired with distractors; that is, the distractors may have had a paradoxical effect of facilitating recall for the FXS group. Perhaps because some males with FXS sample environments in a more gestalt or holistic manner, they recalled the entire computer screen (distractor and card together), as opposed to the TD children who may have been devoting effort to suppressing the distractor at the expense of recalling the attendant card.

In sum, what might be distracting, that is, incidental and unserving of the end goal to a TD child, may actually aid an individual with FXS with encoding and recalling. This may be because the HC does not compress and interleave the novel information in a succinct and meaningful manner. The information encoded with the novel items is given extra vigilance and the memory is therefore stronger. This ongoing vigilance for, and attention to, new information and the inability to compress and accommodate it in long-term store may also explain some of the hyperarousal and anxiety issues seen in the FXS population.

Sequential Processing

Further comparisons focusing on the more sequential memory domain indicate an area of significant deficit in the males with FXS. The FXS group performed worse on tasks relying heavily on the ability to sequence—the verbal auditory learning tasks (both immediate and delayed)—and on the hand movements imitation task (immediate/nonverbal). Although there were no differences between the younger TD MA-matched group and the group with FXS on the sequential card task, when the FXS group was compared to the more developmentally advanced TD reading-matched group, differences were revealed. The males with FXS performed significantly worse on all the twosie and threesie component counts.

The card task results demonstrate that the males with FXS may be sequencing relative to their NV mental age; however, they are not sequencing commensurate to their real-word reading skills. This implies that they may be reading individual words without using sequencing. If they are only memorizing whole words, they may be stuck in phases 1 and 2 of Ehri's phase sequence.

What makes sequencing so difficult? It involves several steps: (a) encoding the information, (b) holding or rehearsing the information in working memory, as an ongoing loop, (c) concatenating incoming components, (d) retrieving the components, and (e) reproducing the string of information. We hypothesize that there were no problems at the first and final levels of encoding and reproduction as the males with FXS performed almost equivalently to the TD children in the onesies condition (col&num). The problems may reside within stages 2, 3, and 4. Attentional resources would surely play a role in the rehearsing of the information, and it is evident that the older TD children have better attentional skills (ES > 1.00). Somewhere along the TD developmental trajectory between the mean age of 5½, and up to 7½ years, the cognitive processes responsible for sequencing and recalling information are developing and surpassing the average performance levels of our sample of males with FXS.

Future Research

Because the cognition involved in sequential memory skills is multistage, complex, and contingent on timing, it lends itself to neural network modeling. A model is currently being designed to simulate and explicate memory processes involved in the Card Task (Johnson-Glenberg, submitted). In addition, more research needs to be conducted with a developmental story in mind. End states are only part of the story. How and when do the working memory skills of the TD population and those with FXS begin to diverge and in which domains? As TD children develop, their memory skills increase and this may be due to several factors. Cowan (1997) posited six that would all be correlated with age and brain growth (and myelination). Memory increase is probably an emergent interaction of multiple factors.

How does understanding the different memory trajectories for the two populations affect the design of cognitive remediation programs for those with FXS? One question of particular interest is how poor sequencing skills might affect reading skills. The reading of new words is contingent on sounding out a sequence of phonemes. If males with FXS display deficits in holding a sequence of information in the phonological loop until they have finished pronouncing a word, they will be very disadvantaged when reading connected text. If sequencing is so disturbed in the males with FXS, then they may only be able to learn via whole word training. But this would limit them in the ability to learn new words and to expand their lexicons independently. One way to circumvent the problems of poor phonological awareness and/or poor sequencing may be with strategies. There are several respected reading programs that add a multimodal component to the learning of letter/sound correspondences. Particularly helpful may be those that stress articulatory awareness. Future research should be devoted to strategy training intervention programs.

How and when do word attack and word identification skills (the reading of real words) begin to diverge? Results from this study demonstrate that the reading of nonwords lags 1.5 years behind the reading of real words for the males with FXS. This significant difference may be due to either phonological awareness or cognitive processing (sequencing) issues or overall working memory deficits. The difference observed in real word and nonword reading in males with FXS is not present in TD readers. Do males with FXS begin very early on to rely on their relatively stronger immediate/simultaneous skills to memorize whole words? And, is this at the expense of putting effort into learning the orthographic–phonemic (letter to sound) correspondences that would be necessary to decode nonwords, and novel words. If so, then the orthographic–phonemic system does not get stimulated at an early age, and it would not have the chance to properly prune. It is also important that future research assess what kinds of clinical interventions have occurred to date with each individual. Several parents of children with FXS reported using flash-card type reading programs with their children; this training would encourage a more whole-word process. Roberts et al. (2005) recommend that future work include "in-depth" measures of (among others) reading, writing, passage comprehension, phonetic decoding, and rhyming

The Developmental Picture and Limitations. This small study did not have the resources to follow participants longitudinally. Tracking individuals' development over time would allow us to ascertain the mental age where the divergence between real word and nonword reading would emerge in males with FXS. Coincidentally, the cognitive correlates could also be mapped. One hypothesis is that the divergence may occur around the time Ehri's (1991, 1998) Phase 2 decoding skills emerge. Phase 2, or the partial alphabetic phase, emerges between 6 and 7 years of age in TD children. However, in a population of TD children the underlying cognitive correlates are also developing traditionally—that is, memory is coming online and phonological processes are developing and expanding in a typical manner. We do not know enough about the ongoing sequential development of memory and phonology in individuals with FXS to say which one of these correlates may first be getting off track, or how far it gets off track, or if both subsystems—once derailed—take each other interactively further off track. All that is known about the complex reading system in this population is that it is compromised. With a clearer developmental timeline for the important cognitive correlates that feed into reading, it may also be possible to administer remediations at "optimal" time-course windows. Remediation is an area that deserves far more future research.

Two other pressing questions fragile X studies should address involve coincidence of autism with FXS and more precise DNA information. This small study did not have the resources to conduct genetic testing, nor to hire experts to administer autism screening measures.

New Tools. There are many new tools being used to more precisely assess how structural and neurochemical dysfunctions can lead to behavioral functioning. Particularly noteworthy is the work with functional magnetic resonance imaging (fMRI). One example of an intriguing memory finding comes from Greicius, Boyett-Anderson, Menon, and Reiss (2004). They found that girls with FXS displayed significantly less activation in the HC and basal forebrain when compared to TD age-matched controls using a visual memory encoding task. This supports the hypothesis that the HC is compromised for immediate memory tasks in some individuals with FXS.

Applications. Again, it may be that individuals with FXS would benefit from the explicit training in strategies, for example, the strategy to verbally mediate hand movements. Using a verbal cue to perform a physical task may have applications in the life skills sector as well. We have hypothesized that pruning problems in the brain may cause some of the cognitive dysfunctions observed in males with FXS. If this is the case, then it would be important to continue to strengthen the connections that are already established, because parts of the brain are plastic throughout life. Cognitive practice can occur at many levels and might take on a game-like format using some of the new software available. It is important to tune training to match a motivating topic in the student's life. This is true even as the student ages.

Using developmental terminology, it would be inappropriate to take the term *end state* literally. The individual has not reached the end of learning even when tested at 38 years of age (the oldest participant in this study). Johnson-Glenberg and Chapman (2004) encouraged parents of children with Down syndrome to continue increasing and stimulating their children's vocabulary into adulthood. Encouragement should be given to the parents of children and the caregivers and educators of individuals with FXS to provide intervention directed toward increasing this population's memory and reading skills throughout the life span.

ACKNOWLEDGMENTS

This research was funded by the FRAXA Foundation and a small grant from the National Institutes of Health (NIH), MRDD-RO3 HD39362-01. Special thanks to Renee Duffy, Amy Shefchik, Yu Cheung Shum, David

Wilson, Len Abbeduto and his dedicated lab group, Jonathan Glenberg, and Sally Miles. Author can be contacted at mina@neuronfarm.com

REFERENCES

Abbeduto, L., Evans, J., & Dolan, T. (2001). Theoretical perspectives on language and communication problems in mental retardation and developmental disabilities. *Mental Retardation and Developmental Disabilities Research Reviews, 7*, 45–55.

Abbeduto, L., Murphy, M. M., Cawthon, S. W., Richmond, E., Weissman, M. D., Karadottir, S., & O'Brien, A. (2003). Receptive language skills of adolescents and young adults with Down or fragile X syndrome. *American Journal on Mental Retardation, 108*(3), 149–160.

Abraham, F., Abraham, R., & Shaw, C. (1990). *A visual introduction to dynamic systems theory for psychology*. Ithaca, NY: Aerial Press.

Adams, M. J. (1990). *Beginning to read*. Cambridge, MA: MIT Press.

Atkinson, R. C., & Shiffrin, R. M. (1968). Human memory: A proposed system and its control processes. In K. W. Spence & J. T. Spence (Eds.), *Psychology of learning and motivation: II* (pp. 162–181). Oxford: Academic Press.

Baddeley, A. (1986). *Working memory*. Oxford: Clarendon Press.

Belmont, J. M., & Butterfield, E. C. (1969). The relations of short term memory to development and intelligence. In L. C. Lipsitt & H. W. Reese (Eds.), *Advances in child development and behavior* (Vol. 4, pp. 71–82). New York: Academic Press.

Boudreau, D. (2002). Literacy skills in children and adolescents with Down syndrome. *Reading & Writing, 15*(5–6), 497–525.

Butler, D. (1979). *Cushla and her books*. Boston: Horn Book.

Byrne, A., MacDonald, J., & Buckley, S. (2002). Reading, language and memory skills: A comparative longitudinal study of children with Down syndrome and their mainstream peers. *British Journal of Educational Psychology, 72*, 513–529.

Campione, J. C., & Brown, A. L. (1977). Memory and metamemory development in educable retarded children. In R.V. Kail, Jr., & W. J. Hagen (Eds.), *Perspectives on the development of memory and cognition* (pp. 367–406). Hillsdale, NJ: Lawrence Erlbaum Associates.

Carrow-Woolfolk, E. (1985). *Test for Auditory Comprehension of Language–Revised*. Allen, TX: DLM Teaching Resources.

Chapman, R. S. (2000). Children's language learning: An interactionist perspective. *Journal of Child Psychology and Psychiatry and Allied Disciplines, 41*(1), 33–54.

Conners, F. A. (2003). Reading skills and cognitive abilities in individuals with mental retardation. In L. Abbeduto (Ed.), *International review of research in mental retardation* (Vol. 27, pp. 71–82). New York: Elsevier.

Conners, F., Atwell, J., Rosenquist, C., & Sligh, A. (2001). Abilities underlying decoding differences in children with intellectual disability. *Journal of Intellectual Disability Research, 45*, 292–299.

Cornish, K. M., Turk, J., Wilding, J., Sudhalter, V., Munir, F., Kooy, F., & Hagerman, R. (2004). Deconstructing the attention deficit in fragile X syndrome: A developmental neuropsychological approach. *Journal of Child Psychology and Psychiatry, 45*(6), 1042–1053.

Cowan, N. T. (1997). The development of working memory. In N. T. Cowan (Ed.), *The development of memory in childhood* (pp. 163–199). Sussex, England: Psychology Press.

Crosby, K. G. (1972). Attention and distractibility in mentally retarded and intellectually average children. *American Journal of Mental Deficiency, 77*(1), 46–53.

Dempster, F. N. (1981). Memory span: Sources of developmental and individual differences. *Psychological Bulletin, 89,* 63–100.

Dykens, E. M., Hodapp, R. M., & Leckman, J. F. (1987). Strengths and weaknesses in the intellectual functioning of males with fragile X syndrome. *American Journal of Mental Deficiency, 92*(2), 234–236.

Ehri, L. (1991). Development of the ability to read words. In R. Barr, P. Mosenthal, & P. Pearson (Eds.), *Handbook of reading research* (Vol. II, pp. 383–417). New York: Longman.

Ehri, L. (1994). Development of the ability to read words: Update. In R. Ruddell, M. Ruddell, & H. Singer (Eds.), *Theoretical models and processes of reading* (4th ed., pp. 323–358). Newark, DE: International Reading Association.

Ehri, L. (1995) Phases of development in learning to read words by sight. *Journal of Research in Reading, 18,* 116–125

Ehri, L. (1998). Grapheme-phoneme knowledge is essential for learning to real words in English. In J. L. Metsala & L. C. Ehri (Eds.), *Word recognition in beginning literacy* (pp. 3–40). Mahwah, NJ: Lawrence Erlbaum Associates.

Ellis, N. R. (1963). The stimulus trace and behavioral inadequacy. In N. R. Ellis (Ed.), *Handbook of mental deficiency* (pp. 134–158). New York: McGraw Hill.

Ellis, N. R. (1970). Memory processes in retardates and normals. In N. R. Ellis (Ed.), *International review of research in mental retardation* (Vol. 4, pp. 241–273). New York, Academic Press.

Elman, J. L., Bates, E. A., Johnson, M. H., Karmiloff-Smith, A., Parisi, D., & Plunkett, K. (1996). *Rethinking innateness: A connectionist perspective on development.* Cambridge, MA: MIT Press.

Ericsson, A. K., & Kintsch, W. (1995). Long term working memory. *Psychological Review, 102*(2), 211–245.

Flavell, J. H., Beach, D. H., & Chinsky, J. M. (1966). Spontaneous verbal rehearsal in a memory task as a function of age. *Child Development, 37,* 283–299.

French, J., & Worcester, D. A. (1956). Critical study of the Columbia Mental Maturity Scale. *Exceptional Children, 23,* 111–113.

Freund, L. S., & Reiss, A. L. (1991). Cognitive profiles associated with fra(X) syndrome in males and females. *American Journal of Medical Genetics, 38,* 542–547.

Gluck, M. A., & Myers, C. E. (2001). *Gateway to memory: An introduction to neural network modeling and the hippocampus and learning.* Cambridge, MA: MIT Press.

Gough, P. B., & Tunmer, W. E. (1986). Decoding, reading, and reading disability. *Remedial and Special Education, 7,* 6–10.

Greicius, M. D., Boyett-Anderson, J. M., Menon, V., & Reiss, A. L. (2004). Reduced basal forebrain and hippocampal activation during memory encoding in girls with fragile X syndrome. *Neuroreport, 15*(10), 1579–1584.

Hodapp, R. M., Leckman, J. F., Dykens, E. M., Sparrow, S. S., Zelinsky, D. G., & Ort, S. I. (1992). K-ABC profiles in children with fragile X syndrome, Down syndrome, and nonspecific mental retardation. *American Journal on Mental Retardation, 97*(1), 39–46.

Howieson, D. B., & Lezak, M. D. (1995). Separating memory from other cognitive problems. In A. D. Baddeley, B. A. Wilson, & F. N. Watts (Eds.), *Handbook of memory disorders* (pp. 411– 426). Oxford: John Wiley & Sons.

Irwin, S. A., Galvez, R., & Greenough, W. T. (2000). Dendritic spine structural anomalies in fragile X mental retardation syndrome. *Cerebral Cortex, 10,* 1038–1044.

Irwin, S., Patel, B., Idupulapati, M., Harris, J., Crisostomo, R., Larson, B., et al. (2001). Abnormal dendritic spine characteristics in the temporal and visual cortices of patients with fragile X syndrome. *American Journal of Medical Genetics, 98,* 161–167.

Ivanco, T. L., & Greenough, W. T. (2000). Fragile X knockout mice show an increase in mossy fiber sprouting in the hippocampus compared to wildtype mice. *Society for Neuroscience Abstracts, 26*(223), 80.12.

Johnson-Glenberg, M. (submitted). *Fragile X syndrome: A neural network model of working memory in males.*

Johnson-Glenberg, M. C., & Chapman, R. S. (2004). Predictors of parent–child language during novel task play: A comparison between typically developing children and individuals with Down syndrome. *Journal of Intellectual Disability Research, 48*(3), 225–238.

Karmiloff-Smith, A., Brown, J. H., Grice, S., & Paterson, S. (2003). Dethroning the myth: Cognitive dissociations and innate modularity in Williams syndrome. *Developmental Neuropsychology, 23*(1 & 2), 229–244.

Karmiloff-Smith, A., & Thomas, M. S. (2002). Developmental disorders. In M. A. Arbib (Ed.), *The handbook of brain theory and neural networks* (2nd ed., pp. 292–294). Cambridge, MA: MIT Press.

Katims, D. (1996). The emergence of literacy in elementary students with mild mental retardation. *Focus on Autism and Other Developmental Disabilities, 11,* 147–157.

Katims, D. S. (2000). Literacy instruction for people with mental retardation: Historical highlights and contemporary analysis. *Education and Training in Mental Retardation and Developmental Disabilities, 35,* 3–15.

Kaufman A. S., & Kaufman, N. L. (1983). *Kaufman Assessment Battery for Children—Interpretive manual.* Circle Pines, MN: AGS.

Maccoby, E. E., & Hagen, J. W. (1965). Effects of distraction upon central versus incidental recall: Developmental trends. *Journal of Experimental Child Psychology, 2,* 280–289.

Mazzocco, M., & Reiss, A. L. (1999). Behavioral neurogenetics approach to understanding the fragile X syndrome. In H. Tager-Flusberg (Ed.), *Neurodevelopmental disorders: Contributions to a new framework from cognitive neurosciences* (pp. 43–63). Cambridge, MA: MIT Press.

McClelland, J. L., & Goddard, N. H. (1996). Considerations arising from a complementary learning systems perspective on hippocampus and neocortex. *Hippocampus, 6,* 654–665.

McClelland, J. L., McNaughton, B. L., & O'Reilly, R. C. (1995). Why there are complementary learning systems in the hippocampus and neocortex: Insights from the successes and failures of connectionist models of learning and memory. *Psychological Review, 102*(3), 419–457.

Miles, S., & Chapman, R. S. (2002). Narrative content as described by individuals with Down syndrome and typically developing children. *Journal of Speech, Language, and Hearing Research, 45,* 175–189.

Miyake, A., Friedman, N. P., Emerson, N. J., Witzki, A. H., Howerter, A., & Wager, T. D. (2000). The unity and diversity of the executive functions and their contribution to "frontal lobe" tasks: A latent variable analysis. *Cognitive Psychology, 41,* 49–100.

Moni, K. B., & Jobling, A. (2001). Reading-related literacy learning of young adults with Down syndrome: Findings from a three year teaching and research program. *International Journal of Disability, Development and Education, 48,* 377–394.

Munir, F., Cornish, K. M., & Wilding, J. (2000). Nature of the working memory deficit in fragile-X syndrome. *Brain and Cognition, 44,* 387–401.

Naus, M. J., Ornstein, P. A., & Aivano, S. (1977). Developmental changes in memory: The effects of processing time and rehearsal instructions. *Journal of Experimental Child Psychology, 23,* 237–251.

Oberle, I., Rousseau, F., Heitz, D., Kretz, C., Devys, D., Hanauer, A., Boue, J., et al. (1991). Instability of a 550-base pair DNA segment and abnormal methylation in fragile X syndrome. *Science, 252,* 1097–1102.

Pascual-Leone, J. (1970). A mathematical model for the transition rule in Piaget's developmental stages. *Acta Psychologica, 32,* 301–345.

Reiss, A., & Freund, L. (1992). Behavioral phenotype of fragile X syndrome: DSM–III–R autistic behavior in male children. *American Journal of Medical Genetics, 43,* 35–46.

Reiss, A. L., Lee, J., & Freund, L. (1994). Neuroanatomy of fragile X syndrome: The temporal lobe. *Neurology, 44,* 1317–1324.

Roberts, J., Long, S., Malkin, C., Barnes, E., Skinner, M., Hennon, E., et al. (2005). A comparison of phonological skills in young males with fragile X and Down syndrome. *Journal of Speech, Language, and Hearing Research, 48,* 980–995.

Scharfenaker, S., O'Connor, R., Stackhouse, T., Braden, M., Hickman, L., & Gray, K. (1996). An integrated approach to intervention. In R. Hagerman & A. Cronister (Eds.), *Fragile X syndrome* (2nd ed., pp. 349–411). Baltimore: Johns Hopkins Press.

Singh, N. N., & Singh, J. (1986). Reading acquisition and remediation in the mentally retarded. In N. R. Ellis & N. W. Bray (Eds.), *International review of research in mental retardation* (Vol. 14, pp. 165–199). New York: Academic Press.

Sobesky, W. E., Hull, C. E., & Hagerman, R. J. (1992). The emotional phenotype in mildly affected carriers. In R. J. Hagerman & P. McKenzie (Eds.), *1992 International Fragile X Conference proceedings* (pp. 99–106). Denver: Spectra/National Fragile X Foundation.

Smith, M. L., & Milner, B. (1981). The role of the right hippocampus in the recall of spatial location. *Neuropsychologia, 19*(6), 781–793.

Thelen, E. (1994). *A dynamic systems approach to the development of cognition and action.* Cambridge, MA: MIT Press.

Thorndike, R. L., Hagen, E. P., & Sattler, J. M. (1986). *The Stanford-Binet Intelligence Scale: Fourth Edition.* Chicago: Riverside.

Verkerk, A. J., Pieretti, M., Sutliffe, J. S., Fu, Y. H., Kuhl, D. P., Pizutti, A., Reiner, O., et al. (1991). Identification of a gene (FMR-1) containing a CGG repeat coincident with a breakpoint cluster region exhibiting length variation in fragile X syndrome. *Cell, 65,* 905–914.

Weiss, B., Weisz, J. R., & Bromfield, R. (1986). Performance of retarded and nonretarded persons on information-processing tasks: Further tests of the similar structure hypothesis. *Psychological Bulletin, 100*(2), 157–175.

Winters, J. J., & Semchuk, M. T. (1986). Retrieval from long-term store as a function of mental age and intelligence. *American Journal of Mental Deficiency, 90*(4), 440–448.

Woodcock, R. W. (1998). *Woodcock Reading Mastery Tests–Revised.* Circle Pines, MN: AGS.

Woodcock, R. W., McGrew, K. S., & Mather, N. (2001). *Woodcock-Johnson Tests of Cognitive Abilities III.* Chicago: Riverside.

9

The Case for Bilingualism in Children With Down Syndrome

Elizabeth Kay-Raining Bird
Dalhousie University, Halifax, Nova Scotia, Canada

Children with Down syndrome (DS) have cognitive and language deficits secondary to a genetic disorder involving trisomy of the 21st chromosome. This is the most frequent of the chromosomal disorders resulting in intellectual disability. Language learning is particularly problematic for these children. Consequently, at least in North America, interventionists often recommend that the language input to these children be limited to a single language. This recommendation, on the surface, may seem logical. However, several factors argue against such a recommendation. First, current research has identified few deficiencies and several cognitive and language benefits of bilingualism (e.g., Bruck, Genesee, & Caravolas, 1997) for typically developing children. Also, there is almost no information available regarding the impact of multilingual contexts on the language-learning success or failure of children with language-learning difficulties, particularly those with concomitant intellectual disabilities. Third, there can be severe negative consequences for children and their families that result from limiting language input to a single language in a society that is increasingly diverse. Finally, there is emerging evidence that children with language impairments (Paradis, Crago, Genesee, & Rice, 2003), including children with Down syndrome (Kay-Raining Bird, Cleave, Trudeau, Thordardottir, Thorpe, & Sutton, 2005; Vallar & Papagno, 1993; Woll & Grove, 1996), can become successfully bilingual.

This chapter first reviews research on typical monolingual and bilingual development with a particular focus on developmental findings in terms of the sequence and rate of language development in bilingual as compared to monolingual children. The metalinguistic consequences of bilingualism are also reviewed. Research that has resulted in a well-defined phenotype of cognitive and language abilities of monolingual children with Down syndrome is then discussed. The literature on bilingualism in children who have language and/or cognitive impairments is reviewed next. Finally, work that has focused on intervention with bilingual populations is discussed. Based on the review of these areas, clinical recommendations are made with respect to bilingual children with Down syndrome. It is hoped that this chapter will provide some assistance to parents and practitioners when making decisions about bilingualism for individuals with Down syndrome and others with cognitive and/or language disabilities, and that it may serve as an impetus for additional much needed research in this area.

MONOLINGUAL ENGLISH DEVELOPMENT

By far, the greatest amount of information available on language development has been obtained from studies of monolingual English-speaking children who are typically developing. For these children, general milestones of development can be identified. First words emerge in production by about 10 to 12 months of age (e.g., Benedict, 1979). By 15 months children have an average productive vocabulary of 10 words. Although children add new words to their productive lexicons quite slowly at first, with lexicons of approximately 50 words at about 18 months of age, the rate of vocabulary acquisition accelerates. Nouns predominate in the early lexicons of most young children learning English and emerge earlier than verbs. By 24 months, productive lexicons contain, on average, over 300 words (Fenson et al., 1993).

By 2 years of age, children are beginning to combine words. Usually, early word combinations involve uninflected word forms. Grammatical morphemes begin to emerge with a mean length of utterance (MLU) of approximately 2.0. By 2½, children's sentences are, on average, 2.5 morphemes in length (Miller, 1981). Children refine their productive morphosyntax over the next few years. Early on, simple sentences predominate. However, multiclausal utterances emerge with MLUs of 3.0 or higher (Paul, 1981). Morphosyntactic complexity, only crudely measured by MLU in later years, continues to increase, reaching on average approximately 3.2

at by 3 years, 5.7 at 5 years (Miller, 1981), 6.5 at 9 years, and 7.0 at 13 years in conversation (Leadholm, Miller, Contrucci, Brittingham, & Odell, 1992). Pragmatic abilities emerge prelinguistically in the ability of children to monitor another's eye gaze to establish joint attention and to use gestures, eye gaze, and vocalizations to make requests or draw another's attention to an interesting object or event. Pragmatic skills expand from an early focus on conversational discourse to narrative and, later, expository discourse: skills that are refined throughout the school years.

Metalinguistics, the ability to explicitly think and talk about language as an object, emerges as young as 2 years of age with early spontaneous uses of metaphoric language and continues to develop in type and complexity through the preschool and school years (van Kleeck, 1994a). By 4 years of age, children are spontaneously rhyming and playing with the sounds in words. By 6 years, they are beginning to segment words into component sounds, a skill referred to as *phoneme awareness,* which has been shown to develop from as well as predict reading skills in children, particularly the ability to sound out (decode) unknown words (Blachman, 1994). Although generalizations such as these can be made, there is considerable individual variability in both rate of development and style of children's language behaviors (Bates, Bretherton, & Snyder, 1988).

BILINGUALISM

Defining bilingualism is not a simple matter. Bilingual children have different experiences with bilingualism. They differ in the languages to which they are exposed, the degree to which they are exposed to each language, the timing of exposure, and the context of exposure. For example, some bilingual children hear two languages in the home from birth, as is the case for children growing up in homes where one parent speaks one language to them and the other parent speaks another language (i.e., the one-parent-one-language context). Other bilingual children are exposed to one of their languages in the home and another outside the home, as when a babysitter speaks a second language to the child only when a parent is at work or when the child attends a day care or preschool program in which a second language is spoken.

As a general principle, the more frequently and consistently one is exposed to a language, the better is one's knowledge of that language. However, the quantity of language exposure varies considerably across individual children, even those growing up in monolingual environments. For example, Hart and Risley (1995) reported considerable individual variability in the number of utterances directed to children in different households, with children who experienced higher levels of child-directed language developing better vocabulary skills than children with less exposure. Also, the most important contributor to the frequency of language exposure in the Hart and Risley (1995) study was socioeconomic status: Families in higher status jobs and with more education and income spoke more frequently to their children. For bilingual children, the amount of exposure to each language can be quite different (Bialystok, 2001). As with monolingual children, effects of exposure frequency have been found for bilingual language learners. Pearson, Fernandez, Lewedag, and Oller (1997), for example, showed that a parental estimate of frequency of input in each language of exposure for bilingual children was highly correlated ($r = .81$) with measured growth over 2 months in that same language. Patterson and Pearson (2004), in their review, reported that frequency effects are discernible only up to fifth grade for simultaneous bilinguals, or until a "critical mass" of language ability has been reached. General measures of exposure, such as the number of years of exposure to a particular language, seem to have less predictive value (Genesee, Paradis, & Crago, 2005) than more specific measures that reflect the degree of current exposure to each language.

The timing of first exposure to a second language also varies (Bialystok, 2001). Children can be exposed to a second language from birth or any time thereafter. The literature in bilingual development differentiates between children who are learning language simultaneously versus those learning it sequentially. Simultaneous bilinguals are those who are exposed to both languages essentially from birth. In Montreal, for example, it is not unusual for children to grow up in a household where both French and English are spoken to the children. Sequential bilingualism occurs when children are exposed to a second language after considerable learning in a first language has already taken place, often defined as after 3 years of age (Hoff, 2005). In Nova Scotia, for example, English-speaking children are able to enter French immersion programs in kindergarten or Grade 6, after they have acquired a considerable proficiency with their first language.

Who speaks which language makes a difference as well. Primary caregivers, usually parents, have the greatest impact on language learning in their children at early ages. Once children enter school, peers and the academic environment have an increasingly important impact in this area. A child's motivation to learn, assessment of need, and perception of usefulness can also influence how proficient they become with a particular language. As metacognitive abilities improve and a child becomes more capable of assessing such factors. Thus, a child who speaks one language in the classroom but another with friends and family may perceive that there is little need to use the classroom language in other contexts and may therefore be less motivated to acquire it. In situations where a true need to use language in order to communicate exists, motivation is often not an issue for children (Genesee et al., 2005).

Another factor that influences language development in bilingual children is the relative status of languages in society. Children may be exposed to a language at home that is not the majority language outside the home. Factors such as how the home language is viewed by the larger community and access to a community of speakers outside the home can have a substantial impact on a child's continued use of the home language as they mature. These same factors also affect parental patterns of language use with the child (see Genesee et al., 2005, for a discussion of these issues).

When bilingual individuals interact, they interweave their languages at times. This is called *language mixing*. Language mixing can occur within and across utterances. As Genesee et al. (2005) state, "[Language mixing] is a typical and ubiquitous pattern of language use among bilingual children and adults" (p. 111). The frequency of language mixing varies widely across individuals (e.g., Nicoladis & Genesee, 1997a), with most bilingual speakers mixing at least some of the time. By 3 years of age, children tend to mix languages at a frequency similar to that found in the input (Nicoladis & Genesee 1997b). Although some researchers argue that a clear separation of languages in talk to bilingual children will assist in the acquisition of two languages (e.g., Lanza, 1997), it is obvious from studies of language mixing that a clear separation is rarely realized (Bialystok, 2001). Indeed, the capacity to define or explain in one language and then switch back to another may be essential at times to ensure communicative success and therefore may enhance learning, especially in the weaker language.

Given the variability of the bilingual experience, it is not surprising that most children who are bilingual have better proficiency in one of their two languages. The better language can be referred to as the dominant language. As a child matures and significant life contexts change, language dominance can also change. In the case of many immigrant families, for example, the language of the home is often the dominant language for the child until school entry. At this point, the language of the larger society can replace that of the home (Romaine, 1996).

LANGUAGE ACQUISITION IN A BILINGUAL CONTEXT

Successful bilingualism is a fact of life for many adults and children around the world. For this reason alone bilingualism should be viewed as a typical path of development. Although early studies were conducted with the assumption that bilingual children would be disadvantaged in their cognitive and language development relative to monolinguals, more recent studies have refuted this contention (Bialystok, 2001; Pacheco, 1983; Payan, 1989). Indeed, research has now provided evidence for many similarities and some differences in the language development of monolingual and bilingual children, as well as some advantages that may result from bilingualism (Cromdal, 1999; Oller, 1983; Pacheco, 1983).

Nicoladis and Genesee (1997a) note that there are three "logical possibilities" regarding the effect of bilingualism upon language learning: It could lead to language delay, it could lead to more rapid language development, or it could have no effect at all. In their review of the literature these authors conclude that general milestones are reached at comparable times for monolingual and bilingual children. That is, both groups say their first words, attain their first 50 words, and begin to combine words at approximately the same times. Also, the MLUs of bilingual and monolingual children are comparable at various ages, and the order and age of acquisition of various syntactic forms are comparable as well. The authors concluded that with regard to general milestones of development, bilingual children's language abilities do not appear to be "remarkably delayed nor remarkably advanced" (p. 264) relative to that of monolingual children. Bialystok (2001) also concludes that the sequence of acquisition of major developmental milestones is similar for monolingual and bilingual children. Genesee et al. (2005) review the literature on "target-deviant forms" (i.e., errors in child productions of grammatical forms). They conclude that, for the most part, bilingual children who are typically developing produce the same types of target-deviant forms with the same frequency as their monolingual counterparts speaking the same language.

An exception to this general conclusion of comparable developmental timelines and accomplishments for monolingual and bilingual children may be in the area of vocabulary acquisition (Bialystok, 2001; Nicoladis & Genesee, 1997a). Some studies have found a delay in standardized measures of vocabulary comprehension (e.g., the Peabody Picture Vocabulary Test) in bilingual children 4 to 7 years old learning a variety of languages, relative to monolingual controls (Ben-Zeev, 1977; Doyle, Champagne, & Segalowitz, 1978; Rosenblum & Pinker, 1983; Umbel, Pearson, Fernandez, & Oller, 1992). In contrast, Pearson, Fernandez, and Oller (1993) reported no statistical differences between the expressive vocabulary skills of younger monolingual and bilingual children (up to the age of 30 months) and potentially better vocabulary comprehension skills in the bilingual children, using measures from the MacArthur Communication Development Inventory (CDI; Fenson et al., 1993). In addition, the rate of expressive vocabulary growth was similar for both groups. Definitive statements with regards to the comprehension data were difficult, given several methodological shortcomings. As Pearson discusses in her 1998 review of the vocabulary literature, such studies are fraught with methodological problems. She argues that young bilingual children's vocabulary skills are best evaluated using a measure that combines knowledge in both languages of exposure. She also calls on the research community to develop bilingual norms, as standardized samples that currently exist are inadequate for the purposes of studying or evaluating bilingual children. Research groups in Canada and the United States are currently pursuing this goal.

Language-specific developmental differences are evident in both monolingual and bilingual children. Depending on such factors as conceptual complexity (Slobin, 1985), cue availability and reliability (Bates & MacWhinney, 1987), and perceptual saliency (Leonard, Eyer, Bedore, & Grela, 1997), linguistic structures can emerge earlier or later in one language relative to another. Linguistic structures that work in a similar manner across languages appear to have similar developmental time frames (Bedore, 2004), whereas those that do not, diverge. For example, past-tense forms have a more protracted development in English than do such forms in Spanish. In contrast, article use reaches a high level of accuracy earlier in English than in Spanish, where the development of articles and clitics is more protracted due in part to the added complexities of gender marking (Restrepo & Gutiérrez-Clellen, 2004). Similarly, Genesee et al. (2005) describe differences in the sequence and timing of negative sentence formation in French- versus English-speaking children. As with monolingual children, these same language-specific patterns of development can be found in bilingual children (Bedore, 2004; Genesee et al., 2005; Restrepo & Gutiérrez-Clellen, 2004).

The language of bilingual children does not look identical to that of monolingual children. Features of one language can be transferred to the other. Müller (1998), for example, reported that children learning German and either French, English, or Italian used syntactic forms from one language while speaking another, although always by applying the simpler form to the more complex language system. Transfer of one language-specific form for use in another language cannot by definition occur in monolingual children. Müller (1998) cautions, however, that many of the errors usually attributed to transference in bilingual children are also observable in the language of monolingual children, although with less frequency. Indeed, in their review of the literature, Genesee et al. (2005) argued that only a small minority of the language-deviant forms observed in bilingual children are the result of true transference. Similar to Müller, they reported that the usual finding is a difference in frequency of a particular error type, rather than qualitative differences in the errors exhibited by bilingual and monolingual children.

Cognitive Advantages of Bilingualism

Contrary to the expectations of early researchers who predicted a deficit in development resulting from bilingualism, recent literature has revealed some advantages resulting from acquiring two languages. Perhaps the most frequently reported finding of a bilingual advantage is that bilingual children exhibit advanced metalinguistic skill relative to their monolingual peers (Bialystok, 2001; Bruck & Genesee, 1995). An advantage in this area is not usually identifiable in the earliest periods of language development, probably in part because many metalinguistic abilities require a level of conscious knowledge and control of language that is cognitively difficult for very young children. Metalinguistic advantages seem to be related to the degree of bilinguality achieved (Cromdal, 1999; Cummins, 1979, 2000). Cummins has hypothesized that a threshold level of bilingualism is necessary before the beneficial effects of bilingualism can be realized. In his model, cognitive advantages are associated with high levels of bilingual proficiency, whereas cognitive disadvantages can be evident at early levels of bilingual attainment. Interestingly, this model is supported by the only study of cognitive advantages of bilingualism conducted with individuals with intellectual disability (ID; Whitaker, Rueda, & Prieto, 1985). It was found that children with mild ID who had a high bilingual proficiency showed cognitive advantages on a wide variety of tasks, relative to a monolingual control group matched for IQ. The authors cautioned, however, that their IQ measure (Wechsler Intelligence Test for Children–Revised, WISC–R) might have been biased against their Latino subjects, resulting in an invalid diagnosis of ID. The specific skill of word consciousness, or knowledge of the arbitrary nature of words, is one of the earliest aspects of metalinguistic ability reported to be enhanced through bilingualism. Children as young as 2 years of age have demonstrated behaviors reflective of word consciousness (van Kleeck, 1994a). In discussing metalinguistic advantages of bilingualism, Bialystok (2001) distinguishes between two component processes of metalinguistics: control and analysis. She defines metalinguistic control as "the ability to selectively attend to specific aspects of a representation, particularly in misleading situations" (p. 131) and metalinguistic analysis as "the ability to represent increasingly complex and abstract structures" (p. 131). It is enhancement of the control component that she argues is most associated with bilingualism, although balanced bilinguals (i.e., those with close to equal capacity in both languages) also demonstrate a metalinguistic analysis advantage.

Whether metalinguistic abilities can lead to more rapid language learning in children is a question few researchers have addressed directly. Tervoort (1979) reported that his daughter developed a French lexicon by using word awareness to consciously contrast Dutch and French homonyms, suggesting that word awareness can lead to a productive vocabulary learning strategy. Nonetheless, it would appear that this strategy is adopted by only a small subset of bilingual children. Pearson (1998), for example, reported that only 2 of the 24 bilingual children she and her colleagues studied for 27 months used a "doublet strategy" in which the child produced words in the weaker language only after having acquired the labeled concept first in the dominant language. Metalinguistic control may also support language acquisition. Control (as conceptualized by Bialystok, 2001) and comprehension monitoring would appear to be overlapping concepts. Comprehension monitoring, of course, is an essential feature of successful communication and necessary for the repair of communication breakdowns. It seems reasonable that children who are better comprehension monitors will profit from it in the language acquisition process. If metalinguistic abilities do contribute to higher rates of language learning or more efficient language learning, then bilingualism may have some important positive consequences for children with language impairments.

LANGUAGE OF MONOLINGUAL CHILDREN WITH DOWN SYNDROME

Language-learning difficulties in monolingual children with DS often exceed expectations, given their cognitive impairments (Chapman, 1995; Chapman, Schwartz, & Kay-Raining Bird, 1991; Chapman, Seung, Schwartz, & Kay-Raining Bird, 1998, 2000; Fowler, 1990). The gap between language and nonverbal cognition emerges in the early period of language development (Cardosa-Martins, Mervis, & Mervis, 1985; Miller, 1992; Mundy, Kasari, Sigman, & Ruskin, 1995). Children with DS have more difficulty with expressive than receptive language (Chapman, 1995; Chapman et al., 1991, 1998, 2000). Vocabulary acquisition is often a strength for these children (Chapman, 1995; Chapman, Kay-Raining Bird, & Schwartz, 1990; Chapman et al., 1991, 1998, 2000). Nevertheless, vocabulary acquisition in production does not keep pace with that in comprehension (Chapman, 1995; Miller, 1992).

The most difficult component of language for most children with DS to acquire is expressive morphosyntax (Chapman et al., 1998, 2000; Thordardottir, Chapman, & Wagner, 2002), although receptive morphosyntactic abilities are also delayed (Chapman et al., 1991). Early delays in morphosyntax are evident in the delayed onset of word combinations (Clements-Baartman & Girolametto, 1995), and divergence relative to mental-age increases with age (Chapman, 1995). Despite this, there is evidence that children with DS continue to develop in morphosyntax throughout adolescence (Chapman et al., 1991, 1998). Although verb development has been studied very little in this population, there is evidence that these children have particular difficulty acquiring both lexical and grammatical verbs, as well as constructing multi-clausal utterances spontaneously (Hesketh & Chapman, 1998). The acquisition of language may be constrained by a variety of factors in children with DS, including auditory memory deficits (Jarrold, Baddeley, & Phillips, 2002; Kay-Raining Bird & Chapman, 1994; Seung & Chapman, 2000), and intelligibility problems (Miller, 1988).

Only one aspect of metalinguistic ability has been studied to any degree in children with DS: phonological awareness. Phonological awareness is the ability to analyze and consciously manipulate the sounds of a language and is demonstrated through, for example, rhyme generation, alliteration, sound elision, and sound blending tasks. Children with Down syndrome appear to have a particular weakness in the development of phonological awareness skills (Cossu, Rossini, & Marshall, 1993; Fowler, Doherty, & Boynton, 1995; Kay-Raining Bird, Cleave, & McConnell, 2000; Laws & Gunn, 2002). Despite this, phonological awareness is correlated with reading decoding skills in children with DS and predicts and supports later decoding development in this population (Cupples & Iacono, 2000; Gombert, 2002; Kay-Raining Bird et al., 2000; Laws & Gunn, 2002). The link between phonological awareness and bilingualism can be questioned. Phonological awareness would be a component of metalinguistic analysis, using Bialystok's (2001) model of metalinguistics. As such, she argues it would be more related to literacy than bilingualism.

BILINGUALISM AND CHILDREN WITH SPECIFIC LANGUAGE IMPAIRMENTS (SLI)

There is a surprising lack of research involving bilingual or multilingual children with language learning problems. Although it is expected that children with language learning difficulties will experience problems learning any language, the specific manifestations of those problems will vary with the language (Crago & Allen, 1996; Nicoladis & Genesee, 1997a).

Several studies have examined the phonology of bilingual children with phonological impairment (PI). Holm, Dodd, Stow, and Pert (1996–1997) assessed the speech of four bilingual children with PI. They concluded that the bilingual children showed evidence of separate phonological systems in each language. Both languages, they argued, were affected by the same (hypothesized) underlying cause. Nonetheless, both shared and language-specific patterns were identifiable in the phonologies of these children. For example, one bilingual subject exhibited difficulty with clusters in both languages. However, this difficulty was manifested by vowel insertion within clusters in English and cluster reduction in Punjabi. MacLeod and McCauley (2003) compared the phonological abilities of five French–English bilingual children with SLI to that of four monolingual French controls with SLI and four younger French language-matched controls with typical development. Results revealed similar phonetic inventories and phonological skills in the French phonologies of the three groups.

However, the bilingual children with SLI tended to produce more phonological errors but also attempted phonetically more complex words than their monolingual SLI counterparts. These studies suggest that bilingual children with PI will manifest symptoms in both languages, but that the structure of a particular language will dictate the specific patterns observed in each language.

Not surprisingly, bilingual children with specific language impairment (SLI) have been shown to perform more poorly than their typically developing age-matched bilingual peers on measures of morphology and syntax, using both group (Håkansson, Salameh, & Nettelbladt, 2003; Jacobson & Schwartz, 2002) and single-subject designs (Restrepo & Kruth, 2000). Eng and O'Connor (2000) have also shown that bilingual children with SLI respond to syntactic elicitation tasks in a manner similar to that of bilingual controls matched for language dominance (Spanish), gender and age. Specifically, the groups displayed similar hierarchies of difficulty in response to stimuli and both groups benefited from predictability in the stimuli. Even so, the bilingual children with SLI demonstrated reduced accuracy relative to the controls, as would be expected with an age match.

Jordaan, Shaw-Ridley, Serfontein, Orelowitz, and Monaghan (2001) have suggested that children with different language disorders may have different bilingual capabilities. However, the two case studies they presented differed in their exposure to two languages, suggesting that input frequency rather than disorder type could explain the observed differences.

Research that compares the development of bilingual and monolingual children with SLI is only beginning to emerge. In the first study of its type, Crutchley, Botting and Conti-Ramsden (1997) reported that bilingual children with SLI scored less well on a variety of English language and reading measures, compared to monolingual controls with SLI. As a result, the authors claimed that bilingualism may act as an "aggravating factor" in SLI. This interpretation, however, was not warranted because no information about the children's experience with bilingualism was provided. It is likely that their results were confounded by the inclusion of children for whom English was not the dominant language. In contrast to the Crutchley et al. results, Paradis et al. (2003) found that French–English bilingual children with SLI exhibited the same type and frequency of morphosyntactic errors as did monolingual French or English age-matched controls also with SLI. All children had received consistent input in two languages from birth to 6 years in a one-parent-one-language environment. Predictably, the specific surface structures that were affected differed across languages for monolingual and bilingual groups. Only eight bilingual children with SLI were included in this study, however, so the results should be viewed as preliminary. Clearly, we are just beginning to understand how bilingualism affects language learning in children with language impairments. Nonetheless, in their review of the literature, Genesee et al. (2005) emphasized five conclusions regarding bilingual children with SLI. They argued that these children: (a) can become bilingual, (b) will experience difficulties in both languages, (c) may have more deficits in the weaker language, (d) will show the same deficit patterns as monolingual children with SLI, and (e) will acquire language at the same rate as monolingual children with SLI.

BILINGUALISM AND INDIVIDUALS WITH INTELLECTUAL DISABILITY

The literature on bilingual individuals with intellectual disabilities (ID) is even sparser than that for bilingual children with SLI. Some articles assume that bilingual individuals with ID exist but focus on intervention techniques. For example, Duran (1985) described procedures she recommends for teaching reading to bilingual individuals with ID. Similarly, Rohena, Jitendra, and Browder (2002) examined the effects of inserting a time delay between stimulus exposure and elicited response when teaching four Spanish–English bilingual adolescents with moderate ID of unknown origin to read new words. Although language acquisition in these adolescents was not the focus of the study, it is obvious that the subjects were becoming bilingual. The subjects exhibited vocabulary comprehension skills in English between 3;5 (years; months) and 5;6 and in Spanish between 4;11 and 8;0.

Several researchers have expressed opinions about the capacity of individuals with ID to become bilingual (Genesee et al., 2005; Rondal, 2000). In a position paper entitled "Bilingualism in Mental Retardation: Some Prospective Views," Rondal (2000) concluded that, despite a severe dearth of data, there is evidence that at least some individuals with ID can become competent in more than one language. He predicted that there would be substantial differences in bilingual capabilities demonstrated by individuals with different syndromes, as well as considerable individual variability within each syndrome. He further suggested that the same profile of language strengths and weaknesses that research has revealed in monolingual individuals with ID would be observable in both languages of bilingual individuals and that, as with the development of a first language, L2 development should be expected to be delayed. Rondal recommended that "systematic L2 exposure" for individuals with ID should be postponed until "roughly 6 or 7 years CA [chronological age]" (p. 63). He further argued that in cases of "'unavoidable' familial bilingualism" (p. 63), input in two languages should be postponed for a number of years and one language should be chosen to be the primary language of input when bilingual input begins. Rondal alluded to the controversy surrounding "the possible dependence of L2 learning on L1 acquisition" (p. 59). It would appear that he based these latter recommendations on the belief that individuals with ID should have a good grounding in their first language before they begin to learn a second one, but apparently did not differentiate between simultaneous and sequential bilingualism in applying this principle. Genesee et al. (2005) also predicted that individuals with ID would achieve some success with bilingualism. They, however, suggested that the degree of success would differ for those in simultaneous versus sequential bilingual environments and recognized the need for supportive environments both at home and in school to ensure optimal growth. However, Genesee et al. seem to come to a similar conclusion as Rondal with regard to children with lower IQs, stating, "We suspect that children with severe cognitive or sensori-perceptual challenges are likely to experience more success with dual language learning if they are preschool age" (p. 53).

BILINGUALISM AND INDIVIDUALS WITH DOWN SYNDROME

With regard to bilingual individuals with Down syndrome, a small but promising body of evidence is emerging. Several case studies suggest that at least some children with Down syndrome can become functionally bilingual. Woll and Grove (1996) discuss the simultaneous development of British Sign Language (BSL) and English in monozygotic twins with Down syndrome growing up with deaf parents. Although their syntactic skills were delayed in both languages, these girls were acquiring skills in each language and used them selectively in appropriate contexts (i.e., BSL with deaf interactants, English with hearing interactants). Vallar and Papagno (1993) provided a case study of a 23-year-old woman with Down syndrome who became successfully trilingual in Italian, English, and French. Interestingly, this woman presents a very different profile of language and cognitive skills from that usually seen in this population: stronger verbal than nonverbal cognitive scores on the Wechsler Adult Intelligence Scale (WAIS) and good phonological awareness skills relative to a control group. One might wonder whether this woman's multilingualism has affected her particular skill profile. For example, are the unusually high phonological awareness skills indicative of a metalinguistic advantage of bilingualism? Such issues were not explored by the authors.

One somewhat disturbing study has shown that professionals tend to counsel bilingual families of children with DS to raise their children monolingually (Thordardottir, 2002). Although this study was conducted in Montreal, anecdotal reports suggest that such council is far more widespread, extending throughout North America and into many European countries as well. Thordardottir (2002) investigated parents' views of bilingualism using an interview format. Ten bilingual families of children with

DS and six bilingual families of TD children participated. She found that most of the families of children with DS were advised to limit their child's exposure to a single language. Not all did. Parents went against such professional advice either because they considered bilingualism an important asset for their child and/or they knew of other children with DS who were being successfully raised bilingual. Parents who chose to raise their child with DS bilingually reported that their child was experiencing success in acquiring two languages.

Recently, the first study to measure bilingualism in children with Down syndrome was completed. Kay-Raining Bird et al. (2005) studied four groups of children: monolingual and bilingual children with Down syndrome and monolingual and bilingual typically developing controls. Groups were matched on nonverbal mental age (DS) or chronological age (TD). Bilingual children were included if they had had intense ongoing input in two languages, English and one other. The second language was usually French. Further, bilingual children were either English dominant or balanced bilinguals (i.e., showing equal ability in both languages). The majority had been exposed to both languages from birth (average percent of life exposure: DS, 91%; TD, 100%). The protocol was designed to assess the language skills of children in both English and the second language using a variety of measures. In English, the Peabody Picture Vocabulary Test–Revised (PPVT-R; Dunn & Dunn, 1981), the Preschool Language Scale–3 (PLS-3; Zimmerman, Steiner, & Pond, 1992), and the CDI (Fenson et al., 1993) were administered and a language sample was collected. Two analogous tests were administered in the second language, the Quebec French equivalent of the PPVT–R (Échelle de Vocabulaire en Images Peabody [EVIP]; Dunn, Theriault-Whelan, & Dunn, 1993) and the Quebec French version of the CDI (Trudeau, Frank, & Poulin-Dubois, 1999). A language sample was also collected in the second language. Both English and second language samples used a common set of toys and were collected in play with a native speaker of the language. Samples were transcribed using the SALT computer program (version 6.1; Miller & Chapman, 2000) and standard measures were generated (MLU, total words, number of different words).

Group statistical analyses revealed several interesting results (Kay-Raining Bird et al., 2005). First, in their dominant language (English) bilingual children with Down syndrome performed at least as well on all measures as did their monolingual counterparts with DS. This suggests that bilingualism did not disadvantage these children in their language development. Second, a pattern of expressive language difficulties and vocabulary comprehension strengths was evident in the English language performance of both groups of children with DS, relative to TD controls. This suggests that bilingualism does not seem to change the profile of language learning in this population, at least in the dominant language. Third, the bilingual children with DS showed a pattern of expressive morphosyntactic weakness (as measured by MLU) in their second language as well, confirming that the expected profile of language strengths and weaknesses is extended to second-language learning. Fourth, all bilingual children with DS exhibited some second-language abilities. As a group, these skills, at least at the vocabulary level, were comparable to those of matched TD controls. However, considerable individual variability existed. Some exhibited considerable capacity in their second language whereas others exhibited very limited skills. Correlational analyses revealed that mental age and chronological age were significantly related to measures of second-language ability. These measures have been shown to predict language development in monolingual children with DS (e.g., Sloper, Cunningham, Turner, & Knussen, 1990). However, Whitaker et al. (1985) have shown that bilingual children with mild ID matched on IQ can have quite different bilingual proficiency. Clearly, cognitive ability is not the only factor to consider when accounting for growth in the second language. Chapman et al. (2000) report that MA, CA, and comprehension were all separate predictors of MLU in monolingual children with DS.

Kay-Raining Bird et al. (2005) stress that their results are preliminary and can only be generalized to children in earlier stages (MLU < 3.5) of language development. Clearly, much more work in this area is needed to understand the implications of bilingualism for children with DS.

ASSESSMENT AND INTERVENTION FOR BILINGUAL CHILDREN WITH COMMUNICATION DISORDERS

In North America, communication disorders are typically assessed and treated by speech-language pathologists (SLP) and audiologists. In both Canada and the United States, professional organizations have released position papers providing guidelines for the clinical management of individuals with communication disorders from culturally and/or linguistically different backgrounds (ASHA, 1985; Crago & Westernoff, 1997). A knowledge and skills document on the same topic has also been released (ASHA, 2004). These documents espouse similar philosophies. They charge professionals to educate themselves regarding issues of cultural and linguistic diversity and to assess and treat all individuals in a culturally and linguistically appropriate manner. They stress the importance (and difficulty) of distinguishing between a difference and a disorder and note that treatment of differences is optional and must be elected by a client or their caregiver. Collaborative efforts are encouraged, to bring together complimentary skills. Collaborations should include bilingual professionals if possible. However, as less than 6% of professionals are self-reported to be bilingual in the United States (ASHA, 2004), the use of trained interpreters, translators, and cultural mediators is also highly encouraged. These papers also argue that assessment and intervention is optimally provided in a child's first language, or bilingually.

Although the body of literature on language development and disorders in English outstrips that for other languages, there are nonetheless many publications describing the nature of language and communication in various cultures, dialects, and languages, and, to a lesser degree, some developmental information is available. These publications can serve as valuable resources for language assessment and intervention (e.g., Battle, 1993; Garry & Rubino, 2001; Heath, 1985; Hickmann, 1997; Kamhi, Pollack, & Harris, 1996; Schieffelin & Ochs, 1986; Slobin, 1985, 1992; Tannen & Saville-Troike, 1985; Taylor, 1986a; van Kleeck, 1994b). Many other publications have suggested modifications to assessment and intervention procedures and materials in order to accommodate individuals from diverse backgrounds (e.g., Adler, 1993; Baca & Cervantes, 1989; Coleman, 2000; Kamhi et al., 1996; Mattes & Omark, 1991; Taylor, 1986b; Taylor & Clarke, 1994; Taylor & Leonard, 1999; Vaugn-Cooke, 1986). Despite these resources, many professionals feel ill equipped to assess and treat children from diverse language and cultural backgrounds. For example, in a recent survey of 811 SLPs, 40% reported that they would be less likely to assess and treat bilingual as opposed to monolingual clients (Kritikos, 2003). A large majority of the SLPs who participated in this survey, even those who were bilingual, reported feeling either "incompetent" or only "somewhat competent" to assess an individual in a language they did not speak, even with an interpreter. One reason for the lack of confidence of many professionals and their consequent tendency to avoid servicing individuals from other language and cultural groups may be the limited number of empirical studies focusing on assessment and intervention. For the present purposes, research involving bilingual children is of particular interest and is next reviewed.

Two studies have focused upon the effects of vocabulary interventions with bilingual children. Perozzi and Sanchez (1992) studied 38 bilingual first graders who were language impaired and Spanish dominant. They taught English pronouns and prepositions to groups of children under two conditions: first-Spanish-then-English, or English only. They found that fewer trials were needed to learn both Spanish and English prepositions and pronouns in the first-Spanish-then-English group than were required to learn English words alone in the English-only group. This suggests that use of the dominant language leads to more efficient vocabulary learning in the second language. This seems logical for situations where the concepts mapped to words are the same across the two languages. Thordardottir, Ellis Weismer, and Smith (1997) studied English vocabulary learning in a

5-year-old bilingual boy with language impairment who was a dominant Icelandic speaker. Intervention was conducted either bilingually (i.e., Icelandic and English) or solely in English. In the bilingual condition, Icelandic productions were responded to and target words were discussed in both languages and directly translated and explained in Icelandic. In the monolingual condition, Icelandic was not used by the therapist and the child was reminded to speak English when he used Icelandic. Results revealed that vocabulary learning did not vary across the two conditions. Given that both conditions supported vocabulary learning equally well, the authors recommended bilingual intervention as a means of socially and linguistically promoting both languages.

Several studies have investigated transference of speech intervention benefits from one language to another in bilingual children. Holm, Ozanne, and Dodd (1997) studied a bilingual Cantonese- and English-speaking child with speech symptoms that the authors claimed had two different bases. The child presented with some consistent error patterns the authors classified as phonological in nature, and other errors that were considered to have a motoric basis. Two different interventions were conducted in English only, each targeting a different posited underlying problem. The phonological disorder was treated using a metaphonology approach, and the motoric disorder with traditional articulation therapy. The authors reported that errors associated with an articulation problem resolved in both languages, but that phonological intervention had an effect only in the treated language (English). Similarly, Holm and Dodd (1999) studied a Punjabi–English-speaking boy who exhibited inconsistent errors that the authors classified as a "motor planning disorder." The child was treated in English only, using a core vocabulary approach. Posttherapy, the child showed increased consistency in his lexical productions in both languages. Given the results of these and similar studies, Holm and Dodd (2001) argued that some, but not all, intervention effects can be expected to generalize across languages. Therefore, depending on the type of disorder (and underlying cause), the number of languages targeted in intervention would need to vary. Specifically, they argued that the effects of therapy targeting articulation and motor planning might be expected to cross language boundaries, whereas therapy targeting phonological disorders might not, therefore requiring dual-language intervention. In contrast, Ray (2002) reported that a minimal pairs approach implemented in English with a trilingual child to reduce the use of phonological processes was effective in increasing intelligibility in all three languages. Thus, this author argued that the effects of phonological interventions can positively impact the untreated languages in a multilingual child. Again, further study is warranted.

CONCLUSIONS AND CLINICAL IMPLICATIONS

In this chapter, language development in monolingual and bilingual children with typical development was compared, followed by a review of the literature on bilingualism in language-impaired children with and without intellectual difficulties, with a specific focus on individuals with Down syndrome. The following discussion addresses the clinical implications of the previous review for children with DS.

The review of the literature on typical language development in monolingual and bilingual children suggests that simultaneous bilingual children can be expected to acquire language milestones in the same sequence and at relatively the same rate as children growing up in a monolingual environment. This does not mean that bilingual children will exhibit identical language behaviors as monolingual children. Analyses of error patterns exhibited by monolingual and bilingual children do show some differences, probably due to cross-language influences. However, the similarities in error patterns far outweigh the differences. Thus, evidence from typical development suggests that successful bilingualism is the norm and that one can expect few negative consequences (relative to monolingual controls) of bilingualism. Of course, bilingual input is not a unitary phenomenon. Many factors such as timing of initial input, frequency and duration of exposure, consistency of exposure, and social status and perceived usefulness of each language all can be expected to effect the rate and ultimate level of achievement in each language.

The typically developing literature also provides us with guidance regarding language mixing. It would appear that using two languages in a single utterance or across utterances in a conversation is a normal practice and is more likely to reflect pragmatic needs or semantic constraints than difficulties in the ability to develop separate language systems. Finally, the review of typical development suggests that bilingualism may result in cognitive advantages, especially in terms of metalinguistic ability, but that these advantages will probably not be discernible until children have attained some competency in both languages. It is not yet clear how metalinguistic ability impacts language learning. It is possible that some aspects of metalinguistic skill (e.g., word consciousness) can result in useful learning strategies for at least some children.

These findings have important implications for children with Down syndrome. It would appear that becoming bilingual is not more difficult than becoming monolingual, at least with regard to simultaneous bilingualism. Consequently, clinicians and families should consider bilingualism for individuals with DS. Research on bilingualism in language-impaired children and emerging evidence of successful bilingualism in children with DS also supports this conclusion. Although the language deficits of children with DS (or SLI) will be apparent in both languages, simultaneous bilingualism does not appear to disadvantage these children relative to monolingual controls.

The literature reviewed provides us with some insights as to how best to approach bilingualism in children with Down syndrome. First, Rondal's (2000) recommendation that second-language input to individuals with ID be delayed at least until the preschool years is not supported. Instead, successful bilingualism seems possible, for children with DS even when input in both languages begins at birth. Also, because clear frequency effects have been found in the typically developing literature, it would seem important to ensure intensive input on an ongoing basis in both languages in order to optimize bilingual success. Presumably, ensuring that adequate time is spent with each language is particularly important for children with DS, given their language learning problems. In order to ensure that children have an opportunity to hear and speak both languages with adequate frequency, it might also be useful to clearly identify when and with whom a particular language is spoken. Because language mixing is a normal component of bilingualism, it should not be viewed as a sign that a child is having difficulty becoming bilingual. Indeed, direct translation of terms or use of the dominant language to explain something may at times facilitate the child's understanding and ability to interact effectively in the weaker language, and thus may enhance learning.

The clinical implications discussed to this point are with reference to simultaneous bilingualism. It is unclear whether the same conclusions can be drawn for sequential bilingualism. Although this is only conjecture, I would suspect that children with DS can experience success with sequential bilingualism as well, if adequate support for learning in both languages is provided and a high frequency of input is available. As De Houwer (1999) states, bilingualism is most often a necessity, not a choice. When bilingualism is a necessity, whether simultaneous or sequential, then the issue is not whether bilingualism should be supported but how best to support it.

Family-centered treatment (FCT) has become accepted practice with young children with language disorders, including children with DS. Several components are key to FCT. First, the family is accepted as a team member. Second, clinical decisions reflect the family's goals and needs. Third, the family is recognized by team participants as the key decision maker, caregiver, teacher, and advocate for the child (McNeilly & Coleman, 2000). Thus, within an FCT model, professionals should help families to identify and clarify their goals and needs with regards to multiple languages. To do so, questions such as the following can be asked: What are the important life contexts for this child and family? What languages are necessary in order for the child to participate fully in these important life contexts? Once decisions about which languages need to be learned have been made, then the team can focus on providing optimal support for each language and within each of the child's important life contexts.

The bilingual intervention research provides some direction with regards to direct intervention. First, it seems that the language of intervention might vary depending on what aspect of language is targeted. For example, it seems that articulation problems, and perhaps phonological problems as well, can be treated in one language, even perhaps the weaker language, and that beneficial effects can be expected to spread to another language. In contrast, teaching vocabulary first in the stronger language appears to be the most efficient route to learning (at least some) concepts and words. Finally, bilingual intervention may help the child recruit language resources in either language in service of intervention goals.

At this point it seems appropriate to stop thinking in terms of restricting children with language and intellectual disabilities to a single language and to focus on learning how to best support them in all the languages they need to know. To this end, further research is critical.

ACKNOWLEDGMENTS

This research was supported by grants 410-97-0819 and 410-2000-1409 from the Social Sciences and Humanities Research Council of Canada. Thanks are extended to my long time mentor and friend, Robin Chapman, and my colleagues Patricia Cleave, Elin Thordardottir, Natacha Trudeau, and Ann Sutton, who have helped shape my thinking about bilingualism over the years.

REFERENCES

Adler, S. (1993). *Multicultural communication skills in the classroom*. Toronto, ON: Allyn & Bacon.

American Speech-Language-Hearing Association. (1985, June). Clinical management of communicatively handicapped minority language populations. *ASHA, 27*(6), 57–60.

American Speech-Language-Hearing Association. (2004). Knowledge and skills needed by speech-language pathologists and audiologists to provide culturally and linguistically appropriate services. *ASHA Supplement, 24,* 152–158.

Baca, L. M., & Cervantes, H. T. (1989). *The bilingual special education interface*. Toronto, ON: Merrill.

Bates, E., Bretherton, I., & Snyder, L. (1988). *From first words to grammar: Individual differences and dissociable mechanisms*. New York: Cambridge University Press.

Bates, E., & MacWhinney, B. (1987). Competition, variation and language learning. In B. MacWhinney (Ed.), *Mechanisms of language acquisition* (pp. 157–194). Hillsdale, NJ: Lawrence Erlbaum Associates.

Battle, D. (1993). *Communication disorders in multicultural populations*. Toronto, ON: Andover.

Bedore, L. M. (2004). Morphosyntactic development. In B. A. Goldstein (Ed.), *Bilingual language development and disorders in Spanish-English speakers* (pp. 163–186). Baltimore: Paul H. Brookes.

Benedict, H. (1979). Early lexical development: Comprehension and production. *Journal of Child Language, 6*, 180–200.

Ben-Zeev, S. (1977). The influence of bilingualism on cognitive strategy and cognitive development. *Child Development, 48*, 1009–1018.

Bialystok, E. (2001). *Bilingualism in development: Language, literacy, & cognition*. Cambridge, UK: Cambridge University Press.

Blachman, B. (1994). Early literacy acquisition: The role of phonological awareness. In G. P. Wallach & K. G. Butler (Eds.). *Language learning disabilities in school-age children and adolescents* (pp. 253–274). Toronto: Maxwell Macmillan.

Bruck, M., & Genesee, F. (1995). Phonological awareness in young second language learners. *Journal of Child Language, 22*, 307–324.

Bruck, M., Genesee, F., & Caravolas, M. (1997). A cross-linguistic study of early literacy acquisition. In B. Blachman (Ed.), *Foundations of reading acquisition and dyslexia: Implications for early intervention* (pp. 145–162). Mahwah, NJ: Lawrence Erlbaum Associates.

Cardosa-Martins, C., Mervis, C. B., & Mervis, C. A. (1985). Early vocabulary acquisition by children with Down syndrome. *American Journal of Mental Deficiency, 90*, 177–184.

Chapman, R. S. (1995). Language development in children and adolescents with Down syndrome. In P. Fletcher & B. MacWhinney (Eds.), *The handbook of child language* (pp. 641–663). Oxford, England: Blackwell.

Chapman, R. S., Kay-Raining Bird, E., & Schwartz, S. E. (1990). Fast mapping of words in event contexts by children with Down syndrome. *Journal of Speech and Hearing Research, 55*, 761–770.

Chapman, R. S., Schwartz, S. E., & Kay-Raining Bird, E. (1991). Language skills of children and adolescents with Down syndrome. *Journal of Speech and Hearing Research, 34*, 1106–1120.

Chapman, R. S., Seung, H. K., Schwartz, S., & Kay-Raining Bird, E. (1998). Language skills in children and adolescents with Down syndrome: II. Production deficits. *Journal of Speech and Hearing Research, 41*, 861–873.

Chapman, R. S., Seung, H.-K., Schwartz, S. E., & Kay-Raining Bird, E. (2000). Language skills of children and adolescents with Down syndrome: III. Predicting production. *Journal of Speech, Language, and Hearing Research, 43*, 340–351.

Clements-Baartman, J., & Girolametto, L. (1995). Facilitating the acquisition of two-word semantic relations by preschoolers with Down syndrome: Efficacy of interactive versus didactic therapy. *Journal of Speech–Language Pathology and Audiology, 19*, 103–111.

Coleman, T. J. (2000). *Clinical management of communication disorders in culturally diverse children*. Needham Heights, MA: Allyn & Bacon.

Cossu, G., Rossini, F., & Marshall, J. C. (1993). When reading is acquired but phonemic awareness is not: A study of literacy in Down's syndrome. *Cognition, 46*, 129–138.

Crago, M., & Allen, S. E. M. (1996). Building the case for impairment in linguistic representation. In M. Rice (Ed.), *Towards a genetics of language* (pp. 261–290). Hillsdale, NJ: Lawrence Erlbaum Associates.

Crago, M., & Westernoff, F. (1997). CASLPA position paper on speech-language pathology and audiology in the multicultural, multilingual context. *Journal of Speech-Language Pathology and Audiology, 21,* 223–224.

Cromdal, J. (1999). Childhood bilingualism and metalinguistic skills: Analysis and control in young Swedish-English bilinguals. *Applied Psycholinguistics, 20,* 1–20.

Crutchley, A., Botting, N., & Conti-Ramsden, G. (1997). Bilingualism and specific language impairment in children attending language units. *European Journal of Disorders of Communication, 32,* 267–276.

Cummins, J. (1979). Linguistic interdependence and the educational development of bilingual children. *Review of Educational Research, 49,* 222–251.

Cummins, J. (2000). *Language, power, and pedagogy: Bilingual children in the crossfire.* Cleavedon, England: Multilingual Matters.

Cupples, L., & Iacono, T. (2000). Phonological awareness and oral reading skill in children with Down syndrome. *Journal of Speech, Language, and Hearing Research, 43,* 595–608.

De Houwer, A. (1999). Two or more languages: Some general points and practical recommendations. *ERIC Digest* (EDO-FL-99-03). U.S. Department of Education, Office of Educational Research and Improvement, National Library of Education, under contract ED-99-CO-0008.

Doyle, A., Champagne, M., & Segalowitz, N. (1978). Some issues in the assessment of linguistic consequences of early bilingualism. In M. Paradis (Ed.), *Aspects of bilingualism* (pp. 13–21). Columbia, SC: Hornbeam Press.

Dunn, L. M., & Dunn, L. M. (1981). *Peabody Picture Vocabulary Test–Revised.* Circle Pines, MN: American Guidance Service.

Dunn, L. M., Theriault-Whelan, C. M., & Dunn, L. M. (1993). *Échelle de vocabulaire en images Peabody*. Toronto, ON: Psychan.

Duran, E. (1985). Teaching functional reading in context to severely retarded and severely retarded autistic adolescents of limited English proficiency. *Adolescence, 20,* 433–439.

Eng, N., & O'Connor, B. (2000). Acquisition of definite article + noun agreement of Spanish–English bilingual children with specific language impairment. *Communication Disorders Quarterly, 21,* 114–124.

Fenson, L., Dale, P., Reznick, S., Thal, D., Bates, E., Hartung, J., Pethick, S., & Reilly, J. (1993). *The MacArthur Communicative Development Inventory.* San Diego, CA: Singular.

Fowler, A. (1990). Language abilities in children with Down syndrome: Evidence for specific syntactic delay. In D. Cicchetti & M. Beeghly (Eds.), *Children with Down syndrome* (pp. 302–328). Cambridge, MA: Cambridge University Press.

Fowler, A., Doherty, B., & Boynton, L. (1995). The basis of reading skill in young adults with Down syndrome. In L. Nadel & D. Rosenthal (Eds.), *Down syndrome: Living and learning in the community*. New York: John Wiley & Sons.

Garry, J., & Rubino, C. (Eds.). (2001). *Facts about the world's languages*. New York: New England Publishing Associates.

Genesee, F., Paradis, J., & Crago, M. (2005). *Dual language development and disorders*. Baltimore: Paul H. Brookes.

Gombert, J.-E. (2002). Children with Down syndrome use phonological knowledge in reading. *Reading and Writing: An Interdisciplinary Journal, 15,* 527–548.

Håkansson, G., Salameh, E.-K., & Nettelbladt, U. (2003). Measuring language development in bilingual children: Swedish-Arabic children with and without language impairment. *Linguistics, 41,* 255–288.

Hart, B., & Risley, T. R. (1995). *Meaningful differences in the everyday experiences of young American children*. Toronto, ON: Paul H. Brookes.

Heath, S. B. (1985). *Ways with words: Language, life and work in communities and classrooms*. Cambridge, England: Cambridge University Press.

Hesketh, L., & Chapman, R. (1998). Verb use by individual with Down syndrome. *American Journal on Mental Retardation, 103,* 288–304.

Hickmann, M. (1997). The acquisition of French as a native language: Structural and functional determinants in a crosslinguistic perspective. *Journal of Speech-Language Pathology and Audiology, 21,* 236–257.

Hoff, E. (2005). *Language development* (3rd ed.). Belmont, CA: Thompson Wadsworth.

Holm, A., & Dodd, B. (1999). An intervention case study of a bilingual child with phonological disorder. *Child Language Teaching and Therapy, 15,* 139–158.

Holm, A., & Dodd, B. (2001). Comparison of cross-language generalization following speech therapy. *Folia Phoniatrica et Logopaedica, 53,* 166–172.

Holm, A., Dodd. B., Stow, C., & Pert, S. (1996–1997). Speech disorders in bilingual children: Four case studies. *OpiL, 22–23,* 45–64.

Holm, A., Ozanne, A., & Dodd, B. (1997). Efficacy of intervention for a bilingual child making articulation and phonological errors. *International Journal of Bilingualism, 1,* 55–69.

Jacobson, P. F., & Schwartz, R. G. (2002). Morphology in incipient bilingual Spanish-speaking preschool children with specific language impairment. *Applied Psycholinguistics, 23,* 23–41.

Jarrold, C., Baddeley, A., & Phillips, C. E. (2002). Verbal short-term memory in Down syndrome: A problem of memory, audition, or speech? *Journal of Speech, Language, and Hearing Research, 45,* 531–544.

Jordaan, H., Shaw-Ridley, G., Serfontein, J., Orelowitz, K., & Monaghan, N. (2001). Cognitive and linguistic profiles of specific language impairment and semantic-pragmatic disorder in bilinguals. *Folia Phoniatrica et Logopaedica, 53,* 153–165.

Kamhi, A., Pollack, K. E., & Harris, J. L. (1996). *Communication development and disorders in African American children*. Toronto, ON: Brookes.

Kay-Raining Bird, E., & Chapman, R. S. (1994). Sequential recall in individuals with Down syndrome. *Journal of Speech and Hearing Research, 37,* 1369–1380.

Kay-Raining Bird, E., Cleave, P., & McConnell, L. (2000). Reading and phonological awareness in children with Down syndrome: A longitudinal study. *American Journal of Speech-Language Pathology, 9,* 319–330.

Kay-Raining Bird, E., Cleave, P. L., Trudeau, N., Thordardottir, E., Sutton, A., & Thorpe, A. (2005). The language abilities of bilingual children with Down syndrome. *American Journal of Speech-Language Pathology, 14,* 187–199.

Kritikos, E. P. (2003). Speech-language pathologists' beliefs about language assessment of bilingual/bicultural individuals. *American Journal of Speech-Language Pathology, 12,* 73–91.

Lanza, E. (1997). *Language mixing in infant bilingualism: A sociolinguistic perspective.* Oxford: Oxford University Press.

Laws, G., & Gunn, D. (2002). Relationships between reading, phonological awareness skills and language development in individuals with Down syndrome: A five year follow-up study. *Reading and Writing: An Interdisciplinary Journal, 15,* 527–548.

Leadholm, B. J., Miller, J. F., Contrucci, V. J., Brittingham, K. V., & Odell, B. C. (1992). *Language sample analysis: The Wisconsin guide.* Madison: Wisconsin Department of Public Instruction.

Leonard, L. B., Eyer, J. A., Bedore, L. M., & Grela, B. G. (1997). Three accounts of the grammatical morpheme difficulties of English-speaking children with specific language impairment. *Journal of Speech, Language, and Hearing Research, 40,* 741–753.

MacLeod, A. A. N., & McCauley, R. J. (2003). The phonological abilities of bilingual children with specific language impairment: A descriptive analysis. *Journal of Speech-Language Pathology and Audiology, 27,* 29–44.

Mattes, L. J., & Omark, D. R. (1991). *Speech and language assessment for the bilingual handicapped.* Oceanside, CA: Academic Communication Associates.

McNeilly, L., & Coleman, T. (2000). Early intervention: Working with children within the context of their families and communities. In T. Coleman (Ed.), *Clinical management of communication disorders in culturally diverse children* (pp. 77–100). Needham, MA: Allyn & Bacon.

Miller, J. (1981). *Assessing language production in children.* Austin, TX: Pro-Ed.

Miller, J. F. (1988). The developmental asynchrony of language development in children with Down syndrome. In L. Nadel (Ed.), *The psychobiology of Down syndrome* (pp. 167–198). Cambridge, MA: MIT Press.

Miller, J. F. (1992). Lexical development in young children with Down syndrome. In R. S. Chapman, (Ed.), *Processes in language acquisition and disorder* (pp. 202–216). Boston, MA: Mosby Year Book.

Miller, J., & Chapman, R. S. (2000). *Systematic analysis of language transcripts* (SALT, version 6.1). Madison, WI: Language Analysis Laboratory.

Müller, N. (1998). Transfer in bilingual first language acquisition. *Bilingualism: Language and Cognition, 1,* 151–171.

Mundy, P., Kasari, C., Sigman, M., & Ruskin, E. (1995). Nonverbal communication and early language acquisition in children with Down syndrome and in normally developing children. *Journal of Speech and Hearing Research, 38,* 157–167.

Nicoladis, E., & Genesee, F. (1997a). Language development in preschool bilingual children. *Journal of Speech-Language Pathology and Audiology, 21,* 258–270.

Nicoladis, E., & Genesee, F. (1997b). The role of parental input and language dominance in bilingual children's code-mixing. In E. Hughes, M. Hughes, & A. Greenhill (Eds.), *Proceedings of the 21st Annual Boson University Conference on Language Development* (pp. 422–432) Somerville, MA: Cascadilla Press.

Oller, J. W. (1983). Testing proficiencies and diagnosing language disorders in bilingual children. In D. R. Omark & J. G. Erickson (Eds.), *The bilingual exceptional child* (pp. 69–88). Boston: College-Hill Press.

Pacheco, R. (1983). Bilingual mentally retarded children: Language confusion or real deficits? In D. R. Omark & J. G. Erickson (Eds.), *The bilingual exceptional child* (pp. 233–254). Boston: College-Hill Press.

Paradis, J., Crago, M., Genesee, F., & Rice, M. (2003). French–English bilingual children with SLI: How do they compare with their monolingual peers? *Journal of Speech, Language, and Hearing Research, 46,* 113–127.

Patterson, J. L., & Pearson, B. (2004). Bilingual lexical development: Influences, contexts and processes. In B. A. Goldstein (Ed.), *Bilingual language development and disorders in Spanish–English speakers* (pp. 77–104.). Baltimore, MD: Paul H. Brookes.

Paul, R. (1981). Analyzing complex sentence development. In J. Miller (Ed.), *Assessing language production in children* (pp. 36–40). Austin, TX: Pro-Ed.

Payan, R. M. (1989). Language assessment of the bilingual exceptional child. In L. M. Baca & H. T. Cervantes (Eds.), *The bilingual special education interface* (pp. 125–152). Toronto, ON: Merrill Publishing.

Pearson, B. Z. (1998). Assessing lexical development in bilingual babies and toddlers. *International Journal of Bilingualism, 2,* 347–372.

Pearson, B. Z., Fernandez, S., & Oller, D. K. (1993). Lexical development in bilingual infants and toddlers: Comparison to monolingual norms. *Language Learning, 43,* 93–120.

Pearson, B., Fernandez, S., Lewedag, V., & Oller, D. K. (1997). Input factors in lexical learning of bilingual infants (ages 10–30 months). *Applied Psycholinguistics, 18,* 41–58.

Perozzi, J., & Sanchez, M. L. C. (1992). The effect of instruction in L1 on receptive acquisition of L2 for bilingual children with language delay. *Language, Speech, and Hearing Services in the Schools, 23,* 348–352.

Ray, J. (2002). Treating phonological disorders in a multilingual child: A case study. *American Journal of Speech-Language Pathology, 11,* 305–315.

Restrepo, M. A., & Gutiérrez-Clellen, V. (2004). Grammatical impairments in Spanish-English bilingual children. In B. A. Goldstein (Ed.), *Bilingual language development and disorders in Spanish-English speakers* (pp. 213–234). Baltimore: Paul H. Brookes.

Restrepo, M. A., & Kruth, K. (2000). Grammatical characteristics of a Spanish-English bilingual child with specific language impairment. *Communication Disorders Quarterly, 21,* 66–76.

Rohena, E. I., Jitendra, A. K., & Browder, D. M. (2002). Comparison of the effects of Spanish and English constant time delay instruction on sight word reading by

Hispanic learners with mental retardation. *Journal of Special Education, 36,* 169–184.

Romaine, S. (1996). Bilingualism. In W. C. Ritchie & T. K. Bhatia (Eds.), *Handbook of second language acquisition* (pp. 571–604). Toronto, ON: Academic Press.

Rondal, J. A. (2000). Bilingualism in mental retardation: Some prospective views. *Child Development and Disabilities, 26,* 57–64.

Rosenblum, T., & Pinker, S. (1983). Word magic revisited: Monolingual and bilingual children's understanding of the word–object relationship. *Child Development, 54,* 773–780.

Schieffelin, B. B., & Ochs, E. (1986). *Language socialization across cultures.* Cambridge, England: Cambridge University Press.

Seung, H.-K., & Chapman, R. S. (2000). Digit span in individuals with Down syndrome and in typically developing children: Temporal aspects. *Journal of Speech, Language, and Hearing Research, 43,* 609–620.

Slobin, D. (Ed.). (1985). *The crosslinguistic study of language acquisition. Volume 1: The data.* Hillsdale, NJ: Lawrence Erlbaum Associates.

Slobin, D. (Ed.). (1992). *The crosslinguistic study of language acquisition* (Vol. 3). Hillsdale, NJ: Lawrence Erlbaum Associates.

Sloper, P., Cunningham, C., Turner, S., & Knussen, C. (1990). Factors related to the academic attainments of children with Down syndrome. *British Journal of Educational Psychology, 60,* 284–298.

Tannen, D., & Saville-Troike, M. (1985). *Perspectives on silence.* Norwood, NJ: Ablex.

Taylor, O. L. (1986a). *Nature of communication disorders in culturally and linguistically diverse populations.* Austin, TX: Pro-Ed.

Taylor, O. L. (1986b). *Treatment of communication disorders in culturally and linguistically diverse populations.* Boston: College Hill Press.

Taylor, O. L., & Clarke, M. G. (1994). Culture and communication disorders: A theoretical framework. *Seminars in Speech and Language, 15,* 103–113.

Taylor, O. L., & Leonard, L. (Eds.). (1999). *Language acquisition across North America: Cross-cultural and cross-linguistic perspectives.* San Diego, CA: Singular Thompson.

Tervoort, B. (1979). Foreign language awareness in a five- to nine-year-old lexicographer. *Journal of Child Language, 6,* 159–166.

Thordardottir, E. (2002, November). *Parents' views on language impairment and bilingualism.* Presented at the meeting of the American Speech-Language-Hearing Association, Atlanta, GA.

Thordardottir, E., Chapman, R. S., & Wagner, L. (2002). Complex sentence production by adolescents with Down syndrome. *Applied Psycholinguistics, 23,* 163–183.

Thordardottir, E., Ellis Weismer, S., & Smith, M. (1997). Vocabulary learning in bilingual and monolingual clinical intervention. *Child Language Teaching and Therapy, 13,* 215–227.

Trudeau, N., Frank, I., & Poulin-Dubois, D. (1999). A Quebec-French adaptation of the MacArthur Communication Development Inventory. *Journal of Speech-Language Pathology and Audiology, 23,* 61–73.

Umbel, V. M., Pearson, B., Fernandez, M. C., & Oller, D. K. (1992). Measuring bilingual children's receptive vocabularies. *Child Development, 63,* 1012–1020.

Vallar, G., & Papagno, C. (1993). Preserved vocabulary acquisition in Down's syndrome: The role of phonological short-term memory. *Cortex, 29,* 467–483.

van Kleeck, A. (1994a). Metalinguistic development. In G. P. Wallach & K. G. Butler (Eds.), *Language learning disabilities in school-age children and adolescents. Some principles and applications* (pp. 53–98). New York: Merrill.

van Kleeck, A. (1994b). Potential cultural bias in training parents as conversational partners with their children who have delays in language development. *American Journal of Speech-Language Pathology, 3,* 67–77.

Vaugn-Cooke, F. (1986). The challenge of assessing the language of nonmainstream speakers. In O. L. Taylor (Ed.), *Treatment of communication disorders in culturally and linguistically diverse populations* (pp. 23–48). Toronto, ON: College-Hill Press.

Whitaker, J. H., Rueda, R. S., & Prieto, A. G. (1985). Cognitive performance as a function of bilingualism in students with mental retardation. *Mental Retardation, 23,* 302–307.

Woll, B., & Grove, N. (1996). On language deficits and modality in children with Down syndrome: A case study of twins bilingual in BSL and English. *Journal of Deaf Studies and Deaf Education, 1,* 271–278.

Zimmerman, I. L., Steiner, V. G., & Pond, R. E. (1992). *The Preschool Language Scale–3.* Toronto, ON: The Psychological Corporation.

10

The Development of Communicative Competence in Vulnerable Populations

Helen L. Johnson
Queens College
Graduate University Center, City University of New York

This chapter presents the musings of a researcher whose focus on child language development has lapsed and been born again. At a time when the study of language development was opening up in important ways, my own work began with a focus on connections between language and thought, as reflected in children's comprehension and production of relational terms (Johnson, 1974; Johnson & Chapman, 1980). The questions about how children think and learn that are addressed by this research, however, did not seem to transfer well to studying language in children who were "at risk" due to family and environmental variables. Although some of the problems of transfer were methodological, the more troubling issues concerned what evaluation researchers are wont to call "utility." In other words, these issues focus on how the data that are gathered will be used, and on the extent to which the data will serve a tangible purpose, or yield some benefit, particularly for the research participants themselves.

For me, as a researcher, confronting the immediacy and urgency of the challenges in the day-to-day lives of vulnerable children forced a reconsideration of the types of questions that needed to be asked. Too often, vulnerable children face broad, almost all-encompassing challenges to healthy development that overshadow specific issues related to their linguistic functioning such as early word learning or comprehension strategies. In this context, questions about basic processes and links between language and thought seemed less critical than questions about variables that appeared to facilitate healthy development in children encountering serious obstacles in their everyday lives. Of most interest were questions that could help to identify variables that were both associated with more optimal functioning and amenable to change. In other words, the value of the research was gauged less in terms of the elegance of its design or theoretical significance, and more in terms of its potential to yield practical insights to guide prevention and intervention, and thereby enhance the lives of the children participating in the research.

Studies of children's language development address the processes of normal development and the processes associated with the emergence of specific language disorders (Chapman, 2000). This dichotomy mirrors the work in the evolving field of developmental psychopathology, in which studies address the mechanisms through which normal developmental processes can result in aberrant outcomes, and through which atypically endowed organisms can achieve normal outcomes (Seifer & Sameroff, 1997). These approaches highlight the complexity of defining organismic and environmental contributions to development, for there is a constant interplay between these forces, with each in turn stretching and limiting the possibilities presented by the other. These competing influences have particular significance in working with children whose developmental prospects are compromised by adverse circumstances. For these children, it is often difficult to ascertain whether problematic functioning reflects intractable organic limits, organic limits that are ameliorable with change, or normal/adaptive responses to environmental circumstances that are themselves maladaptive.

This chapter examines some of the data that have been gathered on the development of communicative competence in vulnerable children, emphasizing children whose vulnerability is associated with prenatal exposure to drugs. Research with these vulnerable populations has highlighted the importance of an interactionist model of development. In doing so, it has resulted in more focus on the processes and factors that contribute to communicative development than on the content of the language and cognition that were developing. The interaction between content and process, however, is central to language development, for the child's understanding of the world is both reflected and shaped by linguistic expression and communicative acts. There is striking evidence of these reciprocal influences in cross-cultural research (Fernald & Morikawa, 1993; Miller, Wiley, Fung, & Liang, 1997). This reciprocity is also the basis for many of the didactic approaches to early language intervention that have been proposed for children living in poverty. Adopting the perspectives on developmental psychopathology that have been applied so fruitfully by Rutter (1979), Sameroff (Sameroff, 1997; Sameroff & Chandler, 1975; Seifer & Sameroff, 1987), and Werner (Werner & Smith, 1982), this chapter emphasizes both the vulnerability of communicative development to adverse environmental circumstances (Beckwith et al., 1994; Johnson, Nusbaum, Bejarano, & Rosen, 1999; Mayes, Bornstein, Chawarska, Haynes, & Granger, 1996; Rodning, Beckwith, & Howard, 1989), and the significance of communicative competence to the resilience that some children demonstrate in the face of such circumstances (Johnson, Glassman, Fiks, & Rosen, 1990). By extending the focus beyond specific language learning to communicative competence, this chapter considers modalities of expression and representation that may prove particularly valuable in working with children with varied strengths, experiences, and needs.

TAKING AN INTERACTIONIST APPROACH

The complex mechanisms through which multiple and multilevel factors reciprocally shape development in vulnerable populations illustrate the strengths and challenges of interactionist models. A critical aspect of the interactionist approach is its highlighting of the ongoing reciprocal influences of child and environment through the course of development, illuminating the mechanisms that underlie developmental change. Indeed, the dynamic interplay between influences is best understood not in a particular moment, but rather as it unfolds over time. This is exemplified in the transactional model first proposed by Sameroff and colleagues, which emphasizes the ongoing nature of influences between *organism, behavior, caregiving environment,* and *societal context*. The individual *organism* brings both unique and universal endowments to the process of development. This combination of temperament, reactivity, and biological capacities generates *behavior* that is more or less effective in expressing and representing the child's needs. This expression and representation validates the child's organismic states and needs at the same time as it is activated and defined through them. The impact of the child's *behavior* on the *caregiving environment* is significant in determining how adequately and appropriately the child's needs are met.

The environment's response to the child's behavior, however, reflects characteristics of the behavior itself, of the environment, and of the compatibility ("goodness of fit," Thomas & Chess, 1977) between the two. In cases of poor compatibility, the organism's task is to adapt and modify its behavior. At the same time, the behavior alters the caregiving environment's response to the child. In optimal circumstances, caregivers will seek to accommodate the particular needs of the child by modifying demands, responses, and resources. In less than optimal circumstances, caregivers will seek to override the particular needs of the child by persisting with expectations and demands that do not mesh well with the child's endowments, and by failing to structure resources in ways that maximize their accessibility for the child. Each exchange in this process reverberates across domains, redefining subsequent transactions. Moreover, throughout these transactions, the responses of the *caregiving environment* are framed within the broader *cultural context,* which includes societal expectations about both child-rearing practices and developmental norms.

THE INTERACTIONIST MODEL IN SITU: THE STORY OF J

What do these transactional exchanges look like in the development of a child? Let's consider J, a boy whose mother was on methadone maintenance during pregnancy and had a progressive degenerative muscular disease. J's organismic characteristics include: intelligence within normal range (assessed by Bayley Scales through age 2, McCarthy Scales at age 3, Wechsler Preschool and Primary Scale of Intelligence [WPPSI] at age 5); "easy" temperament (moderate activity level, positive affect, adaptive responses to environment and change); and severe asthma. Although J experienced moderate narcotics abstinence syndrome (withdrawal) after birth, his neurological evaluations (conducted every 6 months since birth) have all been normal.

From the outset, J was a "vulnerable" child. His prenatal exposure to methadone and other substances of abuse placed him at heightened risk for developmental difficulties. During infancy, however, J's development did not appear to have been compromised by these prenatal factors. He displayed growth and development consistent with general developmental norms, and also significant strengths in social skills and engagement. Despite the limited responsiveness of his mother, J benefited from frequent and extended contact with his grandmother and with clinic staff, with whom he formed close attachments. He was extremely effective at eliciting and sustaining constructive interactions. Ironically, these strengths ultimately restricted J's access to environmental supports.

As J's mother's physical condition deteriorated, she found it increasingly difficult to parent an active, inquiring 3-year-old. Moreover, J's frequent acute asthmatic episodes, which required emergency medical attention, were extremely stressful for his mother. She scolded and berated J, rejected his attempts to engage her in conversation and play, and demonstrated harsh and restrictive parenting. J clearly would have benefited from enrollment in a preschool or day care; time in a more supportive environment would have fostered his cognitive and language development, and his strong interpersonal skills would have enabled him to take advantage of the activities and interactions. Unfortunately, seats in public day care programs are limited, and because J did not display signs of developmental delay or adjustment problems, he was not given priority for enrollment. Moreover, J's mother did not pursue day care placement because she was reluctant to handle transportation arrangements. In fact, by the time J was enrolled in kindergarten, his mother's physical condition confined her to a wheelchair, and she frequently kept J home from school to assist with her own care. Although J's performance on the WPPSI at age 5 was within normal range, he was less attentive and engaging than at prior visits. J also was less responsive to verbal instructions, and exhibited oppositional behavior toward his mother and noncompliant behavior toward clinic staff.

The interactional nature of J's experience is complex. J's organismic characteristics included many strengths, which were reflected in positive social behavior and engagement in the environment. These organismic strengths and constructive behaviors, however, still require support and nurturance from the caregiving environment to continue and thrive. In J's case, both the immediate caregiving environment and the broader societal context failed to provide this support. In fact, by the time he was 5 years old, J's mother was actively restricting his access to environments that might have provided more support. J's case epitomizes the transactional nature of development: Organismic strengths that initially engender positive behaviors, but continually fail to elicit positive responses from the environment, may be rechanneled into behaviors that either demand an environmental response or elicit less resistance. These behaviors shape the subsequent feedback provided by the environment, and in this way revise the child's sense of self in relation to others. For J, the social skills and engagement that initially were focused on seeking constructive interactions were now being redirected into behaviors that reliably achieved a reaction, although negative, from his mother. Conversational skills, game playing, and other social-communicative behaviors that should have been blossoming at age 5 were less characteristic of J than they had been earlier. The combination of his declining positive social engagement and his erratic school attendance predicts the difficulties frequently associated with the stereotypic "drug-exposed" child.

DEVELOPMENTAL VULNERABILITY—AFFECT AND COMMUNICATION

J's emerging behavioral profile reflects the influence of specific risk factors (prenatal drug exposure, asthma, poor parenting skills). More importantly, however, it illustrates the complex interactions between variables in shaping developmental risk and resilience. The significance of these interactions is particularly apparent in the profiles of children who were exposed to drugs through maternal use during pregnancy. The infant born to a drug-abusing mother enters the world with specific characteristics that have been shaped by many factors, including prenatal drug exposure. This infant enters a world in which the mother's involvement with drugs compromises the family's ability to provide consistent and responsive care. This child's developmental prospects are further diminished by societal expectations that this child *will* do poorly. Poor impulse control, impaired social and communicative functioning, and delayed cognitive and academic achievement all fit conventional wisdom's profile of the child born to a drug abuser. Too often, the fact of the mother's drug abuse is accepted as the explanation for the child's developmental difficulties, thereby limiting intervention efforts. My intent here is not to downplay the seriousness of maternal drug abuse for the child, but to suggest that in order to understand its impact, we must look beyond the initial time of exposure and the neonatal period, and examine how perinatal factors operate to shape development over time, through the interactions between the developing child and the environment.

In the lives of real children, maternal substance abuse during pregnancy typically occurs in combination with a variety of other factors—including poverty, maternal depression, limited maternal education, chaotic living arrangements, and family and community violence—known to pose obstacles to healthy development. Over the past 25 years, the research on prenatally drug-exposed children has repeatedly shown the difficulties inherent in trying to separate the effects of these interwoven variables, for in research with children born to methadone-maintained and polydrug abusing women, specific maternal drug habits and neonatal characteristics generally did not directly predict long-term outcome (Bernstein & Hans, 1994; Coles & Platzman, 1993; Hurt et al., 1995; Johnson, Glassman, Fiks, & Rosen, 1987; Johnson et al., 1990; Malakoff, Mayes, & Schottenfeld, 1994). Instead, what emerged was a pattern of effects that are best understood in terms of a transactional model of development similar to the one proposed by Sameroff and his colleagues (Sameroff & Chandler, 1975; Seifer & Sameroff, 1987). In this model, three ongoing levels of organization—the individual organism, the immediate family, and the culture—influence one another recurrently over time to shape developmental course.

Maternal substance abuse during pregnancy affects the developing child both directly, through exposure to the drugs themselves, and indirectly, through the impact of drug use on maternal functioning. Profiles of addicted mothers indicate higher levels of depression and stress and lower levels of self-esteem than in matched non-drug-abusing mothers (Fiks, Johnson, & Rosen, 1985). Diminished feelings of self-efficacy lead addicted women to employ emotion-focused, confrontational coping styles; they show little self-control or planning, and are less likely to seek and utilize social services and support (Kouzekanani & Neely, 1997). These ineffectual coping strategies serve to maintain the isolation that addicts frequently experience. The lack of interpersonal engagement carries over into parenting behavior. Cocaine-abusing mothers have been found to be less attentive and responsive to their infants (Mayes et al., 1996). Moreover, the addicted mother is more likely to have negative perceptions of her child and to view the child as a source of stress (Bernstein & Hans, 1994; Howard, Beckwith, Rodning, & Kropenshke, 1989; Johnson & Rosen, 1990).

At the same time, a disproportionate number of infants exposed to drugs prenatally show characteristics of the "difficult baby" described by Thomas and Chess (1977). In the case of prenatal drug exposure, the intense cry, irritability, and poor consolability, which define the difficult baby in the Thomas et al. paradigm, may actually be symptoms of neonatal narcotics abstinence syndrome (Finnegan, 1976). Regardless of the etiology, however, this behavioral constellation makes the task of providing loving and responsive care for the infant particularly demanding.

Research has also highlighted disruptions in early attentional and self-regulating capacities in drug-exposed infants (Beeghly & Tronick, 1994; Mayes et al., 1996). Taken together, these factors result in a serious mismatch between the mother's limited emotional resources and the infant's intense caregiving needs (Johnson, Diano, & Rosen, 1984). The tension within the dyad generated by this mismatch is likely to limit the mother's emotional responsiveness to her infant. Over time, because the infant's behavior does not consistently encourage or reward maternal efforts, the likelihood of contingent maternal responses is further diminished.

This cycle of ineffective or mismatched parent–child transactions has serious long-term consequences for the child's development. The importance of maternal emotional responsiveness and availability to the infant's development has been well documented (Crockenberg, 1981; Howard et al., 1989). Maternal emotional availability provides the foundation for the attachment relationships that frame the child's development of working models of self in relation to others, which in turn guide socioemotional development (Bretherton & Waters, 1985). The child who does not expect positive and relevant feedback from the environment is likely to become less engaged. This was illustrated in the work of

Field and colleagues, who found that infants of depressed mothers display depressed interactive behavior not only with their depressed mothers, but also with nondepressed adults (Field et al., 1988). Similarly, a child whose caregiver is erratic or abusive may well learn not to engage in extended social interaction—there are no models for it in the child's experience, and interaction carries with it the possibility of negative consequences that are best avoided.

Through early attachment relationships, the infant develops the capacity to focus and sustain attention. The infant's growing awareness of her or his own ability to have an effect on people and objects fosters the evolving sense of self as competent and effective, and motivates further exploration and interaction. By providing the foundation for engagement, exploration and sustained attention, attachment is central to the development of cognition and language as well (Morisset, Barnard, Greenberg, Booth, & Stieker, 1990; Slade, 1987). Robinson and Acevedo (2001) found that the emotional vitality of 6- to 9-month-old infants predicted their language and cognitive skills at 2 years. Meins (1998) highlighted the mechanisms connecting attachment and language in a study of securely and insecurely attached 20-month-olds and their mothers. Securely attached infants had larger overall vocabularies, and proportionately more nouns as opposed to frozen phrases. Importantly, the mothers of securely attached infants were more likely to attribute meaning to their infants' utterances, reflecting the greater responsiveness or attunement that is associated with secure attachment. These findings epitomize the interwoven nature of communication and affect in early experience. They also illustrate the critical role of attachment relationships in the child's communicative and cognitive development. A defining characteristic of the securely attached toddler is the ability to explore and experiment with some degree of independence. The child's knowledge and understanding grow through the child's capacity to resolve the mismatches between what is expected and what is encountered in experience. This capacity to explore novelty and try out new solutions requires the sense of emotional safety and personal competence that define secure attachment.

At the same time as J's case illustrates the impact of repeated negative feedback from the caregiving environment on the development of social and communicative behavior, it also demonstrates how tightly intertwined different aspects of development are. This means that disturbances in maternal emotional availability that make it difficult for the child to get what she or he needs from interactions with the caregiver (Bernstein & Hans, 1994) will compromise subsequent development across multiple domains, encompassing affect, cognition, and language.

THE VULNERABILITY OF COMMUNICATIVE BEHAVIOR

The vulnerability of language development in children growing up in difficult circumstances has been extensively documented. Impairments in language and representational play have been reported for children exposed to maternal depression (Cox, Puckering, Pound, & Mills, 1987), low social support (Coster, Gersten, Beeghly, & Cichetti,1989), and stress (Morriset et al., 1990). Working with a population of premature, low-birth-weight, low-socioeconomic-status infants, Bradley and colleagues (Bradley et al., 1994) found that only 12% displayed "normal" functioning at age 3 years. Bradley et al. suggest that the poor performance of these children is best understood as the outcome of the "double jeopardy" of poor parenting skills and unstimulating environments.

Infants exposed to drugs prenatally actually experience a "triple jeopardy" of drug effects/withdrawal, poor parenting, and chaotic living circumstances. Since the early 1980s, there have been indications of the particular vulnerability of language and social development in this population (Jeremy & Bernstein, 1984; Johnson et al., 1984). The evidence of vulnerability of language in this population strongly reinforces the importance of interaction between organism and caregiving environment in shaping development. Even in studies that have found clear differences between drug-exposed and nonexposed children, the differences suggest environmental influences as much as organismic/neurological ones.

For drug-exposed infants and preschoolers, scores within normal range on standardized measures do not preclude deficits in communicative and social behavior. Beckwith, Rodning, and colleagues reported that drug-exposed toddlers had impairments of representational function and play behavior (Howard et al., 1989; Rodning et al., 1989). These findings occurred despite the absence of significant differences between drug-exposed and matched nonexposed toddlers on standardized developmental assessments.

Malakoff et al. (1994) examined language development in 21 preschoolers, ranging in age from 29 to 70 months. All of the children were living with cocaine-dependent caregivers, and 60% had been exposed to cocaine prenatally. The findings indicated that all but three of the children had some degree of language delay. The severity of the impairment, however, was not related to prenatal cocaine exposure, suggesting that any central nervous system effects associated with prenatal cocaine exposure are less significant to the child's language development than the characteristics of the caregiving environment. Malakoff and colleagues interpret the finding that older children showed a greater degree of delay than younger as evidence of the cumulative effects of inadequate environmental supports. Interestingly, the relationship between receptive and expressive language skills in this population did not follow the normal pattern: Impairments were more severe in receptive than expressive language. The authors point to differences in task demands as one possible explanation for this finding. The naming behavior required for the expressive language task may be simpler and more familiar to these children than the behavior involved in the receptive language task, which requires the children to attend to more than one object at a time, follow verbal instructions and identify the appropriate object.

Although differences in task demands certainly contribute to performance differences, the delays in receptive language warrant further consideration. Delays in receptive language during early development are particularly significant in predicting more long-term problems with language and literacy (Rescorla & Schwartz, 1990), and may be associated with a more general delay in cognitive development. Receptive language delays may reflect gaps in concept development that are attributable to environments that fail to provide stimulation that includes information that is sufficiently clear, consistent, and responsive to the child's interests and needs.

Mentis (1998) reported delays in expressive language, especially the pragmatics of language use, among cocaine-exposed toddlers. Although the findings are based on a very limited sample, they indicate that the drug-exposed children showed less overall engagement in communicative interactions, and "used communication for different and less mature functions." The strong connection between pragmatics and effectiveness in interpersonal situations highlights once again the interactive mechanisms underlying development. The child who is slow to acquire the social and cultural conventions for communication is likely to elicit more non-responsive and/or restrictive feedback from the environment. In the case of children living in adversity, the situation is further complicated by the possibility that the caregiver's behavior may actually be providing models of ineffective or inappropriate communicative strategies. In a striking example of this, Freier (1994) reported strong similarities between the behavioral modulations of drug-exposed infants and their mothers, noting that the infants recreated the mood swings and outbursts they observed in their mothers. In such instances, normal adaptive processes can result in deviant outcomes (Sameroff, 1997), and disorders attributed to the organism may in fact reflect normal developmental and interactional processes operating in atypical circumstances.

A more fine-grained analysis of the nature of the differences in communicative behavior between drug-exposed and non-exposed toddlers is offered by Bland-Stewart, Seymour, Beeghly, and Frank (1998), who focused on the development of semantic knowledge in a group of 22 African American 2-year-olds, half of whom had been prenatally exposed to cocaine.

Bland-Stewart and colleagues point out that semantic knowledge offers a particularly meaningful perspective on communicative development, because it illuminates "the emergence of language form, semantic content, and the interaction between form and content" (p. 172).

The drug-exposed and nonexposed toddlers did not differ on the Bayley Scales of Infant Development (BSID) or the Sequenced Inventory of Communication Development–Revised Edition (SICD–R), or in structural features of language such as length of utterance and distribution of utterance types. However, the drug-exposed toddlers' utterances demonstrated more restricted and delayed semantic development. Although the drug-exposed and nonexposed toddlers appear to follow a similar sequence in their semantic development, the drug-exposed toddlers "appear to follow this sequence at a somewhat slower pace than do their non-exposed peers." Again, as in the research of Malakoff et al. and Beckwith et al., although the results of standardized (and more global) assessments failed to differentiate drug-exposed from nonexposed children, Bland-Steward et al. found that assessments of specific aspects of language functioning revealed differences. Indeed, the findings of all three research groups reveal differences that are significant because of their links to cognitive functioning and because of their similarity to findings with children who are at risk due to other environmental factors, such as maternal depression and poverty. As Malakoff and colleagues (1994) commented, "The magnitude and ongoing nature of the negative effects of the caregiving environment and mother-child interaction may be such that they 'wash out' any effects due specifically to prenatal exposure" (p. 352).

The special vulnerability of communicative behavior, then, is essentially interactional in nature. The interaction between the infant's organismic vulnerability and the environment's inadequate and unresponsive practices results in delays in development. There are many organismic characteristics associated with maternal poverty, depression, and substance abuse. Infants born to women in these circumstances are more likely to be exposed to complications during labor and delivery, to be born small, and to be born prematurely. From the outset, such infants come to experience in the world slightly less prepared to engage effectively. At the same time, mothers dealing with poverty, depression, and substance abuse are less likely to have the emotional resources necessary for providing responsive care, and for engaging in sustained and nondirective communicative interactions.

COMMUNICATION INPUT FROM VULNERABLE PARENTS

The challenges to healthy development encountered by vulnerable children frequently compromise the functioning of their caregivers as well.

There is reliable evidence that the stresses in daily living faced by women raising children in poverty affect the tone of parenting (Duncan, Yeung, Brooks-Gunn, & Smith, 1998). Conger and colleagues (Conger et al., 1992) found that financial concerns were associated with increased harshness in maternal parenting behavior. Werner and Smith's seminal longitudinal study (1982) indicated that exposure to adverse social conditions is ten times more likely than perinatal complications to result in poor development. When the resources available to families are limited, both directly and by virtue of support networks that are themselves impoverished and overextended, an increased amount of energy must be directed toward fulfilling the basic tasks of daily living (Okongwu, 1995). This necessary focus on securing and maintaining basic living needs restricts the emotional resources and time available for parenting.

The child's everyday activities and experiences provide the input, or raw material, from which the child constructs systems of communication and structures of language. Over the years, there has been extensive consideration of the salient features of that input—its quantity, well-formedness, and responsiveness to the child's interests. Special emphasis has been placed on the quality of input that low-income and poverty mothers provide to support communicative development. Hess (1999) has suggested that children living in abusive or impoverished environments are likely to experience fewer responsive and facilitative interactions with adults. An earlier study by Hoff-Ginsburg (1991) offered an important perspective on the source of these differences. Hoff-Ginsburg examined the quantity and amount of maternal language to children in several settings. The findings indicated that different settings elicited different types of maternal communication—more directive language occurred in functional settings such as feeding, and more inquiry and open-ended language in play settings such as book reading. There were not significant socioeconomic differences in maternal behavior within settings. However, in comparison to middle-income mothers, lower-income mothers spent proportionately more of their time in functional activities such as feeding. In this way, the environmental pressures that compel low-income mothers to focus much of their time and attention on survival issues limit these mothers' ability to engage their children in settings and interactions associated with enhanced language development. To the extent that socioeconomic differences in maternal communicative behavior are explained by differences in "setting," these differences themselves reflect the lack of environmental supports—such as books, quiet space, uninterrupted time—for both mother and child.

Hart and Risley (1995) have suggested that the academic difficulties experienced disproportionately by children growing up in poverty are largely explained by differences in the quantity of language addressed to children, and that differences in early language development are precursors of reading disorders. A recent study in the United Kingdom by Locke, Ginsborg, and Peers (2002) examined the language and cognitive abilities of 240 low-income children just entering preschool. Locke and colleagues found that the children performed significantly lower than middle-income children on measures of receptive and expressive language. Indeed, more than half met the criteria for diagnosis of moderate, moderate to severe, or severe language delay. It is important to note that although the level of the low-income children's language performance was significantly lower than that of middle-income norms, their cognitive performance was not. The authors suggest that low-income children may have limited exposure to activities that "draw their attention to structural features of language." The importance of environmental input is also emphasized by Huttenlocher and colleagues (Huttenlocher, Vasilyeva, Cymerman, & Levine, 2002), whose data indicate that this influence extends through infancy into early childhood, and operates through both home and classroom language input. In sum, research indicates that environment shapes language development both by providing content and topics for communication and by directing attention to critical aspects of communication systems and processes.

COMMUNICATION, EXPRESSION, AND RESILIENCE

Too often, appreciation of the impact of environmental influences leads to a lack of consideration for what the child brings to experience generally, and to the process of communicative development specifically. A critical piece in this development is the child's quest for personal expression. Naming the people, objects, events, and feelings in one's world are central to the development of self. The child moves into language to accomplish this, and expression is a central function of communication from the start. The seminal work of Bloom and colleagues (Bloom, Margulis, Tinker, & Fujita, 1996; Bloom & Tinker, 2001) has documented the importance of expression in early language, beginning with infants in the "first words" period. Although communication is an interactive and social behavior, at its core there are thoughts, feelings, wishes, and questions that the infant seeks to share. As Bloom and Tinker remark, "Somehow, the child has to be kept in the picture as the major player, as the *agent* of the practices that contribute to the acquisition process" (Bloom & Tinker, 2001, p. 5).

The significance of this agency is magnified in dealing with vulnerable children, in terms partly of our understanding of their developmental strengths and challenges, but in terms of their opportunities to maximize the realization of their potential as well. The experience of personal effectiveness in a communicative exchange provides a basis for continued engagement, and for an emerging sense of self as competent and worthy.

Bloom's data indicate that even very young speakers are not simply responders; they initiate communicative exchanges because they have things that they want to talk about. The response of the caregiving environment is critical in shaping subsequent communicative behavior. The child whose communications are acknowledged, understood, and valued is motivated to maintain effort and sustain attention. When early communicative efforts meet with success, the child is motivated to sustain and expand expression. When they do not, the child comes to expect less, or at least less positive, results from communicative exchanges. These exchanges hold out less promise of personal expression, and the motivation to engage and attend to them is thereby diminished.

There is a great deal of evidence that these less than optimal communicative exchanges occur with disproportionate frequency in the lives of vulnerable children. The environmental circumstances that place stress on children entail stress for their families as well. Children living in these difficult circumstances face many obstacles, but these obstacles in and of themselves do not determine the scope of what is developmentally possible for these children. At each juncture, organic, cognitive, emotional, and social characteristics of the child interact with features of the family and broader caregiving environment to shape the next phase. In each of these transactional exchanges, the agency of the child is critical. The child whose attempts to communicate or enact feelings are not validated becomes less engaged. Over time, the lack of engagement has multiplicative effects on social, language, and cognitive development. Although we frequently frame our research questions in terms of the effect of one discrete variable on another, isolating the effects of variables through sophisticated data analysis techniques does not mirror their operation in the lives of children and families, and attributes a level of precision of measurement that may not be warranted with variables that are fundamentally diffuse and complex. As Chapman notes:

> At the end of the 20th Century, the Cartesian mind–body distinction that has conveniently separated our domains of discourse, and associated explanations, in biology and behavior, body and mind, and brain and cognition, is dissolving in the repeated demonstrations of interactivity at every analytic level, from the environmental contributions to directional orientation in embryos to genes turned on or off by cellular contexts to the observable biological effects in the brain of mind, thinking, or experiencing. (Chapman, 2000, p. 44)

Acknowledging the permeability of boundaries between domains of functioning changes the nature of questions regarding risk and resilience. The interactionist approach leads us past seeking to determine whether J's emerging behavioral profile reflects the impact of specific risk factors (his prenatal drug exposure, his asthma, his mother's poor parenting skills), or the cumulative risk (cf. Sameroff) created by these combined factors. Rather, although attributing some validity to each of these approaches, the interactionist approach focuses on the complexity of endowments and supports that define the individual child. In this way, highlighting strengths and vulnerabilities can guide the pinpointing of opportunities to redirect the developmental trajectory to more positive paths.

How does this redirection begin? We must come back once more to the recognition that at each point in time, children bring with them, always, content and meaning, thoughts and feelings, to be expressed. The teachers in my graduate education classes often comment that a particular child doesn't participate effectively in written or oral language activities "because he doesn't have anything to talk about." This is not an adequate description of any child. The challenge is to provide ways for children with unusual or nontraditional experiences to draw on them within the context of classroom experiences. One classroom strategy to address this concern is illustrated in Dyson's (1994) powerful documentation of a third-grade classroom that encouraged children to write and read personal stories. Dyson recounts an incident in which the teacher suggests to William, a student, that parents and teachers visiting the classroom may not like his plan to write "I like to get in fights." In response, William replies, "'That's too bad they don't like it,' he says, 'I'm gonna *express* myself'" (Dyson, 1994, p. 155). In this classroom, children do use language and literacy activities for personal expression, and their work covers some topics and words that violate traditional expectations for classroom behavior. Dyson highlights the impact of these classroom activities on children's communicative development. The sustained participation in a classroom environment that supports and values personal expression increases the overall level of the children's communicative behavior—language is used to express and work through feelings that previously would have been handled physically, and the quality of the children's writing improves significantly as well. The experience of self as effective communicator is reinforced by responses from peers, and acceptance, although not without revision, from teacher.

Learning to talk, the child continually asks, "Can you hear me? Do you read me? Send message, over and out" (Chapman, 1991, p. 47). Assurance that messages have been received, and will be sent, provides the child with a safe base for exploring and engaging the world. In this way, communicative development provides a foundation that supports the child's path through increasingly complex experiences. Communication enables the child to share discoveries, insights, and feelings, and to request clarification and help moving through confusing or demanding experiences. For the vulnerable child, this support is particularly essential. Experiencing self as an effective communicator in a somewhat alien environment fosters the child's inclination to push on, and move further ahead, with resilience. The challenge for the adults who work with these children is to provide meaningful and consistent opportunities for personal expression that both validate and extend the child's world.

REFERENCES

Beckwith, L., Rodning, C., Norris, D. Phillipsen, L., Khandabi, P., & Howard, J. (1994). Spontaneous play in two-year-olds born to substance-abusing mothers. *Infant Mental Health Journal, 15,* 189–201.

Beeghly, M., & Tronick, E. Z. (1994). Effects of prenatal exposure to cocaine in early infancy: Toxic effects on the process of mutual regulation. *Infant Mental Health Journal, 15,* 158–175.

Bernstein, V. J., & Hans, S. L. (1994). Predicting the developmental outcome of two-year-old children born exposed to methadone: The impact of social-environmental risk factors. *Journal of Clinical Child Psychiatry, 23,* 349–359.

Bland-Stewart, L. M., Seymour, H. N., Beeghly, M., & Frank, D. A. (1998). Semantic development of African-American children prenatally exposed to cocaine. *Seminars in Speech and Language, 19,* 167–187.

Bloom, L., Margulis, C., Tinker, E., & Fujita, N. (1996). Early conversations and word learning: Contributions from child and adult. *Child Development, 67,* 3154–3175.

Bloom, L., & Tinker, E. (2001). The intentionality model and language acquisition. *Monographs of the Society for Child Development, 66*(Serial No. 267).

Bradley, R., Whiteside, L., Mundfrom, D., Casey, P., Kellerher, K., & Pope, S. (1994). Early indications of resilience and their relation to experiences in the home environments of low birthweight, premature children living in poverty. *Child Development, 65,* 346–360.

Bretherton, I., & Waters, E. (1985). Growing points in attachment theory. *Monographs of the Society for Research in Child Development, 50*(Serial No. 207).

Chapman, R. S. (1991). *Learning to talk.* Dodgeville, WI: Fireweed Press.

Chapman, R. S. (2000). Children's language learning: An interactionist perspective. *Journal of Child Psychology and Psychiatry, 41,* 33–54.

Coles, C. D., & Platzman, K. A. (1993). Behavioral development in children prenatally exposed to drugs and alcohol. *International Journal of the Addictions, 28,* 1393.

Conger, R. D., Conger, K. F., Elder, G. H., Jr., Lorena, F. O., Simmons, R. L., & Whitbeck, L. B. (1992). A family process model of economic hardship and adjustment in early adolescent boys. *Child Development, 63,* 526–541.

Coster, W., Gersten, M. S., Beeghly, M., & Cichetti, D. (1989). Communicative functioning in maltreated toddlers. *Developmental Psychology, 25,* 1020–1029.

Cox, A. D., Puckering, C., Pound, A., & Mills, M. (1987). The impact of maternal depression in young children. *Journal of Child Psychology and Psychiatry, 28,* 917–928.

Crockenberg, S. (1981). Infant irritability, mother responsiveness and social support influences on the security of infant–mother attachment. *Child Development, 52,* 857–865.

Duncan, G. J., Yeung, W. J., Brooks-Gunn, J., & Smith, J. R. (1998). How much does childhood poverty affect the life chances of children? *American Sociological Review, 63,* 406–423.

Dyson, A. H. (1994). "I'm gonna express myself": The politics of story in the children's worlds. In A. H. Dyson & C. Genishi (Eds.), *The need for story* (pp. 220–239). New York: Teachers College Press.

Fernald, A., & Morikawa, H. (1993). Common themes and cultural variations in Japanese and American mothers' speech to infants. *Child Development, 64,* 637–656.

Field, T., Healy, B., Goldstein, S., Perry, S., Bendell, D., Schanberg, S., Zimmerman, E. A., & Kuhn, C. (1988). Infants of depressed mothers show "depressed" behavior even with non-depressed adults. *Child Development, 59,* 1569–1579.

Fiks, K., Johnson, H. L., & Rosen, T. S. (1985). Methadone-maintained mothers: Three year follow-up of parental functioning. *International Journal of Addictions, 20,* 651–660.

Finnegan, L. P. (1976). Clinical effects of pharmacological agents on pregnancy and the fetus and the neonate. *Annals of the New York Academy of Science, 281,* 74–89.

Freier, K. (1994). In vitro drug exposure and maternal–infant interaction: The complexities of the dyad and their environment. *Infant Mental Health Journal, 5,* 176–188.

Hart, B., & Risley, T. (1995). *Meaningful differences in the everyday experiences of young children.* Baltimore: Paul H. Brookes.

Hess, L. J. (1999). Let's talk and play: A study of poverty mothers and toddler daughters. *Infant-Toddler Intervention, 9,* 1–16.

Hoff-Ginsburg, E. (1991). Mother-child conversation in different social classes and communicative settings. *Child Development, 62,* 782–796.

Howard, J., Beckwith, L., Rodning, C., & Kropenshke, V. (1989). The development of young children of substance-abusing parents: Insights from seven years of intervention and research. *Zero to Three, 9,* 8–12.

Hurt, H., Brodsky, N. L., Betancourt, L., Braitman, L. E., Malmud, A. E., & Gianetta, J. (1995). Cocaine-exposed children: Follow-up through 30 months. *Developmental and Behavioral Pediatrics, 16,* 29–35.

Huttenlocher, J., Vasilyeva, M., Cymerman, E., & Levine, S. (2002). Language input and child syntax. *Cognitive Psychology, 45,* 337–374.

Jeremy, R. J., & Bernstein, V. J. (1984). Dyads at risk: Methadone-maintained women and their four-month-old infants. *Child Development, 55,* 1141–1154.

Johnson, H. L. (1974). The meaning of *before* and *after* for preschool children. *Journal of Experimental Child Psychology, 19,* 243–260.

Johnson, H. L., & Chapman, R. S. (1980). Children's judgement and recall of causal statements: A developmental study of *because, so,* and *and. Journal of Psycholinguistic Research, 9,* 243–260.

Johnson, H. L., Diano, A., & Rosen, T. S. (1984). 24-month neurological follow-up of children of methadone-maintained mothers. *Infant Behavior and Development, 7,* 115–123.

Johnson, H. L., Glassman, M. B., Fiks, K., & Rosen, T. S. (1987). Path analysis of variables affecting 36-month outcome in a population of multi-risk children. *Infant Behavior and Development, 10,* 451–465.

Johnson, H. L., Glassman, M. B., Fiks, K., & Rosen, T. S. (1990). Resilient children: Individual differences in developmental outcome of children born to drug abusers. *Journal of Genetic Psychology, 15,* 523–539.

Johnson, H. L., Nusbaum, B. J., Bejarano, A., & Rosen, T. S. (1999). An ecological approach to development in children with prenatal drug exposure. *American Journal of Orthopsychiatry, 69,* 448–456.

Johnson, H. L., & Rosen, T. S. (1990). Mother-infant interaction in a multi-risk population. *American Journal of Orthopsychiatry, 60,* 281–288.

Kouzekanani, K., & Neely, M. A. (1997). Coping styles of female cocaine addicts. *Substance Abuse, 18,* 165–171.

Locke, A., Ginsborg, J., & Peers, I. (2002). Development and disadvantage: Implications for the early years and beyond. *International Journal of Language and Communication Disorders, 37,* 3–15.

Malakoff, M. E., Mayes, L. C., & Schottenfeld, R. S. (1994). Language abilities of preschool-age children living with cocaine-using mothers. *American Journal on Addictions, 4,* 346–354.

Mayes, L. C., Bornstein, M. H., Chawarska, K., Haynes, O. M., & Granger, R. H. (1996). Impaired regulation of arousal in 3-month-old infants exposed prenatally to cocaine and other drugs. *Development and Psychopathology, 8,* 29–42.

Meins, E. (1998). The effects of security of attachment and maternal attribution of meaning on children's linguistic acquisitional style. *Infant Behavior and Development, 21,* 237–252.

Mentis, M. (1998). *In utero* cocaine exposure and language development. *Seminars in Speech and Language, 19,* 147–165.

Miller, P. J., Wiley, A. R., Fung, H., & Liang, C.-H. (1997). Personal storytelling as a medium of socialization in Chinese and American families. *Child Development, 68,* 557–568.

Morisset, C. E., Barnard, K. E., Greenberg, M. T., Booth, C. L., & Stieker, S. J. (1990). Enviromental influences on early language development: The context of social risk. *Development and Psychopathology, 2,* 127–149.

Okongwu, A. (1995). Looking up from the bottom to the ceiling of the basement floor: Female single-parent families surviving on $22,000 or less a year. *Urban Anthropology, 24,* 313–362.

Rescorla, L., & Schwartz, E. (1990). Outcome of toddlers with specific expressive language delay. *Applied Psycholinguistics, 11,* 393–407.

Robinson, J. L., & Acevedo, M. C. (2001). Infant reactivity and reliance on mother during emotion challenges: Prediction of cognition and language skills in a low-income sample. *Child Development, 72,* 402–415.

Rodning, C., Beckwith, L., & Howard, J. (1989). Characteristics of attachment organization and play organization in prenatally drug-exposed toddlers. *Development and Psychopathology, 1,* 277–289.

Rutter, M. (1979). Protective factors in children's responses to stress and disadvantage. In M. W. Kent & J. E. Rolf (Eds.), *Principles in psychopathology: Social competence in children* (pp. 49–74). Hanover, NH: University Press of New England.

Sameroff, A. J. (1997, April). *Developmental contributions to the study of psychopathology.* Invited address, Society for Research in Child Development, Washington, DC.

Sameroff, A. J., & Chandler, M. J. (1975). Reproductive risk and the continuum of caretaking casualty. In F. D. Horowitz, E. M. Herherington, S. Scarr-Salapatek, &

G. M. Siegel (Eds.), *Review of child development research* (Vol. 4, pp. 187–244). Chicago: University of Chicago.

Seifer, R., & Sameroff, A. J. (1987). Multiple determinants of risk and invulnerability. In E. J. Anthony & B. J. Cohler (Eds.), *The invulnerable child* (pp. 51–69). New York: Guilford.

Slade, A. (1987). Quality of attachment and early symbolic play. *Developmental Psychology, 23,* 78–85.

Thomas, A., & Chess, S. (1977). *Temperament and development.* New York: Brunner/Mazel.

Werner, E. E., & Smith, R. S. (1982). *Vulnerable but invincible: A study of resilient children.* New York: McGraw-Hill.

11

Could Verbs Be Hubs?

Christine Dollaghan
University of Pittsburgh

VERBS (AND HUBS)

Until rather recently the language acquisition literature could fairly be described as "noun-o-centric"; although the importance of verbs had long been acknowledged, there were relatively few empirical investigations of them until a small group of investigators, including Robin S. Chapman, focused specifically on verbs in the late 1970s. Robin's work (e.g., Chapman, 1978; Chapman & Kohn, 1978) provided important evidence on typically developing children's comprehension of action words and verbs; she also conducted one of the first analyses of the verbs that caregivers use with their very young children (Chapman, Dollaghan, Kenworthy, & Miller, 1983). The ensuing years have witnessed an explosion of interest in children's verb acquisition and use (e.g., Ambalu, Chiat, & Pring, 1997; Gillette, Gleitman, Gleitman, & Lederer, 1999; Hesketh & Chapman, 1998; Olguin & Tomasello, 1993; Tomasello, 1992; Tomasello, Akhtar, Dodson, & Rekau, 1997), but in many ways it seems that the more we have learned about verbs, the more mysterious they have become.

The literature on verbs in children with specific language impairment (SLI) is a case in point. Thordardottir and Ellis Weismer (2001) summarized a rather large body of contradictory evidence on the seemingly straightforward question of whether such children's difficulties with verb morphology are matched by deficits in the size and/or nature of their verb lexicons (e.g., Leonard, Miller, & Gerber, 1999). As Thordardottir and Ellis Weismer as well as Conti-Ramsden and Jones (1997) noted, some studies have suggested that children with SLI have disproportionately small verb lexicons; others have not. Some have suggested that children with SLI use too many semantically "light" verbs and/or "general all-purpose" (GAP) verbs; others have not. It is certainly possible that differences in participant characteristics and methodologies can account for many of these discrepant findings, but it is also possible that our analytical approaches and/or our verb typologies are not adequate for the task. I took this chapter as an opportunity to explore some alternative approaches to thinking about the nature, role, and acquisition of verbs in typical and atypical child language using ideas derived from the growing literature on "small-world" networks. Examining features and processes of development that may be common to seemingly disparate domains suggested some new analyses and yielded some unexpected findings. Although this work is frankly exploratory, I think that it illustrates how the broader developmental perspective that Robin Chapman has always advocated can inform our efforts to understand children's language deficits.

My introduction to the idea of small-world networks came in a course on genetics at the Jackson Laboratories in Bar Harbor, ME, a few years ago. Several of the course instructors described work by investigators such as Watts and Strogatz (1998) and Barabási (2002) to characterize the structure and growth of complex systems in a variety of domains. Intriguing results suggested that many kinds of complex networks (ranging from biochemical reactions to social interactions) share certain properties that contribute to their efficiency and robustness, and that these properties emerge naturally as networks "grow" according to a few simple principles. As I began to read in this literature, I was struck by its potential relevance to the complex, self-organizing network of children's language. Although papers have recently described the applicability of the small-world model to relationships among approximately 75% of the 10^7 words in the British National corpus (Ferrer i Cancho & Solé, 2001), among words in a 30,000-entry online thesaurus (Motter, de Moura, Lai, & Dasgupta, 2002), and even specifically to the frequency of verbs and verb conjugation paradigms in large English corpora (Perebeynoss & Khidekel, 2004), at the time when I conducted the analyses below I was unaware of efforts to apply these ideas to children's language. I have since learned that Michael Vitevitch has submitted a manuscript in which the lexicons of children and adults were analyzed using the small-world perspective (M. S. Vitevich, personal communication, June 13, 2005). The findings described here, then, represent some very early steps toward analyzing the utility of the small-world framework for understanding the developing language systems of children.

The starting point for these analyses was an unpublished descriptive study of the verbs produced by a large ($n = 241$), sociodemographically diverse group of children, 36–38 months of age, during 15-min conversations with their caregivers (Dollaghan et al., 2000). We have described these participants and reported on other aspects of these language samples in several previous reports (e.g., Dollaghan et al., 1999). Briefly, participants were children who had been enrolled by age 2 months in a longitudinal study of otitis media and child development (see Paradise et al., 2001, for details); they were free of biological and other suspected threats to developmental outcomes, such as low birth weight, neonatal asphyxia, serious illness, and multiple birth. They were all monolingual speakers of English, and the demographic characteristics of the sample were representative of the Pittsburgh, PA, area. The cumulative experience of otitis media in these 241 children was insufficient to qualify them for the randomized trial component of the larger study; it ranged from none to 45% of days between 2 and 24 months of age. It should be noted that the cumulative duration of otitis media in this sample has not been associated with developmental outcomes in cognition, language, speech, hearing, or behavior at age 3 (Paradise et al., 2000, 2001), at age 4 (Paradise et al., 2003) or at age 6 years (Paradise et al., 2005). Thus, these 241 children constitute a demographically representative sample of three-year-olds free of known biological risks to development.

The language samples were audio-recorded as children and their caregivers played with a consistent set of toys at the end of an assessment session involving measures of hearing, cognition, vocabulary comprehension, and articulation. Samples were transcribed by research assistants using the Systematic Analysis of Language Transcripts (SALT) program (Miller & Chapman, 1999); percentages of interrater agreement for utterance boundaries, mean utterance length, and measures of lexical production exceeded 85%.

We had expected it to be a reasonably straightforward matter to analyze the verbs appearing in the SALT Word Root lists in order to quantify conversational verb use by this sample of 3-year-olds, but we soon encountered a degree of what might be termed "form-class homonymy" for which we were unprepared. Across the 241 samples we found 555 different word roots that could potentially be verbs; fully 70% of these had alternative form-class assignments, either as nouns (e.g., *bump, fry*), adjectives (e.g., *cool, fake*), adverbs (e.g., *even*), or some combination of these (e.g., *back*). Interestingly, analyses of adult corpora by Widdows (2003) have revealed a reliable asymmetry between English verbs and nouns in this regard; more than half of verbs also occurred as common nouns, but only 13% of common nouns also occurred as verbs. Although we did not ask whether the 241 corpora exhibited a similar noun–verb asymmetry, it seems reasonable to consider form-class ambiguity as another variable that might contribute to the apparently later and slower acquisition of verbs than nouns by young children (e.g., Childers & Tomasello, 2002; Tardif, Shatz, & Naigles, 1997). In addition, the degree of form-class homonymy we found raises some interesting questions about the category structure of early lexicons. The "Action Word" list on the MacArthur Communicative Development Inventory: Words and Gestures (Fenson et al., 1993), for example, lists a number of presumably early-acquired words (e.g., *bite, bump, clean, drink, hug, kiss, ride, swing, walk*) that children seem likely to encounter in more than one form-class context (e.g., *Give Grandma a kiss* vs. *Kiss Grandma; Let's clean up the blocks* vs. *Here's a clean diaper*). Doherty (2004) argued that children as old as 10 years have significant difficulties learning secondary meanings of homonyms for nouns that have familiar as well as unfamiliar referents. How then do much younger children represent form-class homonyms in their early lexicons, and when and how do these representations change as children become aware of the cues (linguistic or otherwise) suggesting that a word can act as, say, a verb as well as a noun (e.g., Kelly, 1992; Naigles & Hoff-Ginsberg, 1995)? Is there a cost to maintaining the alternative form-class assignments for a word in immediate memory for children who are unable to use these cues (e.g., Merriman & Marazita, 1995)? Form-class homonymy (termed *zero derivation*) has been discussed with reference to models of the structure of the adult lexicon (e.g., Don, 2004) and has recently been recognized as an important nuisance variable in behavioral and cognitive imaging studies designed to compare processing of nouns and verbs (e.g., Tranel et al., 2005; Tyler et al., 2004). Although several investigators have addressed the extent to which young children are willing to use verbs in argument structures and with morphological markers other than those in which they have heard them (e.g., Bedore & Leonard, 2000; Brooks, Tomasello, Dodson, & Lewis, 1999; Oetting, 1999; Olguin & Tomasello, 1993), questions about the effect of form-class homonyms on processing and acquisition of verbs have apparently rarely been addressed. Efforts to understand verb acquisition by children with language impairments might also benefit from additional attention to the phenomenon.

The finding of form-class homonymy in the potential verb roots we compiled, although interesting, meant that we had to examine the context of each potential verb for evidence that it should be counted as a verb. In an effort to ensure that our analyses included only unambiguous uses of verbs we imposed the following exclusion rules:

1. We excluded verbs in four specific contexts that we judged as more likely to reflect memorized routines rather than verb phrase formulation (*Thank you, You're welcome, Let's, I don't know, I love you*).
2. We excluded cases in which a potential verb was used with cues that clearly indicated that it was being used as a noun, adjective, or adverb (e.g., *He's a cook*).

3. We excluded past participle forms if they occurred in constructions that could be analyzed as either truncated passives or adjectival complement constructions (e.g., *broken* was excluded if it occurred in the utterance *It was broken*, but was included in the utterance *It was broken by the dog*).
4. We excluded indeterminate uses, in which contextual cues did not disambiguate the word's form class (e.g., In *I cook* the word *cook* can be glossed as either a noun or a verb).

In deference to the young age of these participants, we did credit bare stems as verbs if they were produced in direct response to "What doing?" questions (e.g., Adult: *What are you doing?* Child: *Cook*). Contractions (e.g., *'ll*) were counted with their full forms (*will*). Finally, variants of the verbs *be* (*am, is, are*) and *do* (*do, did, don't*) that have different vowels were counted as different verbs.

For this chapter, I focused on the verb use of children at the tails of this large distribution of expressive skills, defined simply by their mean utterance length in morphemes (MLU). Accordingly, the more detailed analyses described here were conducted on the 10 children with the highest, and the 10 children with the lowest, MLUs. Summary information on these 20 participants appears in Table 11.1.

The MLUs of the 10 children at the bottom of the distribution ranged from 1.25 to 1.76, placing them more than two standard deviations (*SD*s) below the mean according to Miller and Chapman (1981) and more than 1.64 *SD*s below the mean of the entire sample (Dollaghan et al., 1999). However, they had normal-range standard scores (≥ 77) on either a measure of cognitive development (General Cognitive Index, McCarthy Scales of Children's Abilities; McCarthy, 1972) a measure of vocabulary comprehension (Peabody Picture Vocabulary Test–Revised; Dunn & Dunn, 1981), or both. These children are designated as language delayed in what follows, but to indicate that this designation was based strictly on their developmentally inappropriate utterance lengths and not on other diagnostic indicators of language disorder they are labeled as "LD-MLU."

Conversely, the 10 children at the upper end of the distribution had MLUs placing them more than 1.65 *SD*s above the mean relative to Miller and Chapman (1981) and more than 2.38 *SD*s above the mean relative to the mean of the entire sample. Their scores on measures of cognition and vocabulary comprehension also were at and in some cases well above the normal range. The children in this group apparently were quite efficient language learners; referring to them as having normal language development (NL) indicates that they did not have language deficits rather than that their language skills were average. As shown in Table 11.1 (and consistent with many other reports comparing children with typical and atypical

TABLE 11.1
Demographic Information, Mean Scores, and (Standard Deviations) for the Specific Language Delay (LD-MLU) and Normal Language Development (NL) Groups

	LD-MLU (*n* = 10)		*NL* (*n* = 10)	
Age in months	36.6	(0.8)	36.8	(0.6)
GCI[a]	91	(9)	118	(9)
PPVT[b]	88	(18)	112	(18)
Total number of verbal utterances[c]	157	(52)	194	(31)
MLU in morphemes[c]	1.57	(0.17)	4.49	(0.15)
Total number of words (TNW)[c]	274	(102)	787	(131)
Number of different words (NDW)[c]	74	(24)	179	(15)
Percent males	60	—	10	—
Percent White	80	—	100	—

[a]Standard score (*M* = 100; *SD* = 15), General Cognitive Index of the McCarthy Scales of Children's Abilities (McCarthy, 1972).
[b]Standard score (*M* = 100; *SD* = 15), Peabody Picture Vocabulary Test–Revised (Dunn & Dunn, 1981).
[c]From 15-min conversational sample audio-recorded during play with caregiver.

language skills), the NL group produced utterances that not only were longer but contained more total words (word tokens) and more different words (word types) than did the LD-MLU group.

Applying the verb coding rules already described to these 20 transcripts yielded a total of 2240 verb uses and 141 different verbs. As shown in Table 11.2, the NL group used substantially greater numbers of both verb types and verb tokens than did the LD-MLU group and in fact the groups did not

TABLE 11.2
Means and (Standard Deviations) for Verb Measures for the Specific Language Delay (LD-MLU) and Normal Language Development (NL) Groups

	LD-MLU		*NL*	
Total number of verbs (TNV)	32	(15)	192	(37)
Number of different verbs (NDV)	14	(6)	41	(6)
NDV/Number of different words	0.18	(0.04)	0.23	(0.03)

overlap on raw frequencies of verb production (i.e., all LD-MLU children used fewer than 55 verb tokens and all NL children produced more than 145 verb tokens). However, as noted by Thordardottir and Ellis Weismer (2001) and other investigators (Owen & Leonard, 2002; Watkins, Kelly, Harbers, & Hollis, 1995), it is difficult to interpret comparisons of raw frequencies that originate from language samples and utterances of different lengths. After controlling for such differences by indexing each child's number of different verbs to his or her number of different words, the group differences were much less striking; as shown in Table 11.2, the two groups have similar ratios of different verbs to different words (0.18 and 0.23 in the LD-MLU and NL groups, respectively).

Another way to approach a group comparison is to focus on the most frequently used verbs in each group, as has been done in a number of previous investigations (e.g., Conti-Ramsen & Jones, 1997; Kelly, 1997; Rice & Bode, 1993; Thordardottir & Ellis Weismer, 2001). Table 11.3 lists the verbs that were among the 20 most frequently used by both groups and by the

TABLE 11.3
Verbs in the 20 Most Frequent of Both Groups, of the Group With Normal Language Development (NL) Only, and of the Group With Specific Language Delay (LD-MLU) Only

In 20 Most Frequent Verbs of Both Groups	*In 20 Most Frequent Verbs of NL Group Only*	*In 20 Most Frequent Verbs of LD-MLU Group Only*
be (am, 'm)	call	cook
be (are, 're)	got	cut
be (is, 's)	have	did
can/can't	make	know
come	see	look
do	will	sit
don't		
eat		
get		
go		
need		
play		
put		
want		

Note. Order of verbs is alphabetical within columns.

individual groups. The idea that children in the LD-MLU group lack certain important early verbs is not well supported by this table. Fourteen of the 20 verbs used most frequently by the NL group were also among the 20 verbs used most frequently by the LD-MLU group, and there seem to be more semantic and syntactic similarities than differences in the verbs that were among the 20 most frequent verbs for one group but not for the other. This finding is consistent with results of a similar analysis of verbs reported by Thordardottir and Ellis Weismer (2001), although their participants were substantially older and their methods for verb identification were somewhat different.

If verbs are as crucial to grammatical development as is usually assumed (e.g., Forbes & Poulin-Dubois, 1997; Tomasello, 1992), the lack of striking differences between the NL and LD-MLU groups in either verb diversity or in specific verbs is surprising. I began to think about whether the groups differed in the way they deployed their verbs, which led me to the work on self-organizing complex networks mentioned at the beginning of this chapter.

HUBS (AND VERBS)

Albert-László Barabási's 2002 book, titled *Linked: The New Science of Networks,* suggested some interesting possibilities for approaching this hypothesis. Barabási notes that interactions among the components of many highly organized complex systems in diverse domains are characterized well by mathematical functions known as power laws in which a small number of units or nodes is involved in the bulk of the interactions in the system and the large majority of units participate in relatively few, a phenomenon consistent with the "80/20 rule" that has often been described in the popular press (e.g., 80% of crime is committed by 20% of criminals, 80% of an organization's work is done by 20% of its employees, etc.; Barabási, 2002, p. 66). The small number of highly connected units, known as hubs, gradually come to dominate the events in the networks of which they are a part and are believed to contribute to both efficiency and robustness of complex networks. Barabási proposes that hubs emerge as a natural consequence of two laws (growth and preferential attachment) that govern the development of complex networks; he suggests that the emergence of power laws and hubs is one indication that a relatively chaotic system is in transition to a relatively organized system. In fact, Barabási describes the emergence of hubs as "a hint of self-organization and order" (p. 78).

I began to wonder whether certain verbs in children's lexicons might act as hubs, and whether the existence of "hub verbs" might differentiate the NL and LD-MLU groups better than had the ratio of verbs to other words or the specific verbs used. If there are parallels between the complex networks characterized by power laws that have been identified in other domains and the emergence of a well-organized system of syntactic utterance production, we might predict a relatively equal division of labor among verbs in utterances produced by the LD-MLU children, in whose nascent syntactic systems the principles of growth and preferential attachment had not had much time to operate. By contrast, we might hypothesize that a small number of verbs (something close to the quintessential "80/20" imbalance) would dominate the utterances resulting from the more highly developed and organized syntactic systems of the NL children.

Because I was interested in the relationship between hub verbs and expressive syntax, I first used SALT to exclude all one-word utterances so that the samples comprised all and only the multiword utterances produced by each child. Table 11.4 shows that the same relationships hold between the NL and LD-MLU groups when the samples are restricted to multiword utterances; that is, utterance length, volubility, and absolute numbers of verb types and tokens are substantially higher in the NL than in the LD-MLU group, but the ratio of verb types to word types is again similar in the groups.

I next ranked the verb types in each child's multiword utterances by frequency of occurrence and identified the verbs representing the top 20% of that child's verb lexicon (i.e., repertoire of different verbs). For example, subject LD-MLU1 used 14 different verbs in multiword utterances; 20% of this child's inventory would comprise 3 different verbs (14 × 0.20 = 2.8, rounded to the nearest whole number). Thus after ranking the 14 verbs in his inventory according to their frequency of use in multiword utterances, I identified his "top 20%" as the three verbs used most frequently, in this case *want*, *is*, and *sit*. I then counted the number of multiword utterances in the transcript that contained these top 20% verbs and divided by the total num-

TABLE 11.4
Means and (Standard Deviations) for Multiword Utterances by Group (Specific Language Delay, LD-MLU; Normal Language Development, NL)

	LD-MLU		*NL*	
Total utterances	61	(27)	159	(31)
MLUm	2.78	(0.31)	5.36	(0.27)
Total words	101	(56)	573	(123)
Different words	44	(19)	155	(17)
Total verbs	26	(15)	191	(36)
Different verbs	13	(5.5)	41	(6.6)
Different verbs/different words	0.30	(0.09)	0.26	(0.04)

ber of multiword utterances to derive the proportion of the child's multiword utterances that were constructed with one of the top 20% verbs. In the case of subject LD-MLU1, the 3 top-20% verbs were used in 23 of his 64 multiword utterances, or a proportion of 0.36. By contrast, subject NL1 had an inventory of 42 different verbs in her multiword utterances; she used her eight top-20% verbs (*go, is, put, can, need, get, play, look*) in 131 of her 170 multiword utterances, or a proportion of 0.77.

The results of these calculations were striking, as shown in Fig. 11.1. The deployment of verbs in multiword utterances by the NL group was consistent with the "80/20" distribution expected of a system with emergent organization. Specifically, in the NL group the proportion of multiword utterances containing a top-20% verb ranged from 0.64 to 0.92, with a mean proportion of 0.75 (*SD* = 0.09). By contrast, children in the LD-MLU group appeared to use their top-20% verbs in a much more egalitarian (or randomly distributed) fashion. In the LD-MLU group the proportion of multiword utterances containing a top-20% verb ranged from 0.05 to 0.36, with a mean proportion of 0.18 (*SD* = 0.09). In short, "hub verbs" seem to characterize the syntactic utterance production of children in the NL group but not of children in the LD-MLU group, at least at 36 months of age. The sharp discontinuity between the groups in proportional use of top-20% verbs contrasts with the lack of differentiation between the groups on more

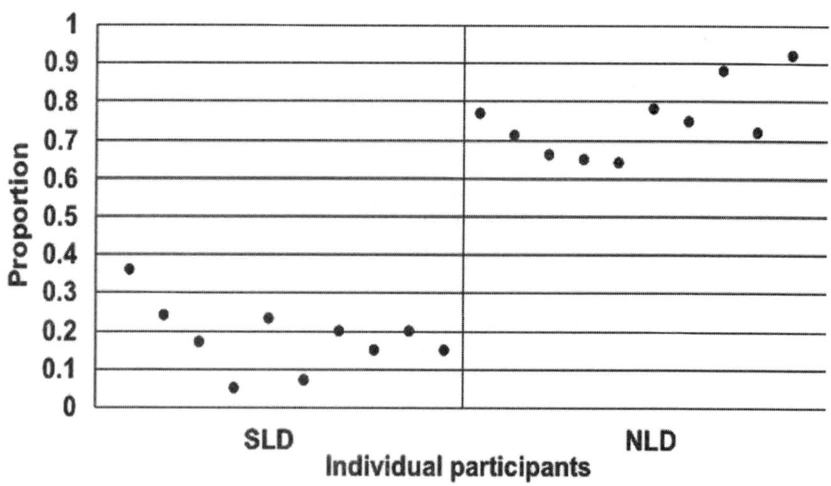

FIG. 11.1. Proportion of multiword utterances containing "top-20%" verbs for the 10 children with specific language delay (LD-MLU) and for the 10 children with normal language development (NL).

traditional measures of verb diversity such as the proportion of different words that were verbs, which is plotted in Fig. 11.2.

Table 11.5 shows a compilation of the specific verbs that were among the top 20% for both groups, for the NL group only, and for the LD-MLU group only. Again it appears that it is not the specific verbs that differentiate the NL and LD-MLU groups, but rather the extent to which their top-20% verbs play a dominant role in their multiword utterances.

Why do hub verbs characterize the syntactic productions of children in the NL but not the LD-MLU groups? One relatively uninteresting reason for which the groups might differ has to do with the difficulties that auxiliary and copula forms of the verb *be* pose to children with language deficits (e.g., Hadley & Rice, 1996); perhaps treating the three phonological variants of *be* (*am/'m; is/'s; are;'re*) as different verbs skewed the identification of top-20% verbs and/or the proportion of multiword utterances containing top-20% verbs in favor of the NL children who were more likely to have mastered these forms. To examine this possibility I collapsed all *be* forms so as to count them as a single verb and reanalyzed the data. Interestingly, however, this maneuver increased rather than decreased the fit of the data to the idealized 80/20 distribution, increasing the average proportion of top-20% verb uses by the NL group from 0.75 ($SD = 0.09$) to 0.82 ($SD = 0.09$) while having little impact on the proportion of top-20% verb uses by the LD-MLU group, which increased from 0.18 to 0.19.

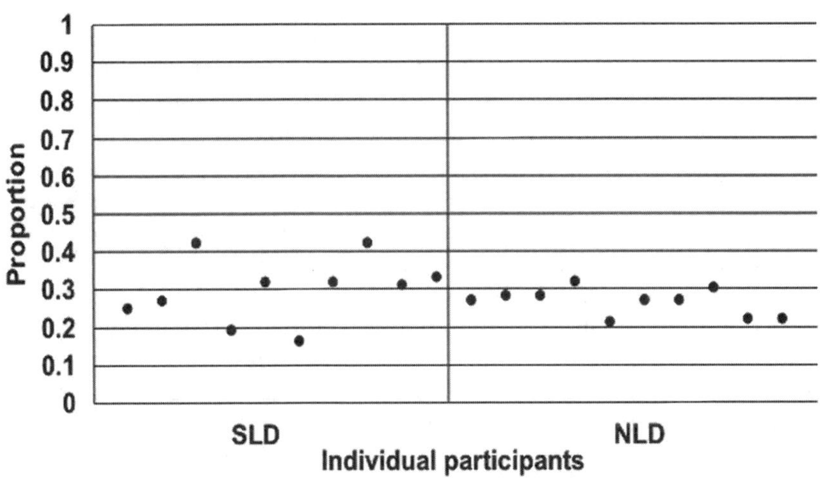

FIG. 11.2. Proportion of different words that were verbs for the 10 children with specific language delay (LD-MLU) and for the 10 children with normal language development (NL).

TABLE 11.5
Verbs in the Top 20% by Frequency of Use in Multiword Utterances, for Both Groups, for the NL Group Only, and for the LD-MLU Group Only

Top 20%, Both Groups Only	*Top 20%, NL Group Only*	*Top 20%, LD-MLU Group Only*
be (am, 'm)	be (are, 're)	cook
be (is, 's)	do	did
can	don't	turn
come	have	
eat	let	
get	make	
go	put	
look	stay	
need	think	
play	will	
sit		
want		
work		

Note. Order of verbs is alphabetical within columns.

No doubt there are other alternative explanations for the results of this exploratory study that can and should be pursued. The two small groups compared here differed not only on expressive language measures but also on measures of cognition and receptive vocabulary; the question of whether conceptual and/or lexical knowledge contributed to the difference in verb use remains for future investigation. But if we assume that the hub verbs observed in the syntactic systems of the NL group in this study are something more than epiphenomena, is there a basis for hypothesizing that they might actually facilitate (and not just reflect) syntactic utterance production? The literature on hubs in other complex systems suggests that the answer is yes. Specifically, the emergence of hubs has been proposed to change complex networks in which the connections among nodes are distributed either randomly or regularly (i.e., nearest neighbor networks; Ferrer i Cancho & Solé, 2001), into small-world networks, in which the widespread direct connections of the few key hub nodes to nodes at the far reaches of the network provide shortcuts by which even a very large network can be traversed with relatively few intervening connections (Barabási, 2002; Ferrer i Cancho & Solé, 2001; Motter, de Moura, Lai, &

Dasgupta, 2002; Watts & Strogatz, 1998). A network in which hubs have emerged is thus a network that despite its complexity can be accessed rapidly and efficiently. In addition, a law of preferential attachment is proposed to govern the addition of new nodes to at least some (cf. Raghavan, 2003) complex networks, such that new nodes are more likely to be connected to nodes that are themselves highly connected (such as hubs) than to nodes with fewer connections. This means that the network "scales"; regardless of its ultimate size and density, the shortest path between any two nodes (known as the path length coefficient *L*; Watts & Strogatz, 1998) is predicted to comprise no more than approximately three connections, an obvious benefit when temporal demands are high.

With respect to children acquiring language, the concepts of small worlds and hubs thus seem to suggest some new ways to think about lexical and verb diversity and the relationship between lexical items and utterance production. For example, rather than focusing only on the broad semantic (e.g., "light vs. heavy"; state vs. motion) and syntactic (e.g., argument structure; morphological regularity) characteristics inherent to verbs, it might be useful to think about their connections not just to lexical items with similar characteristics but to lexical items that may seem quite disparate. These ideas might also motivate some alternative hypotheses about how best to address the difficulties experienced by children with language delays and disorders. For instance, rather than using a priori category schemes to identify target verbs for language intervention or simply trying to increase the numbers of verbs known or used by the child, it might be useful to consider taking a verb already in use and attempting to facilitate its status as a hub by increasing or strengthening its connections to disparate lexical items and/or to a broader range of syntactic constructions. Similarly, rather than trying to reduce complexity for the child by targeting verbs (and other lexical items) that are unambiguous, it might actually be beneficial to target at least some words with multiple meanings, because these will generally be more widely connected to other lexical items and thus more likely to act as potential hubs. Analyses by Widdows (2003) of the British National Corpus are interesting in this regard; he hypothesized that storing verb–noun form-class homonyms together in a single vector would facilitate processing of verbs (at least by machine). Findings such as this suggest that it might be beneficial to explore the value of explicitly drawing children's attention to the existence and distributional features of verb–noun homonym pairs in an effort to forge links that could enable a more rapid and robust deployment of verbs in syntactic constructions.

These ideas are nothing more than speculations at this point. We don't know whether the emergence of hubs can be facilitated in children's language and not only in computer simulations. More basically, we don't know whether the disparity in hub verbs between 3-year-olds with normal and delayed language development that was described in this chapter will turn out to characterize larger samples of children, or whether it reflects anything more than the groups' relative facility in verb phrase construction (e.g., Hadley, 1998). But the idea that certain verbs may act as hubs in the complex network of children's language, organizing lexical and syntactic relationships to enable the high speed and low error rate necessary for competent real-time conversational participation, seems to raise some interesting hypotheses for future investigation. Examining not only the raw or relative frequency of verb types used by a child but also the extent to which hub verbs characterize his or her syntax production might provide some new insights into the processes and conditions underpinning both typical and atypical language development.

My intent with this exploratory study was to follow one of the guiding themes of Robin Chapman's work: the value of grounding the study of child language disorders firmly in models of normal developmental processes. In this case the developmental processes considered are quite general ones; they will undoubtedly be refined as "the new science of networks" (Barabási, 2002) progresses. Whether or not the "small-world" perspective ultimately leads to an accurate conceptualization of child language development, it seems likely to motivate some productive new approaches to difficult questions about child language delays and disorders.

EPILOGUE

Robin Chapman, in addition to her influential work as a psycholinguist, also understands that words serve many functions besides the utilitarian. Her love of words extends to poetry, and in that spirit I offer the following "found" poem:

Be Do

Drink Eat

Play

Sleep

(Alphabetized verb lexicon of a child with delayed language)

ACKNOWLEDGMENTS

This work was supported by grants from NICHHD (J. L. Paradise, Principal Investigator) and from NIDCD (C. Dollaghan, Principal Investigator). Special thanks to Denise Balason, Tammy Nash, Stephanie Nixon, Brenda Smolky, Heather Rusiewicz, and Heather Starmer, with whom the initial verb analyses of the sample of 241 children were conducted.

REFERENCES

Ambalu, D., Chiat, S., & Pring, T. (1997). When is it best to hear a verb? The effects of the timing and focus of verb models on children's learning of verbs. *Journal of Child Language, 24,* 25–34.

Barabási, A.-L. (2002). *Linked: The new science of networks.* Cambridge, MA: Perseus.

Bedore, L. M., & Leonard, L. B. (2000). The effects of inflectional variation on fast mapping of verbs in English and Spanish. *Journal of Speech, Language, and Hearing Research, 43,* 21–33.

Brooks, P. J., Tomasello, M., Dodson, K., & Lewis, L. B. (1999). Young children's overgeneralizations with fixed transitivity verbs. *Child Development, 70,* 1325–1337.

Chapman, R. S. (1978). Comprehension strategies in children. In J. F. Kavanagh & W. Strange (Eds.), *Speech and language in the laboratory, school, and clinic* (pp. 308–327). Cambridge MA: MIT Press.

Chapman, R. S., Dollaghan, C., Kenworthy, O. T., & Miller, J. F. (1983). Microcomputer testing and teaching of verb meaning: What's easy and what's hard? In A. Cherry Wilkinson (Ed.), *Classroom computers and cognitive science* (pp. 95–119). New York: Academic Press.

Chapman, R. S., & Kohn, L. L. (1978). Comprehension strategies in two and three year olds: Animate agents or probable events? *Journal of Speech and Hearing Research, 21,* 746–761.

Childers, J. B., & Tomasello, M. (2002). Two-year-olds learn novel nouns, verbs, and conventional actions from massed or distributed exposures. *Developmental Psychology, 38,* 967–978.

Conti-Ramsden, G., & Jones, M. (1997). Verb use in specific language impairment. *Journal of Speech, Language, and Hearing Research, 40,* 1298–1313.

Doherty, M. J. (2004). Children's difficulty in learning homonyms. *Journal of Child Language, 31,* 203–214.

Dollaghan, C. A., Campbell, T. F., Paradise, J. L., Feldman, H. M., Janosky, J. E., Pitcairn D. N., & Kurs-Lasky, M. (1999). Maternal education and measures of early speech and language. *Journal of Speech, Language, and Hearing Research, 42,* 1432–1443.

Dollaghan, C., Balason, D., Nash, T., Rusiewicz, H., Nixon, S., Smolky, B., & Starmer, H. (2000, November). *Verb lexicons of 3-year-old children.* Poster session presented at the annual meeting of the American Speech-Language-Hearing Association, Washington, DC.

Don, J. (2004). Categories in the lexicon. *Linguistics, 42,* 931–956.

Dunn, L. M., & Dunn, L. M. (1981). *Peabody Picture Vocabulary Test–Revised.* Circle Pines, MN: American Guidance Service.

Fenson, L., Dale, P. S., Reznick, J. S., Thal, D., Bates, E., Hartung, J. P., Pethick, S., & Reilly, J. S. (1993). *MacArthur Communicative Development Inventories: User's guide and technical manual.* San Diego: Singular.

Ferrer i Cancho, R., & Solé, R. V. (2001). The small world of human language. *Proceedings of the Royal Society of London B, 268,* 2261–2265.

Forbes, J. N., & Poulin-Dubois, D. (1997) Representational change in young children's understanding of familiar verb meaning. *Journal of Child Language, 24,* 389–406.

Gillette, J., Gleitman, H., Gleitman, L., & Lederer, A. (1999). Human simulations of vocabulary learning. *Cognition, 73,* 135–176.

Hadley, P. A. (1998). Early verb-related vulnerability among children with specific language impairment. *Journal of Speech, Language, and Hearing Research, 41,* 1384–1397.

Hadley, P. A., & Rice, M. L. (1996). Emergent uses of BE and DO: Evidence from children with specific language impairment. *Language Acquisition, 5,* 209–243.

Hesketh, L. J., & Chapman, R. S. (1998). Verb use by individuals with Down syndrome. *American Journal on Mental Retardation, 103*(3), 288–304.

Kelly, D. J. (1997). Patterns in verb use by preschoolers with normal language and specific language impairment. *Applied Psycholinguistics, 18,* 199–218.

Kelly, M. H. (1992). Using sound to solve syntactic problems: The role of phonology in grammatical category assignments. *Psychological Review, 99,* 349–364,

Leonard, L. B., Miller, C., & Gerber, E. (1999). Grammatical morphology and the lexicon in children with specific language impairment. *Journal of Speech, Language, and Hearing Research, 42,* 678–689.

McCarthy, D. (1972). *McCarthy Scales of Children's Abilities.* San Antonio, TX: Psychological Corporation.

Merriman, W. E., & Marazita, J. M. (1995). The effect of hearing similar-sounding words on young 2-year-olds' disambiguation of novel noun reference. *Developmental Psychology, 31,* 973–984.

Miller, J. F., & Chapman, R. S. (1999). *SALT: Systematic Analysis of Language Transcripts* [Computer program]. University of Wisconsin–Madison: Language Analysis Lab.

Motter, A. E., de Moura, A. P. S., Lai, Y.-C., & Dasgupta, P. (2002). Topology of the conceptual network of language. *Physical Review E, 65, 065102,* 1–4.

Naigles, L. R., & Hoff-Ginsberg, E. (1995). Input to verb learning: Evidence for the plausibility of syntactic bootstrapping. *Developmental Psychology, 31,* 827–837.

Oetting, J. B. (1999). Children with SLI use argument structure cues to learn verbs. *Journal of Speech, Language, and Hearing Research, 42,* 1261–1274.

Olguin, R., & Tomasello, M. (1993). Twenty-five-month-old children do not have a grammatical category of verb. *Cognitive Development, 8,* 245–272.

Owen, A. J., & Leonard, L. B. (2002). Lexical diversity in the spontaneous speech of children with specific language impairment: Application of D. *Journal of Speech, Language, and Hearing Research, 45,* 927–937.

Paradise, J. L., Dollaghan, C. A., Campbell, T. F., Feldman, H. M., Bernard, B. S., Colborn, D. K., Rockette, H. E., Janosky, J. E., Pitcairn, D. L., Kurs-Lasky, M., & Smith, C. G. (2000). Language, speech sound production, and cognition in 3-year-old children in relation to otitis media in their first 3 years of life. *Pediatrics, 105,* 1119–1130.

Paradise, J. L., Feldman, H. M., Campbell, T. F., Dollaghan, C. A., Colborn, D. K., Bernard, B. S., Rockette, H. E., Janosky, J. E., Pitcairn, D. L., Sabo, D. L., Kurs-Lasky, M., & Smith, C. G. (2001). Early versus late tympanostomy tube placement for persistent otitis media: Developmental outcomes at age 3 years. *New England Journal of Medicine, 344*(16), 1179–1195.

Paradise, J. L., Dollaghan, C. A., Campbell, T. F., Feldman, H. M., Bernard, B. S., Colborn, D. K., Rockette, H. E., Janosky, J. E., Pitcairn, D. L., Kurs-Lasky, M., Sabo, D. L., & Smith, C. G. (2003). Otitis media and tympanostomy tube insertion during the first three years of life: Developmental outcomes at the age of four years. *Pediatrics, 112*(2), 265–277.

Paradise, J. L., Campbell, T. F., Dollaghan, C. A., Feldman, H. M., Bernard, B. S., Colborn, D. K., Rockette, H. E., Janosky, J. E., Pitcairn, D. L., Kurs-Lasky, M., Sabo, D. L., & Smith, C. G. (2005). Developmental outcomes at age six following early or delayed insertion of tympanostomy tubes for persistent otitis media. *New England Journal of Medicine, 353,* 576–586.

Perebeynoss, V., & Khidekel, S. (2004). Frequency of language units as a reflection of their systemic and functional properties. *Journal of Quantitative Linguistics, 11,* 3–25.

Raghavan, P. (2003, January–February). Networks: Not a small world after all. *American Scientist Online.*

Rice, M. L., & Bode, J. V. (1993). GAPS in the verb lexicons of children with specific language impairment. *First Language, 13,* 113–131.

Tardif, T., Shatz, M., & Naigles, L. (1997) Caregiver speech and children's use of nouns versus verbs: A comparison of English, Italian, and Mandarin. *Journal of Child Language, 24,* 535–565.

Thordardottir, E. T., & Ellis Weismer, S. (2001). High-frequency verbs and verb diversity in the spontaneous speech of school-age children with specific language impairment. *International Journal of Language and Communication Disorders, 36,* 221–244.

Tomasello, M. (1992). *First verbs: A study of early grammatical development.* Cambridge, England: Cambridge University Press.

Tomasello, M., Akhtar, N., Dodson, K., & Rekau, L. (1997). Differential productivity in young children's use of nouns and verbs. *Journal of Child Language, 24,* 373–387.

Tranel, D., Martin, C., Damasio, H., Grabowski, T. J., & Hichwa, R. (2005). Effects of noun–verb homonymy on the neural correlates of naming concrete entities and actions. *Brain and Language, 92,* 288–299.

Tyler, L. K., Bright, P., Fletcher, P., & Stamatakis, E. A. (2004). Neural processing of nouns and verbs: The role of inflectional morphology. *Neuropsychologia, 42,* 512–523.

Watkins, R. V., Kelly, D. J., Harbers, H. M., & Hollis, W. (1995). Measuring children's lexical diversity: Differentiating typical and impaired language learners. *Journal of Speech and Hearing Research, 38,* 1349–1355.

Watts, D. J., & Strogatz, S. H. (1998). Collective dynamics of "small-world" networks. *Nature, 393*(4/June), 440–442.

Widdows, D. (2003, May). Unsupervised methods for developing taxonomies by combining syntactic and statistical information. In *Human Language Technology, Conference of the North American Chapter of the Association for Computational Linguistics.* Edmonton, Canada, pp. 276–283.

12

Documenting Progress in Language Production: The Evolution of a Computerized Language Analysis System

Jon Miller
University of Wisconsin–Madison

The publication of *Assessing Language Production in Children* (Miller, 1982), affectionately known as the Blue Book, marked the culmination of 10 years of work developing language assessment techniques that would yield descriptive and quantitative data documenting the developing language of hard-to-test children. This book included major contributions by Robin Chapman and Rhea Paul. The cornerstone of this work was the collection and analysis of language samples (LSA). The process, which includes defining the elicitation context, recording a sample, orthographic transcription conventions, analyses with reference to normal language development, and interpretation was spelled out in detail. The focus was on collecting conversational samples that were naturalistic and spontaneous with limited adult influence in order to compare the spoken output of children with a variety of disabilities with what we hear from typically developing children. This approach reflected the research methodology of that time, which focused on early development from first words to about age 5 and emphasized the use of normal development as a standard against which to evaluate language from children with disabilities.

Transcription was done by hand using tape recorders for playback. Cassette tapes and secretarial transcription machines were just coming into use. The transcription machines were a huge breakthrough in improving accuracy through controlled repetition of segments, reducing wear on tape recorders and in general saving transcription time. Computers were not yet on the scene, so the process required vigilance to maintain consistency of the transcription format.

The focus of analysis was on syntax, because that is the area in which most research on normal development had so far taken place. Detailed explanation was provided for calculating mean length of utterance (MLU), number of different words, 14 grammatical morphemes, and Assigning Structural Stage. One major contribution to this work was provided by my colleague Robin Chapman, who was the first to survey and integrate work being done by a variety of researchers and condense it into a series of tables that outlined what was known about developmental course and synchrony of syntactic acquisition. These charts came to form the bases of the Assigning Structural Stage analyses, which were developed to provide clinicians with a set of guidelines for manually transcribing and comparing the verbal output of children with disabilities to the levels or stages of acquisition as represented in these tables. Rhea Paul later extended this approach to include a summary of what was known about the normal course of complex sentence development, using a similar format. Our research documenting the high correlation between age and MLU allowed us to include, for the first time, age–MLU charts, to assign an age to a specific MLU. These charts were developed using predicted age from the regression analysis formula (Miller & Chapman, 1981). What these early attempts to codify language sample analysis aimed at was a systematic way to compare the forms produced by children with disabilities to forms produced at various levels of development by typical children, to identify the level within a sequence at which the child was functioning in order to determine the existence and extent of a delay, and to then follow the typical sequence as a curriculum guide for teaching language forms.

Even in 1982, however, we knew there was more to language than syntax. The work of Lois Bloom (1970) brought syntactic form and utterance content/function together for the first time and reminded us that form alone was not sufficient to characterize language development. Interpretation of language sample analyses relied on clinicians' knowledge of these developmental data. This topic was addressed in the Blue Book in Robin Chapman's exemplary chapter on semantic relations, which helped bring an expanded focus to analysis.

Although our field and our practice has come a long way since 1982, some things have not changed. We still look to the normal developmental sequence to serve as a guidepost for identification of language delay. We still use the developmental sequence as a blueprint for our intervention plan. The four basic aspects of the Language Sample Analysis (LSA) process—sampling, transcription, analysis, and interpretation—are the same today as they were in 1982. Issues then were, what constituted an utterance and a word, and how many utterances were required for a valid sample of a child's language? These remain as issues today. As a clinical process, LSA required a significant amount of time, knowledge of language development, and consistency in sampling, transcription, and analysis. One of the intents of the Blue Book was to at least provide a resource on language development to aid in interpretation and sampling, and to provide transcription and analysis rules to promote consistency.

COMPUTING CIRCA 1982: THE BEGINNINGS OF COMPUTER-ASSISTED LSA

The computing facility at the University of Wisconsin's Waisman Center in 1982 housed a mainframe computer occupying a space the size a small house: 1,500 square feet. It was a Harris computer, maintained by several computer operators who wrote code for specific tasks and updated the operating system with the Harris Company. Computers were expensive then. Successful computer facilities required staff who bridged hardware and software, working hand in glove with manufacturers. Word processing programs did not yet exist, although it was possible to get various computer languages to produce English text by inserting the appropriate codes. Computer science students hung around computing facilities, gaining experience by working on various code writing projects or serving as an night operators. These machines required 24-hour-a-day monitoring and maintenance.

Shortly after the Blue Book was published, an undergraduate computer science student working in the Waisman computing facility began to work with me to determine whether a computer could do analyses that involved primarily counting, such as computing mean length of utterance, (MLU), type-token ratios (TTR), and number of different words in a speech sample (NDW). After 2 weeks we had a printout of these analyses run on several different transcripts. The possibility that a computer might be able to take on many of the time-consuming counts involved in LSA became our holy grail. It quickly became apparent that the computer could count and sort word and utterance units identified by spaces or punctuation, but could not determine a noun from a verb or identify a bound morpheme without coding. So began an odyssey that has been all-consuming for the past 20+

years. Evolution in computing and the availability of personal computers, which have become smaller and faster, with increased processing speed, have aided our development of LSA software. We have reduced the time required, and increased the consistency of transcription and accuracy of analysis. The project, "how to get the computer to do as much of the process as possible to improve clinical and research access to LSA," was born.

SYSTEMATIC ANALYSIS OF LANGUAGE TRANSCRIPTS: THE SALT PROGRAM

The SALT program was originally developed for use by students and researchers, because computers were not generally available to individuals. As PCs became readily available, however, the possibility that speech-language pathologists in the field might be able to use the software for day-to-day clinical work began to take shape. Because SLP professionals were trained in the collection and analysis of language, the SALT program would provide a powerful assist to this time-consuming process. The goal was to develop a standardized method of transcription that incorporated the entire sample: the language of the child and the communication partner. The early samples were collected using conversation between mother and child to capture spontaneous language, as researchers in typical development, such as Roger Brown and his students, had. Our approach to the transcription format was to focus on creating an accurate orthographic record of the recorded sample with minimal coding so the result was a readable transcript accessible to anyone including clinicians, teachers, parents, and researchers. The result was a basic transcription format for recording the utterances of each speaker, with coding options for adding specific analyses users required. This approach allowed the user to create analyses in addition to using analyses we created. This basic transcription process could be accomplished with minimal training. Advanced coding for more detailed analyses could be subsequently completed. The transcription process and the coding process were separated so users did not code for analyses that may not be used. Only codes required for identifying bound morphemes, utterance punctuation speaker identifiers, and so on were used to save transcription time and effort while providing a range of standard analyses.

The approach to analyzing transcripts was equally open-ended. A set of standard analyses was created. These were analyses that could be done accurately without further coding of the basic transcript, for example, MLU, NDW, and TTR. New standard analyses were later added, as they proved informative. Language features such as speaking rate, verbal fluency, and discourse were analyzed by calculating words per minute, mazes (repetitions and revisions), percent responses to questions, and turn length. Errors at the morpheme, word, or utterance level as well as omissions of morphemes and words were also added. These measures provided access to syntax, semantics, discourse, rate and fluency, and error measures. Currently there are a number of exploratory analyses available in SALT, which allows the user to explore the transcript in detail. These include distributional characteristics for utterance length as well as vocabulary lists of all words in the transcript (including lists of question words, conjunctions and pronouns, and lists of bound morphemes with their word roots). These options place the user in charge of examining the transcript from a variety of perspectives to get the most out the language sample. These exploratory analyses were created to allow clinicians the opportunity to examine the unique features of the language of individual children.

CURRENT RESEARCH EXAMPLES: TRANSCRIPTION AND ANALYSIS

Our current research, funded by IES and NIH Program Project grants, examines factors affecting the variability in reading and school achievement among bilingual, Spanish–English speaking children. Performance on a variety of standardized tests of oral language, reading, and achievement, as well as data from classroom observation and reading intervention programs, are collected each year. Our project is collecting and analyzing oral narratives in each language from 1,450 children in kindergarten through third grade twice a year, creating more than 5,000 transcripts a year for 3 years.

Processing over 5,000 transcripts a year posed a daunting task requiring the development of new tools to facilitate data management and to insure the accurate coding and analysis of each transcript. In the past, individual transcripts were analyzed, using SALT (Miller & Chapman, 1983–2004) or similar LSA software, for various language measures, for example, MLU, number of different words, and TTR. Measures involving human judgment, such as inserting codes for specific word, morpheme, or utterance features, usually required manual categorizing and counting. Coding for features across utterances, narrative structure analysis, for example, was done globally with scores tallied independent from the transcript file being scored. Coding and summarizing data in this way was both time-consuming and error-prone. To avoid these problems, we focused on developing new tools for the automatic processing of large numbers of transcripts. This new development involved designing a database to facilitate data management and expanding the capabilities of the SALT software.

Problem 1: Data Management

Solution: We created a database using Microsoft Access for storing key information from the language samples, including demographic information and analysis data. Utilities were built into this database for creating SALT transcript files containing the sample identification and demographic information previously typed into the beginning of each transcript. Language variables imported from SALT and reading scores imported from spreadsheets sent to us from another site were stored in this database. Routines were created for selecting data for further analysis based on a variety of criteria, including the pairing of English/Spanish samples collected from the same child at the same time.

Problem 2: The Morphology of Spanish

The highly inflected morphology of Spanish can significantly affect the postinflected root word/stem. It is necessary to identify the root form in order to credit Spanish speakers for exhibiting use of morphological forms as well as to avoid overinflation of the total number of different words.

Solution: We created a dictionary-style lookup file to automatically identify the root forms when SALT analyzes the transcript.

Problem 3: Reducing the Time Required for Hand-Coded Analyses

Solution: New features were added to the SALT software for creating customized code lists to facilitate hand-coded analyses. With this new feature, codes can be inserted at the word and utterance level with minimal keystrokes. Routines were created to categorize and count these codes, with the result added to the standard SALT analyses. Scoring narrative structures for seven categories required adding scoring lines to the end of each transcript. Routines were added to SALT to insert the scoring template and to extract these scores from each transcript.

Problem 4: Eliminating the MANUAL Transfer of Language Scores Into Statistical Software for Group Analyses

Solution: Routines were added to the SALT software to select specific language variables from a large number of transcripts in a format that could then be directly imported into statistical software packages for analysis.

Problem 5: Matching Transcript Length So Analyses Are Equivalent

In the past this was accomplished by only transcribing a specified number of utterances, for example, 100. It has become clear that several options were needed to meet specific research needs. For example, matching the number of utterances may bias against delayed children for MLU and number of different word measures. A specified number of utterances may be useful for developing expectations for single groups of speakers by age. When comparing language production for the same elicitation context, for example, retelling the same story, using the entire transcript is of interest, making meaningful measures of total talking such as number of utterances or words, or the transcript duration.

Solution: Several options were added to SALT for matching transcripts based on length in words, utterances, and duration. These choices may be selected in conjunction with the "analysis set," the type of utterances to be included in the analysis. For example, unintelligible, incomplete, or abandoned utterances are usually not included for analysis as the frequency of these utterances varies across speakers and assumptions about words and utterance criteria are not met.

Problem 6: Studies of Vocabulary Use Require Methods to Identify Specific Words

A measure of the number of different words has been available for some time and has proven to be a robust measure of developmental progress. Evaluating the vocabulary used in the same context, retelling a story, for example, requires both searching transcripts for specific vocabulary to create frequency lists summed across transcripts as well as creating word lists from sets of transcripts. We were interested in comparing children's vocabulary use in English and Spanish.

Solution: Routines were added to the SALT software for documenting vocabulary diversity or frequency extracted from existing vocabulary lists or word lists generated from sets of transcripts. Word lists created from the complete version of a story could be used to search hundreds of transcripts to create frequency lists documenting vocabulary use. Alternately, total vocabulary use lists can be created to evaluate the words children actually use to retell a story.

DOCUMENTING VOCABULARY KNOWLEDGE USING NARRATIVE LANGUAGE SAMPLES

Researchers have been interested in vocabulary development for more than 100 years. Early work focused on changes in vocabulary size relative to advancing age. Estimates of children's vocabulary size from this research varied widely. For example, first graders have reported vocabularies ranging from 2,562 to 26,000 words (Stahl, 1999). Across studies, differences have been attributed to three major sources: (a) the definition of what constitutes a "word," (b) the corpus or dictionary used to estimate total word stock, and (c) the criterion or testing method to determine word knowledge. Nagy and Herman (1987) recalibrated earlier estimates for "word" definition and dictionary use and found adjusted yearly vocabulary growth of 2,000 to 3,600 words a year with a median figure of around 3,300. Anglin (1993) documents accelerating word learning across Grades 1, 3, and 5, where children 1.5 years to first grade are estimated to learn 5.52 words per day. From first to third grade, children acquire 12.13 words per day. Children in third to fifth grade attain 27.96 words per day. He noted the greatest change in learning rate to be derived words, which consist of one root word, and one or more derivational affixes. Adding a derivational affix is thought to result in an entirely different, although semantically related word, for example, *er* added to *preach: preacher*. Derived words account for about 1 word per day up to Grade 1, 5 words up to Grade 3, and more than 14 words a day of the almost 28 words estimated to be learned each day up to Grade 5. We can conclude from this that children learn new words at an amazing rate, that the rate of learning is different for different types of words, and that word learning accelerates dramatically after children enter school.

Children learn new words from context, both oral (Carey, 1978; Dollaghan, 1985) and written (Nagy, Herman, & Anderson, 1985). The role of parental language input has been attributed to larger vocabularies and more advanced language development (Hart & Risley, 1992, 1995; Huttenlocher, Haight, & Bryk, 1991). Exposure to difficult words in context results in their use earlier than expected relative to conceptual complexity (Huttenlocher, Vasilyeva, Cymerman, & Levine, 2002). Children learning two languages are faced with the especially difficult task of learning the vocabulary to represent their knowledge in both languages. Vocabulary relies on incidental learning in oral contexts prior to school entry. School provides opportunity for direct instruction of vocabulary as well as opportunity for learning from written context through reading as reading skills advance. Variability in word learning for bilingual children may be attributed to the amount of exposure to the second language. Opportunities for exposure may include listening to stories being read to them, conversational participation, and family and community language use. The age and extent of exposure to the second language will increase the opportunity for incidental vocabulary learning. Where such opportunities are lacking, vocabulary acquisition will suffer.

The role of lexical learning relative to other aspects of language development, such as syntax, has long been a matter of speculation. Bates and Goodman (1997) argued that vocabulary learning drives the acquisition of syntax. Pinker (1994), on the other hand, has suggested that vocabulary learning is dependent on syntax . Vocabulary learning requires exposure to the language representing the objects, actions, and relations the child experiences, as well as the cognitive skills to derive meaning from incidental exposure. The degree to which knowledge of the syntax of the language mediates learning awaits further research, but it is clear that children can use their knowledge of affixes to decipher the meanings of words that are new (Anglin, 1993). Vocabulary acquisition is viewed as crucial to the acquisition of literacy skills. Moreover, when children are faced with the difficult task of learning the words to represent their experience in two languages they can be at risk for learning to read in either language.

Vocabulary acquisition has been studied through a variety of methods, including but not limited to: (a) parent-report measures (Fenson et al., 1993), (b) self-report measures (Anderson & Freebody, 1983), (c) studies of word definition ability, both orally and in writing, (d) studies of word use in sentences, and (e) studies using oral answers to multiple choice questions presented orally and in writing (Anglin, 1993; Beimiller & Slonim, 2001). All of these approaches to measuring vocabulary knowledge are aimed at deriving estimates of the child's vocabulary size either by careful selection of the words from dictionaries representing all words in the language, or by a preselected set of words identified as those learned early in development.

Alternatively, however, vocabulary use could be investigated in the context of a specific sample of language, such as retelling a story. Using this method, we have devised a study in which children are required to listen to a story, observe the story's picture sequence, choose words, construct sentences, and organize the sequence of propositions in order to produce a coherent narrative. This task could be considered a test of vocabulary use in context. If every child retells the same story, then we can examine word use relative to the story model. The consistency of vocabulary used to tell the story and the variability seen when children use alternate word forms to represent the same story construct can both be examined. For bilingual children, the use of Spanish vocabulary when retelling the story in English can be compared with the use of English vocabulary when retelling the story in Spanish.

MEASURES OF VOCABULARY KNOWLEDGE IN NARRATIVES

All measures of vocabulary are based on sampling. This is true whether estimating total vocabulary, new words learned each day or year, parts of speech, or frequency of occurrence. Samples of words can be gathered from tests reflecting subsets of the words in the language delivered orally or through reading. Such tests can produce recognition or comprehension knowledge using a multiple-choice format. Or they can generate word knowledge by requiring definitions or using words correctly in sentences. Alternatively, vocabulary size has been estimated by recording samples of speech in conversation or narratives (Beimiller & Slonim, 2001). The size of the sample is then used as an index of talking during waking hours, and different words are taken as an estimate of vocabulary (Smith, 1941; Templin, 1957; Werner & Kaplin, 1952). Computer programs to analyze language samples have allowed efficient analysis of the vocabulary used in language samples elicited from conversations, narratives and expository texts (Miller & Chapman, 1983–2004). Miller (1987, 1991, 1996; Miller & Klee, 1995) documented that the number of different words (NDW) is highly correlated with age in children from 3 to 13, $r = .72$. This general index of vocabulary diversity can index developmental progress in vocabulary. However, to document specific vocabulary use in a language sample, we will need to get children to talk about the same content and work out ways to index vocabulary against some standard vocabulary list. Children, for example, could tell the same story providing insight into the words necessary for an accurate rendition of the content. The standard could be generated from the story script itself, listing all of the content words used to refer to the characters, actions, and relationships in the story. This seems rather straightforward if we assume that the script words are the only words available to children to retell the story. We must further assume that to get the story right, these specific words need to be used. Alternative words would lead to somewhat different versions of the story.

Another way to look at characterizing children's vocabulary would be to investigate the words children actually used in telling the story. Assuming children's vocabulary increases dramatically each year, and given enough children telling the story, developmental expectations for vocabulary use could be generated. This approach could yield important insights into the vocabulary learning process, or at least a description of the words children use to tell a story in their first and second language. Questions addressed in this line of research include: Is there any order to vocabulary acquisition with advancing age? Is variability in vocabulary use related to reading progress? And finally, is vocabulary growth related to progress in acquiring English syntax or narrative structure?

Three measures of vocabulary were used to address the questions posed in this study.

1. The *number of different words* (NDW) calculated by SALT using the total transcript of the narrative.
2. The *Number of Script Vocabulary* (NSV) used by subjects at each grade. A list of 87 words was identified from the story script. This list was then used by SALT to identify how many of those words were used in each subject's narrative. SALT also used this list to

calculate the percentage of transcripts containing each word and word use frequency.

3. *Peer Vocabulary* (PV) was generated by creating a master list of all the different words used by all the children at each grade. Then the lists were organized in story relevant categories. Finally SALT calculated the word groups used by children at each grade. Working out this analysis produced some unexpected results that may be revealing about word use in English, or the variability in exposure to English specifically, or opportunities to learn vocabulary through incidental learning. Outcomes of this analysis will be measures of consistency and variability of word use to indicate to the same referent.

Number of Different Words

The number of different words, root words, or lexemes revealed significant increases with each year of advancing grade. Children used almost 70 different words in retelling the story in kindergarten and about 100 by the time they reached the third grade. This finding is consistent with past research. There is a significant and moderately high correlation between grade and NDW.

Script Vocabulary

The result of the Script Vocabulary analysis was somewhat surprising. The script vocabulary list contained 87 different word roots/lexemes. The number of script vocabulary used by the subjects in retelling the story was relatively small, even though they were using an increasing number of different words and their narrative structure scores were increasing with advancing grade.[1] Calculating the number of script words used by 70% of the subjects at each grade revealed that the kindergarteners use an average of 5 script words, increasing to 12 script words by the third grade. Apparently the children did not refer to the major story referents using the script vocabulary. The intent of this measure was to document the number of words from the script used by the majority of children to retell the same story. Because the script words came from a complete adult version of the story, we expected more of these words to be used by increasing numbers of children with advancing grade. What words were these children using to retell stories with increasingly complex narrative structures? We sought solution to this question by investigating the vocabulary the children used with the Peer Vocabulary measure.

---

[1]Narrative structure scores came from the Miller, Andriacchi, and Nockerts (2003) Narrative Structure Scheme, a rubric scoring seven categories derived from story grammar, adding coherence, referencing, and mental states.

Peer Vocabulary

The total vocabulary list generated from the stories of all subjects was organized into the 87 categories designated by the script vocabulary. This amounted to creating a list of synonyms for each word. In some cases the group of words for a single referent was quite large. The gopher in *Frog, Where are You?* (Mayer, 1960) was referred to as a gopher, groundhog, beaver, squirrel, chipmunk, mole, rat, raccoon, rabbit, mouse, hamster, skunk, badger, otter, muskrat, bunny, hog, warthog, weasel, koala, and a gerbil. All of the words used by children to refer to a story referent were included in a category as long as the word shared most of the semantic features. The analysis was rerun accepting any referent within the category for the target. The results indicated that children were making reference to script vocabulary categories but using a variety of words. By the third grade, almost 40 of the script vocabulary categories were referred to, versus 12 if the exact vocabulary was required. It seems children have a sense of the story and are using the vocabulary they have available to retell the story events. It is also striking that children are using their own vocabulary and not just repeating the story verbatim, so that although working memory is surely operating, children are integrating their experience with the story and using their own words to produce a unique rendition of the narrative.

These vocabulary measures are undergoing continuing development to capture lexical choice. It is evident that there is a great deal to be learned beyond vocabulary size about how children represent a unique set of events presented in novel stories, and how this ability changes with development. Vocabulary learning mechanisms, rate of learning, vocabulary size, and selection for specific referents are important targets of this work. This work will ultimately inform research on children with a variety of language disorders and perhaps differentiating children with a variety of brain syndromes.

THE FUTURE

Current versions of LSA software allow investigators to study larger samples of children, calculating more measures across language levels. Studies of children with SLI over the past 5 years report an average of sample size of 15. Although samples this size may satisfy effect size estimates to address specific research questions, much larger samples are necessary to model how a variety of measures of language performance relate to one another, change over time, or describe different types of language disorder. Our current more efficient LSA methods allow investigators to collect and analyze samples from large numbers of children. Our current research project is processing 6,000 transcripts a year. It takes an average of 30–40 minutes to transcribe and code a frog story narrative. Using SALT we calculate standard measures, for example, MLU, NDW, WPM, errors, and omissions, as well as the coded analyses, a subordination index, and a narrative structure score. The ability to run all of the analyses at the same time from each transcript allows us to process all of the samples in each language at each data point at the same time. This means that 1,500 transcripts are analyzed at the same time, with the scores for each analysis entered into a rectangular data array that is be ported to statistical analysis software directly. This eliminates any hand data entry, assuring accuracy of the analyses. Advances in LSA efficiency make it possible to conduct longitudinal studies of large numbers of children. Large numbers will be required to document differences in language performance across sampling contexts, for example, conversation, event narratives, storytelling or story retelling, and a variety of expository tasks for children across geographical areas, socioeconomic status (SES) conditions, experience with English, preschool and school experience, reading, and school achievement.

Technology will continue to advance, making high-quality digital recording more accessible. It would be possible to use cell-phone or PDA (personal digital assistant) technology to record and transmit language samples from the field. Speech recognition technology may get to the point of automatically producing a text version of the language sample. These advances would provide opportunity to collect larger samples of language from a broader range of children with and without disabilities. Databases can be complied to be used for comparing individual children. SALT can already perform such comparisons for conversation and narrative samples, using the SALT reference database of 356 samples from children 3–13 years of age. Data sets from more children in a variety of sampling conditions would increase the clinical utility of LSA. A major question we will face is, "How should these databases be constructed?" To answer this question we will require more research on what makes a difference for children's language learning, for example, SES, race, language exposure, geography, and schooling. Will large data sets ever be considered "standardized" in the same sense as a standardized test?

The language sample analysis process seems to be a never-ending work in progress. As new problems emerge, solutions are sought by creating new analyses to better document the complexities of the processes of language development and to characterize disordered performance. In this endeavor, despite the many technological changes and innovations we have embraced, the basic perspective with which we began continues to inform this work: Understanding the role of the normal acquisition of language in greater depth and detail informs practice with children with disabilities. The capacity that SALT and other technical advances provide in this work will, we hope, allow more rapid advances in this direction, but will not change the basic course of our efforts, to map out the typical sequence of language acquisition, so that children who fall behind can be led along an increasingly clear path.

ACKNOWLEDGMENTS

This work was supported in part by grants HD39521 "Oracy/Literacy Development of Spanish-Speaking Children" and R305U010001 "Biological and Behavioral Variation in the Language Development of Spanish-Speaking Children," both jointly funded by the National Institute of Child Health and Human Development and the U.S. Department of Education's Institute of Education Sciences, David Francis PI, Jon Miller Co-PI.

REFERENCES

Anderson, R., & Freebody, P. (1983). Reading comprehension and the assessment and acquisition of word knowledge. *Advances in Reading/Language Research, 2,* 231–256.

Anglin, J. (1993). Vocabulary development: A morphological analysis. *Monographs of the Society for Research in Child Development, 58,* 10.

Bates, E., & Goodman, J. (1997). On the inseparability of grammar and the lexicon: Evidence from acquisition, aphasia and real-time processing. *Language and Cognitive Processes, 12*(5/6), 507–586.

Biemiller, A., & Slonim, N. (2001). Estimating root word vocabulary growth in normative and advantaged populations: Evidence for a common sequence of vocabulary acquisition. *Journal of Educational Psychology, 93*(3), 498–520

Bloom, L. (1970). *Language development: Form and function in emerging grammars.* Cambridge, MA: MIT Press.

Carey, S. (1978). The child as word learner. In M. Halle, J. Bresnan, & G. A. Miller (Eds.), *Linguistic theory and psychological reality* (pp. 264–293). Cambridge, MA: MIT Press.

Dollaghan, C. (1985). Child meets word: "Fast mapping" in preschool children. *Journal of Speech & Hearing Research, 28*(3), 449–454.

Fenson, L., Dale, P. S., Reznick, J. S., Thal, D. J., Bates, E., Hartung, J. P., et al. (1993). *The MacArthur Communicative Development Inventories: User's guide and technical manual.* San Diego, CA: Singular.

Hart, B., & Risley, T. (1992). American parenting of language-learning children: Persisting differences in family-child interactions observed in natural home environments. *Developmental Psychology, 28*(6), 1096–1105.

Hart, B., & Risley, T. (1995). *Meaningful differences in everyday experiences of young American children.* Baltimore: Paul H. Brookes.

Huttenlocher, J., Haight, W., & Bryk, A. (1991). Early vocabulary growth: Relation to language input and gender. *Developmental Psychology, 27*(2), 236–248.

Huttenlocher, J., Vasilyeva, M., Cymerman, E., & Levine, S. (2002). Language input and child syntax. *Cognitive Psychology, 45*(3), 337–374.

Mayer, M. (1960). *Frog, Where are you?* New York: Puffin.

Miller, J. (1987). A grammatical characterization of language disorder. In *Proceedings of the First International Symposium on Specific Speech and Language Disorders in Children* (pp. 100–113). London: AFASIC Press.

Miller, J. (1991). Quantifying productive language disorder. In J. Miller (Ed.), *Research on child language disorders: A decade of progress* (pp. 211–220). Boston: College Hill Press.

Miller, J. (1996). The search for a phenotype of disordered language performance. In M. Rice (Ed.), *Toward a genetics of language* (pp. 297–314). Hillsdale, NJ: Lawrence Erlbaum Associates.

Miller, J., Andriacchi, K., & Nockerts, A. (2003). *A Narrative Scoring Scheme: A rubric for quantifying narrative structure.* Language Analysis Laboratory, University of Wisconsin–Madison.

Miller, J., & Chapman, R. (1983– 2004). Computer programs for the systematic analysis of language transcripts SALT. Research Version 8. Language Analysis Laboratory, Waisman Center, University of Wisconsin–Madison.

Miller, J., & Klee, T. (1995). Quantifying language disorders in children. In P. Fletcher & B. MacWhinney (Eds.), *Handbook of child language* (pp. 545–572). Oxford, England: Basil Blackwell.

Miller, J. F. (1982). *Assessing children's language production: Experimental procedures.* Baltimore: University Park Press.

Miller, J. F., & Chapman, R. S. (1981). The relation between age and mean length of utterance on morphemes. *Journal of Speech and Hearing Research, 24,* 154–161.

Nagy, W. E., & Herman, P. A. (1987). Breadth and depth of vocabulary knowledge: Implications for acquisition and instruction. In M. G. McKeown & M. G. Curtis (Eds.), *Nature of vocabulary acquisition* (pp. 19–36). Hillsdale, NJ: Lawrence Erlbaum Associates.

Nagy, W. E., Herman, P. A., & Anderson, R. C. (1985). Learning words from context. *Reading Research Quarterly, 20,* 233–253.

Pinker, S. (1994). *The language instinct.* New York: Morrow.

Smith, M. K. (1941). Measurement of the size of general English vocabulary through the elementary grades and high school. *Genetic Psychology Monographs, 24,* 311–345.

Stahl, S. A. (1999). *Vocabulary development.* Cambridge, MA: Brookline Books.

Templin, M. (1957). *Certain language skills in children: Their development and interrelationships* (Institute of Child Welfare, Monograph Series No. 26). Minneapolis: University of Minnesota Press.

Werner, H., & Kaplin, E. (1952). The acquisition of word meanings: A developmental study. *Monographs of the Society for Research in Child Development, 15,* 1.

13

Narrative Abilities in Children With Language Impairments

Donna M. Boudreau
Portland State University

The process in which children evolve from a prelinguistic stage of development to fully competent language users is one that continues to intrigue theorists, practitioners, and parents alike. The newborn infant emerges into the world seemingly devoid of any knowledge, skill, or abilities, and in the first 5 years of life acquires a complex language system that includes thousands of lexical referents, the ability to apply structural rules to formulate grammatically accurate sentences, and knowledge of how to use language with others to serve a broad range of pragmatic functions.

One area of both theoretical and clinical interest is the development of discourse skills in children. The ability to understand and produce connected language is a critical developmental process for children, signifying the evolution of linguistic abilities that are no longer tied to the here and now, but can refer to events represented at both different places and points in time. Discourse genres include conversations, personal events, stories, explanations, and expository information (Hughes, McGillivray, & Schmidek, 1997; McCabe & Bliss, 2003). Narrative abilities, which include both personal events and fictional stories, have received the most attention in the literature (McCabe & Bliss, 2003; Peterson & McCabe, 1992). Narratives have been defined as "units of spoken text beyond the sentence level" (Roth, Speece, Cooper, & De La Paz, 1996), as well as "a series of action and events that unfold over time, according to causal principles (Mar, 2004, p. 1415). What is common across definitions is the concept of connected utterances that are temporally related about events that are causally connected. Thus, narrative discourse is much more than an individual sequence of sentences (Graesser, 1997). Constructing and understanding narratives require two related levels of skill: micro-level knowledge, or the linguistic structures used to share and understand ideas, and macro-level knowledge, or more global levels of organization of how narratives are structured (Liles, 1993). There is agreement that narrative skills draw on linguistic, cognitive, and pragmatic skills, world knowledge, and memory, making this level of language use often more difficult than word or sentence level tasks (O'Brien & Albrecht, 1992). Additionally, research also suggests that narrative skills are distinct from other components of language (syntactic, semantic, and phonological levels) (Hemphill, Uccelli, Winner, & Chang, 2002).

The origins of narrative development unfold in parent–child interactions (Eisenberg, 1985; Haden, Haine, & Fivush, 1997). Early in development, a single utterance may serves as a reflection of a previously experienced event (McCabe & Peterson, 1991). Children as young as 2 years of age recount information about new and onetime experiences in interactions with caregivers (Miller & Sperry, 1988; Peterson, 1990). Although early exchanges between parent and child include topics beyond the here and now, the adult provides maximal contextual support to allow the child to participate in this interaction. Here is an example from a parent–child exchange with an 18-month-old:

P: Tell Daddy what we did today.
C: (No response, looks between mother and father).
P: Did we go some where?
C: Go?
P: What did we go see today?
C: Zoo!
P: Tell Daddy what we saw at the zoo. Do you remember?
C: Daddy, zoo!
P: That's right, we went to the zoo. But who was jumping around and swinging their arms? Do you remember? And you kept laughing?
C: Monkeys!
P: That's right, we saw the monkeys at the zoo. And what did we do after we went to the zoo? Do you remember?
C: Hot dogs!
P: That's right! We met Julie and Madeline for lunch today.

Sharing of personal events is the earliest form of narrative genre to develop, and early narrative construction is a cooperative exchange between parent and child (Haden et al., 1997). In the example provided, the parent provides contextual support to help the child retrieve details from memory. At the same time the parent models the use of multiple utterances on a given topic, the temporal sequence of how events occurred, and pragmatically relevant behaviors such as amount of background knowledge that can be assumed and the choice of topic to be shared. Although children can tell about events with little scaffolding provided, they are often difficult to understand for unfamiliar adults because they lack orientating context (Peterson, 1990). Although personal narratives represent the most common narrative genre used by children into kindergarten (Preece, 1987), children are simultaneously developing knowledge about fictional stories. Fictional stories reflect a more creative form of narrative discourse (Hughes et al., 1997), and even sharing of personal narratives is thought to move beyond reporting events to take on more of a storytelling form over time (Hudson & Shapiro, 1991).

Narratives have been shown to play a critical role in social success, with clear connections to life experiences both socially and perceptually as they follow protagonists in goal-directed behavior that often contain obstacles, and emotional responses to these obstacles (Bruner, 1986; Graesser, Singer, & Trabasso, 1994; Nelson, 1986; Rice, Sell, & Hadley, 1991; Roth et al., 1996). Narrative skills have been linked to academic success as well, with the ability to use language in a decontextualized way serving an important transition between oral and written language (Bishop & Edmundson, 1987; Roth et al., 1996; Snow & Dickinson, 1990; Tabors, Snow, & Dickinson, 2001; Westby, 1991).

THEORETICAL MODEL OF NARRATIVE DEVELOPMENT

How do children make the transition from early use of gestures and single words to the ability to connect utterances on a topic in culturally and linguistically competent ways? Early work by Johnson-Laird (1983) focused on the notion of a mental model, which he suggests is a representation of the information within the narrative, including causal relations, goals, and spatial and temporal information. In this framework, the speaker or listener maintains an overall perspective, and selects linguistic items to shift the listener's attention as the narrative unfolds (Liles, 1993). The construction of a narrative is the spoken discussion of what is represented mentally (Lahey & Bloom, 1994), whereas comprehension requires the ability to hold information in memory in order to see relationships across utterances, to integrate new information that adds or modifies current information, and to discard information held or received that is irrelevant or no longer necessary.

The Child Talk model of language processing posited by Chapman and colleagues (Chapman et al., 1992) provides a context in which to understand the development of discourse level skills and the role that the child's early experiences play in the development of narrative abilities. This model suggests that language is learned through repeated shared experiences, with language mapped onto these events. Language is thus context specific early in its history, and is part of a broader representation that includes actions, events, situations, feelings, and goals (Chapman et al., 1992). This model theorizes that events, along with related words and sentence frames, are stored in memory in modular or encapsulated ways. It is through the social context of participating in exchanges about events, as well as listening to and hearing stories, that children develop expectations for how stories are constructed and shared, often referred to as narrative schema. Schema theory relates to an abstract architecture thought to influence the organization of mental representations in both comprehension and production of narratives (Mandler, 1978; Rumelhart, 1975), which becomes part of implicit rather than explicit knowledge (Duchan, 2004). It is well known that children enjoy repeated readings of favorite stories, and learn the language of these familiar events. Within these interactions, children are learning language forms that are initially context specific, and are only gradually generalized to other situations and functions (Chapman et al., 1992). Over time, children begin to see the patterns of stories, which include the temporal and causal relationships that are repeatedly present in these experiences, and learn literate language forms that can be used to represent decontextualized events. Children are also increasing the complexity of the underlying mental model that is constructed, using information from past experiences stored in memory (Lahey & Bloom, 1994). Research shows that these early experiences lay the foundation for understanding and producing more complex connected discourse. Studies of young children have demonstrated that both quantity and quality of interactions around descriptions of past events are significantly related to children's abilities to share past events (Haden et al., 1997; McCabe & Peterson, 1991; Peterson, Jesso, & McCabe, 1999). Additionally, studies that have examined parent–child shared book reading exchanges with young children lend support to the relationship of experiences and interactions in the development of narrative skill. Research has shown that children are able to comprehend and retell stories that are most closely aligned structurally to the types of stories heard at home, and that exposure to well-formed stories helps children internalize a schema for how stories are constructed (Goldman & Rakestraw, 2000; Heath, 1982, 1986; Morrow & Brittain, 2003; Pritchard, 1990; Teale, 2003).

NARRATIVE ABILITIES IN CHILDREN WITH LANGUAGE IMPAIRMENT

Applying our understanding of a developmental skill to populations of children developing atypically provides an opportunity to evaluate theoretical perspectives against varied development trajectories. The prevalence of specific language impairment (SLI) in children is estimated to be approximately 7.4% of the population of monolingual English-speaking children, based on epidemiological research (Tomblin et al., 2001). SLI is characterized by language difficulties in the absence of mental retardation, neurological impairments, or hearing loss (Aram, Morris, & Hall, 1993). Characteristics of language impairments include difficulties in the development of semantics, acquisition of morphology and syntax, and pragmatic/social skills (for a review, see Leonard, 1998; Watkins, 1997).

Performance on narrative tasks from preschool children through school age serves to distinguish children with LI from typically developing peers (Liles, 1993; Liles, Duffy, Merritt, & Purcell, 1995). In addition to difficulties in comprehension of connected discourse (Bishop & Adams, 1992; Crais & Chapman, 1987; Ellis Weismer, 1985), across studies children with LI have been shown to experience difficulty in the use of linguistic structures in productive narrative tasks, including utterance length, cohesive adequacy, lexical diversity, correct use of morphological structures, complex syntax, and fluency (Bishop & Edmunson, 1987; Clifford, 1995; Liles, 1985; Liles & Purcell, 1987; Paul & Smith, 1993; Pearce, McCormack, & James, 2003; Reilly, Losh, Bellugi, & Wulfeck, 2004). Additionally, children with LI also experience difficulty in constructing or retelling narratives, including fewer information units, propositions, utterances, and story grammar components; as well as difficulty with text cohesion (Boudreau & Hedberg, 1999; Crais & Chapman, 1987; Graybeal, 1981; Liles, 1985, 1987; Merritt & Liles, 1987; Paul, 1996; Purcell & Liles, 1992; Ripich & Griffith, 1988; Strong & Shaver, 1991). However, unlike analyses of linguistic components of narratives, research shows that children with SLI perform comparably to age-matched peers on some types of structural analyses as well. For example, although Boudreau and Hedberg (1999) found a significant difference between preschool children with SLI (SLI) and age-matched peers in overall story grammar components included in a story retelling of "Frog, Where Are You?" (Mayer, 1969), comparisons of the inclusion of events key to plot line (initiating event, problem, and resolution) revealed no significant differences between groups. Consistent with these findings, Liles (1985) found that while all children with LI demonstrated difficulties with intersentential cohesion, there was a subgroup of children with LI in her project that successfully answered questions about story grammar knowledge. Finally, Reilly et al. (2004) examined the performance of children with SLI in comparison to chronologically age-matched peers and a group of children with unilateral focal brain lesion. Although children with SLI performed consistently more poorly on measures of linguistic structure, they performed similarly to typically developing peers in establishing and maintaining a search theme (i.e., specific mention of the missing frog and frequency of mention of subsequent search). Additionally, for the oldest age group included in the study, children with SLI included an equal number of story components, and used an equal number of evaluative devices categorized as cognitive inferences, which included inferences to character motivation, causality, and mental state (Reilly et al., 2004).

NARRATIVE DIFFICULTIES: A PERFORMANCE ISSUE?

Despite documented difficulties in both comprehension and production of narratives, few descriptive studies have attempted to account for the problems children with LI experience on discourse-level tasks. A developmental model might attribute the basis of narrative skills to differences in quality and quantity of early experiences of children with SLI; however, there is a paucity of research that has examined the discourse of parent–child interactions with this population. In shared book reading exchanges, studies have shown that parents of children with language delays maintain responsibility for the interactions around text to a greater degree than families of typically developing preschool children, such as asking a larger number of questions, taking more conversational turns, including lower levels of "abstract language use," and engaging in more directive behavior (Evans & Schmidt, 1991; Sulzby & Kaderavek, 1996; van Kleek & Vander Woude, 2003). However, these modifications appear compensatory, and have been attributed to the potential need of children with language difficulties for ongoing mediated assistance to understand the story, or clarification by mothers of their child's incorrect responses to questions posed during story reading (van Kleek & Vander Woude, 2003).

Historically, linguistic difficulties in children with SLI have often been argued as a competence issue, reflecting limitations in the development of specific grammatical rules and structures (Bishop, 1994; Clahsen, 1989, 1999; Gopnick & Crago, 1991). This perspective has been extended to problems children with LI experience on narrative tasks as well, with difficulties in macro- and micro-level aspects of narrative performance attributed to limitations in linguistic skills, as well as difficulty internalizing organizational framework of narrative structure (Liles,

1987). However, this theoretical account appears inadequate for several reasons. From a developmental perspective, both experience and children's abilities to draw from those experiences are critical to discourse level skills. A competence-based model does not account for the significant contribution of early social exchanges to narrative abilities.

Second, a model that presupposes deficits in both macro- and micro-level knowledge is insufficient in that it does not consider the interactions between linguistic and cognitive skills, world knowledge, and memory that discourse level tasks draw on. Lahey and Bloom discuss the idea that narrative skill "involves being able to hold in mind a complex model of relations among events while using language to express these relations" (Lahey & Bloom, 1994, p. 358), a task that is dependent on the integration of abilities at a number of levels. Additionally, research that has examined narrative performance in children with SLI has revealed varied results, depending on the structural analyses employed or the developmental stage of the participants (Boudreau & Hedberg, 1999; Liles, 1985; Reilly et al., 2004). Liles found a subgroup of children with SLI who did not seem to present with difficulties on macro-level knowledge of narrative (Liles, 1985). Finally, the context in which a narrative is elicited (such as medium used in the narrative event presented, or naive versus informed listener) has resulted in differences in overall content, although general organizational patterns appear to be consistent (Merritt & Liles, 1989; Ripich & Griffith, 1988). These studies fail to confirm difficulty in macro-level skills as a general characteristic of children with LI.

More recent research has begun to examine language performance on comprehension and production tasks within a theoretical model of a limited capacity system (Adams, Bourke, & Willis, 1995; Baddeley & Hitch, 1974; Ellis Weismer, Evans, & Hesketh, 1999; Ellis Weismer & Hesketh, 1993, 1996; Gathercole & Baddeley, 1990a, 1990b, 1993; Gathercole, Willis, Emslie, & Baddeley, 1992; Miolo & Chapman, 1999; Montgomery, 2000, 2001). Although theoretical premises differ, a central tenet to the idea of a limited capacity system is that for all cognitive activity, there is a limited amount of resources on which to draw to complete a task. Resources are shared among different cognitive operations, and trade-offs may occur when the system is strained (Lahey & Bloom, 1994). In this framework, performance may be compromised when demands of a task exceed available resources—a more dynamic relationship than previously considered. Despite evidence of the influence of resource demands on language performance at a word and sentence level, limited research has examined this relationship with discourse-level tasks (Evans, 1996; Stine & Wingfield, 1990). Evans (1996) examined the influence of discourse demands within conversational language samples of a small group of school-aged children with LI. This study examined the turn-transitions between speakers, as it was theorized that the verbal and nonverbal constraints of this point of conversational interaction (i.e., avoiding speaker overlap, remaining on topic, appropriate use of paralinguistic and nonverbal cues) would place the greatest amount of processing demand in the interaction. Results revealed that for a subgroup of participants with expressive language impairments, grammatical errors occurred most frequently in across-turn utterances, a pattern that was not replicated in the subgroup of children with expressive-receptive language impairments. However, both subgroups experienced at least minimal increases in grammatical errors (primarily omissions of bound morphemes) in the production of utterances with the greatest discourse demands (Evans, 1996). In another study comparing elderly adults to university-aged students, participants listened to passages that varied in length and propositional density (or idea units), and were immediately asked to recall each passage. Results revealed that low-density texts as well as shorter texts were recalled proportionally better than texts with higher propositional density or length (with younger participants recalling a greater proportion of propositions than the elderly adults) (Stine & Wingfield, 1990). These findings support a need to consider contextual factors and task demands when measuring discourse-level skills in children with LI.

The notion of difficulties on discourse level tasks reflecting variability in underlying cognitive capacity supports a developmental model of narrative acquisition, moving beyond developmental skills to consider the contribution of other cognitive processes to narrative performance. Early parent–child interactions provide a context for acquiring language and knowledge of narrative structure, both of which are critical to narrative performance. If children use language to represent ideas about the world, which is consistent with a mental model framework, they must draw from past experiences, in which they have learned the language of events and expectations about how events are structured. This knowledge is stored in long-term memory (LTM), and must be brought to some level of consciousness to allow for it to be acted on (Lahey & Bloom, 1994). It is the interaction of information in LTM, which includes linguistic knowledge and schema for narratives, as well as an understanding of world and pragmatic knowledge, that is drawn on when a child is asked to complete a narrative task. Strengths in any of these areas that contribute to narrative understanding or production will reduce the amount of resources that must be allocated to that aspect of the task. The early interactions that provide the basis for learning language and narrative schema are thus important to reducing demands on available resources.

CURRENT PROJECT

Our current work addresses discourse-level skills in children with LI, in an attempt to account for at least some of the difficulties experienced on narrative tasks within a framework of a performance issue in a limited capacity model. Narratives may be especially vulnerable to effects of processing demands, as the ability to understand or produce a narrative requires the speaker/listener to hold information in working memory, while at the same time acting on this information. Working memory has been described as "the capacity to hold information 'on-line' for imminent use in the service of some goal," and can be new information received or information drawn from LTM (Crosson, 2000, p. 399). Working memory allows us to maintain information in memory until it is needed for some purpose. Previous research has provided evidence of more limited working memory skills in children with SLI than their typically developing peers (Ellis Weismer et al., 1999; Montgomery, 1995). We hypothesized that narrative performance (comprehension and production) would vary in children with LI as a function of task demands, and that a measure of processing capacity such as working memory would be significantly related to narrative performance.

Methods

We recently completed a pilot project of school aged children with LI (n = 18), ranging in age from 6;8 to 8;8. All children had been identified as having language impairment in the absence of significant cognitive deficits, hearing problems, or neurological impairments based on SLP referral and follow up assessment. All children were monolingual speakers of English. The Block Design and Picture Completion subtests of the Weschler Intelligence Scale for Children–III (WISC–III) (Weschler, 1991) were administered as indices of nonverbal cognition. Two children scored more than 1 *SD* below the mean on nonverbal cognitive subtests administered; however, these children were included in light of current recommendations regarding the need to reevaluate exclusionary criteria for SLI based on nonverbal cognitive functioning (Tager-Flusberg & Cooper, 1999). Language scores on the Test of Language Development (Primary or Secondary, depending on children's age) (Newcomer & Hammill, 1997a, 1997b) revealed scores of at least one standard deviation or more below the mean on at least one language quotient on the TOLD, with the majority of participants performing 1½ *SD* or more below the mean across language quotients

Assessment Measures and Procedures

Children were seen individually on two occasions for approximately 1 hr each session at their elementary school. In addition to language and cognitive measures previously discussed, children also engaged in a 12-min conversational language sample. Working memory skills were assessed using the Competing Language Processing Task (Gaulin & Campbell, 1994), which consists of asking children increasingly longer sets (one to six sentences) of short questions, in which they must indicate whether the sentences are true or false by responding with yes or no (e.g., *Hotdogs can bark. Balloons can float*). After completing each individual set in this fashion, children are asked to recall the last word in each sentence for the individual set of sentences. This task was administered using live voice.

To evaluate narrative abilities, four experimental stories were developed. Picture books developed by the same author/illustrator and judged as not highly familiar to children were utilized as the basis for the experimental stories constructed. They included *Kermit the Hermit* (Peet, 1965b), *Ella the Elephant* (Peet, 1964), *Chester the World Pig* (Peet, 1965a), and *Cyrus the Unsinkable Sea Serpent* (Peet, 1975). Each of the original stories was 48 pages in length. Two of the stories related to animals (a pig and elephant) and two of the stories related to ocean creatures (a crab and a sea monster). From these original stories, new stories were constructed by reassembling pages from each book and rewriting text to correspond to the new story line constructed. Each new story was 14 pages in length and consisted of 26 utterances. Stories were systematically varied on linguistic and structural complexity to comprise stories with the following characteristics: linguistically simple/structurally simple (LS/SS); linguistically simple/structurally complex (LS/SC); linguistically complex/structurally simple (LC/SS); and linguistically complex/structurally complex (LC/SC). Linguistically matched stories were comparable on MLU and proportion of simple to complex utterances. Linguistically simple stories had a mean MLU of 8.46 (8.42 and 8.50, respectively), and 65% of utterances were complex. Comparatively, linguistically complex stories had a mean MLU of 11.08 (10.85 and 11.31, respectively), and 85% of utterances were complex. Structurally matched stories consisted of either a simple plot line with one protagonist (simple structure) or contained an embedded plot structure with two protagonists, each following an independent goal with resulting attempts, consequences, and resolutions (complex stories). All four stories consisted of four episodes. Narrative tasks were counterbalanced over the two sessions; however, the two animal or ocean creature stories were never completed in the same day in an attempt to avoid carryover or interference . Stories were recorded on a high-quality analog tape recorder, and children listened to each story via headphones while viewing the pages of the book. At the completion of each story, the storybook was removed, and participants were prompted to tell the story "for a friend who hadn't seen or heard the story." The starter phrase "Once upon a time, there was ..." was provided for each story. Upon completion of the retelling, children were then asked nine comprehension questions that addressed the individual story. Each set of questions included 4 items targeting actual information from the story (i.e., who/what), 2 questions that addressed emotional content of how a character felt in response to an event in the story (e.g., "How did X feel when ...") and 3 questions that addressed a child's understanding of protagonist(s)'s goals and the ability to draw inferences (e.g., why ...).

Results

We compared performance across the four conditions, to determine whether stories that were either linguistically or structurally more complex resulted in poorer narrative comprehension or production. We measured both linguistic and structural aspects of narratives. Linguistic analyses included mean length of utterance, lexical diversity (number of different words produced), and verbal fluency (total number of words produced). Structural analyses included calculating the total number of utterances produced, the number of propositions or idea units that were included in each story (see example in Appendix A), and the story grammar components recalled as a proportion of the total possible story grammar components (Stein & Glenn, 1979) that could be included (see example in Appendix B) . On all of these variables, comparisons among the four condition were completed using repeated-measures analysis of variance (ANOVA).

For the linguistic analyses, results revealed that MLU did not differ across the four conditions. Thus, despite stories varying in linguistic complexity, participants did not differ in the average length of utterances produced in their retelling. However, we found that the structurally simple stories resulted in greater lexical diversity and a larger total number of words produced than the structurally complex conditions. These differences between the most complex condition (linguistically complex/structurally complex) and the structurally simple conditions were significant for three of four analyses completed (see Fig. 13.1).

In comparing performance among conditions on structural complexity, there was a significant difference among conditions on the total number of utterances included. Fewer utterances were produced in the structurally complex conditions, although the degree of difference observed was statistically significant only between the most complex condition (LC/SC) and one of the structurally simple stories (LC/SS). For overall propositions included, children produced a greater number in their retelling of structurally simple stories, regardless of the linguistically complexity each contained. Again, differences were statistically significant between the most complex condition (LC/SC) and one of the two structurally simple stories (LC/SS). Finally, for proportion of story grammar components included, there was a significant group effect among conditions. Although children included a greater proportion of story grammar components in the structurally simple conditions, statistical comparison in post hoc

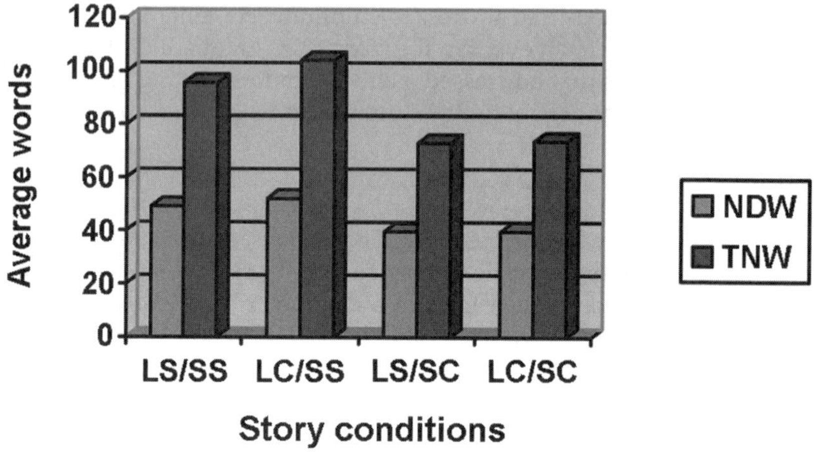

FIG. 13.1. A comparison of number of different words and total number of words between conditions.

analyses were significant for only one set of comparisons (LS/SC and LC/SS) (see Fig. 13.2).

The final set of analyses among conditions examined the effects of story complexity on children's comprehension of the story. Although results of this analysis revealed a significant group effect, none of the post hoc comparisons were significant. Table 13.1 provides mean scores for

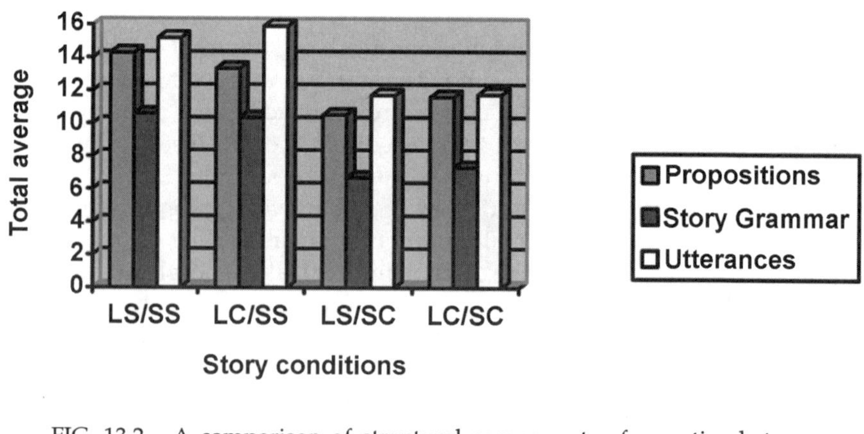

FIG. 13.2. A comparison of structural components of narrative between conditions.

TABLE 13.1
Mean and Standard Deviation (in Parentheses) in Response to Comprehension Questions Across Conditions

	LS/SS	*LC/SS*	*LS/SC*	*LC/SC*
Comprehension questions	7.0	6.89	6.17	5.89
	(1.68)	(1.81)	(1.50)	(2.19)
How	1.78	1.5	1.33	1.11
	(.43)	(.78)	(.59)	(.83)
WH	5.17	5.0	4.77	3.94
	(1.15)	(1.07)	(1.06)	(1.63)
Why	1.33	1.67	1.00	1.22
	(.59)	(.78)	(.69)	(.81)

each condition, for total performance, and for subtypes of comprehension questions posed.

The last question we investigated in this project was the relationship between working memory and narrative abilities. If difficulties on narrative tasks reflect demands on resource capacity, we would expect a relationship between working memory skills and narrative performance for those story conditions that exceed available resources. Findings revealed that working memory was significantly related to both linguistic and structural measures primarily on the most complex story condition (see Table 13.2). The relationship of working memory to narrative comprehension revealed a different picture, with significant correlations with the two story conditions that were either structurally OR linguistically complex. Working memory was weakly correlated with both the simple and the complex condition.

DISCUSSION

Narrative abilities are a complex language skill, representing one form of discourse processing. To engage in narrative tasks, children must construct a mental model of an event, with the complexity of the mental model formed increasing with age and experience (Lahey & Bloom, 1994). Both narrative comprehension and production require the child to maintain a mental representation in memory. In productive tasks, the child must draw on LTM to access knowledge of appropriate structure or schema, and maintain a mental representation of the event while formulating linguistically correct utterances that reflect this representation. Similarly, in comprehending narratives, the child must construct, maintain, and modify a men-

TABLE 13.2
Correlations Between Measures of Working Memory and Narrative Variables

	LS/SS		*LC/SS*		*LS/SC*		*LC/SC*	
	r	*p*	*r*	*p*	*r*	*p*	*r*	*p*
MLU	.173	.506	.394	.106	.168	.519	.264	.324
NDW	.496	.043*	.415	.087	.025	.924	.668	.005**
TNW	.413	.099	.412	.090	.052	.843	.596	.015*
Total utterances	.254	.325	.314	.204	–.138	.597	.518	.040*
Story grammar	.468	.058	.304	.235	.085	.746	.604	.013*
Propositions	408	.104	.305	.218	.280	.276	.558	.025*
Comprehension questions	.274	.272	.508	.031*	.541	.021*	.315	.204

$^*p < .05$; $^{**}p < .01$.

tal representation of the event from language received, including temporal and causal relationships. Both comprehension and production of narratives include demands on linguistic and cognitive abilities, processing capacity, world knowledge, and memory.

The foundations of narrative skills are established in early parent–child interactions, in which adults scaffold the exchange to allow the child to contribute to the interaction. Through repeated experiences, children develop a schema for narratives and learn the language of these events. This provides the basis of knowledge and skills that are critical to understanding and constructing narratives. Research with young children supports the significant contribution of early exchanges, both in parent-mediated discussion of past events and in shared book reading, to the acquisition of narrative abilities. The development of linguistic and structural knowledge of narratives serves to lessen demands on other cognitive capacities, such as processing and memory.

This pilot project attempted to account for at least some of the difficulty children with language impairments experience in narrative production and comprehension from a limited capacity model. It was theorized that a child's abilities to comprehend or produce a narrative may be much more dynamic than has been considered in research to date. Results from this project support our initial hypothesis regarding the influence of task demands on discourse level tasks. When processing load was systematically increased, it resulted in poorer performance on both macro- and micro-level aspects of narrative skill, as well as narrative comprehension. It can be theorized that complex narratives strained available processing resources to a greater degree than simple narratives, resulting in poorer performance overall. It is assumed that capacity limitations influence performance only when resource demands exceed resources available (Just & Carpenter, 1992). Thus, the deterioration of performance on most complex story conditions appears to represent tasks in which available resources were exceeded.

Interestingly, the complexity of narrative structure, which was increased by interweaving two main protagonists among several complete episodes, was more detrimental to narrative performance than increased complexity of linguistic structures. Children performed more poorly on micro-level analyses (number of different words, total number of words) and macro-level analyses (length of story, number of propositions, proportion of story grammar structures) in stimulus stories that were structurally complex, irrespective of the language demands of the task. From a theoretical framework, we might account for these findings in several different ways. First, at least some theories of capacity limitations in working memory (WM) suggest that trade-offs occur between storage and processing when the demands of the task are high (Baddelely & Hitch, 1974; Just & Carpenter, 1992), although more recent work questions whether storage and processing are truly related systems (Towe, Hitch, & Hutton, 1998). In the current investigation, we did not attempt to empirically evaluate whether processing and storage are independent or related systems, but rather completed a preliminary investigation to determine whether performance is influenced when available resources are taxed. It could be theorized, however, that linguistically complex utterances may initially place a greater demand on resources to process the semantic and syntactic structures, but that once interpreted, storage of this information should not be any greater than the events communicated using linguistically simple utterances. Graesser (1997) suggests that more shallow levels of code, such as syntax or word knowledge, "are addressed only to the extent they help clarify how meaning representations are constructed" (p. 166). In contrast, structurally complex narratives likely place a demand on both storage and processing resources. Specifically, unlike the following of a single protagonist, in which a listener must modify/update information on the protagonist's pursuit of a goal, a structurally complex narrative commands that the listener engage in modification of a mental representation for two (or more) sets of characters. Thus, overall storage demands would be greater in these conditions than structurally simple narratives. Given the purpose and design of the study, we can only speculate about these issues. However, as performance within the two structurally complex narrative conditions were highly similar, irrespective of linguistic complexity of the condition, it may be that the demand on WM skills in processing complex narrative structure is particularly high.

A final question investigated in this pilot project was the relative contribution of working memory to narrative discourse. Despite previous research failing to account for performance on discourse level tasks by WM skills (Caspari & Parkinson, 2000), more recent work by Moser and Johnston (2004) revealed a strong and significant relationship between verbal working memory and narrative structure within a single narrative task. In our current project, we examined the relationship of working memory to each story condition. Results revealed a significant relationship between working memory skills and the linguistically and structural complex condition only for both micro- and macro-level aspects of narrative, with the exception of MLU. Thus, only when processing demands were the greatest did it appear that WM played a critical role, with poorer WM abilities associated with poorer performance overall. Failure to see a significant relationship between WM and MLU is likely a function of the stability of this variable across conditions. Working memory was significantly related to narrative comprehension only in the mixed linguistic/structural story condition. Failure to find a significant relationship between working memory and comprehension in the most complex condition may reflect more limited variability overall in this condition as a function of its complexity

Clinical Implications

For children with language impairments who may experience difficulty on discourse level tasks, addressing narrative abilities in speech and language intervention is both warranted and critical. In light of the developmental importance of early interactions that facilitate decontextualized language skills, as well as a sense of story structure, working with families to incorporate discussions of past events and involvement in repeated readings of familiar stories is critical. Research has shown the positive impact of direct training of parents to increase the quality of interactions in discourse-levels tasks. For children who have been identified as demonstrating narrative difficulty, more direct intervention is warranted. The majority of research on intervention to date has focused on explicitly teaching children the underlying structural framework or stories (e.g., story schema or grammar), with resulting improvements observed in children's abilities to construct, retell, or comprehend narratives (Gardill & Jitendra, 1999; Gurney, Gersten, Dimino, & Carnine, 1990; Hayward & Schneider, 2000; Klecan-Aker, 1993). In intervention studies to date, however, attention often focuses on how to make internal narrative structure explicit to children, with little consideration given to the intervention materials utilized in the teaching context, or to how the context in which narrative structure is taught may influence intervention outcomes. Results from this pilot project support the importance of carefully analyzing the linguistic and structural demands of a text used in narrative intervention, which would allow clinician's to select materials that match a child's current linguistic abilities and structural knowledge of stories. The differential influence on performance as a function of linguistic and/or structural complexity suggests these aspects should be considered in intervention planning. Thus, if the goal in a literature-based intervention is improved knowledge/use of more complex *linguistic* structures, for example, then it will be critical to choose stories that are at a level of structural complexity well within a child's skill level so that resources are not being designated to the construction of a complex mental representation, which is likely to draw a great deal of available resources. Similar considerations should be given when targeting comprehension/use of narrative structure in intervention.

CONCLUSIONS

Narrative abilities are developmental skills that are important for social and academic success. Understanding the variables that contribute to the acquisition of discourse-level skills is an important area of research, both theoretically and clinically. Our findings suggest that difficulties in narrative production and comprehension for children with language impairments are in part a performance issue; we are currently continuing this line of research to better understand the interaction of cognitive processes and knowledge and skill that support narrative performance. Future work that examines more closely the early parent–child exchanges in narrative events such as sharing of personal events and shared book reading, and the unique contributions of these exchanges to later narrative performance for children with language delays, is also critical.

ACKNOWLEDGMENTS

Completion of this chapter was supported by a grant from the National Institutes of Health (NIH) National Institute on Deafness and Communication Disorders (5 RO3 DC005920-02). Thank you to the following students for their help in data transcription and analyses: Katie Milesnick, Kristin Schultz, Jennifer Jablonski, Kerry Conrad, and Miranda Kruswall. The assistance of speech-language pathologists from Portland and Beaverton public schools, as well as the contributions of children and families that participated, are greatly appreciated.

APPENDIX A:
PROPOSITIONAL ANALYSES FOR FRANK THE CRAB

1. There was a crab.
2. Name was Frank.
3. Liked to find stuff.
4. Couldn't fit in his house.
5. Would do anything to find junk.
6. There was a bird.
7. The bird told Frank about a can.
8. Frank wanted the can.
9. Frank went hunting for it.
10. There was a boy.
11. The boy saw Frank.
12. Frank tried to hide in a hole.
13. The boy found Frank.
14. The dog found Frank.
15. The boy threw frank in the water.
16. Frank tried to swim.
17. He couldn't swim to the top.
18. Frank was scared.
19. Frank was sad.
20. He wanted to go home.
21. Frank was very tired.
22. He saw a big trunk.
23. Frank got inside the trunk.
24. There was a shark.
25 The shark wanted to eat frank.
26. Frank was afraid of the shark.
27. The shark poked his nose in the trunk.
28. The shark shook the trunk.
29. Frank didn't think he would get back home.
30. Frank peeked out.
31. He saw a worm on a hook.
32. He knew someone was fishing.
33. Frank decided to hold on to the fishing line.
34. Frank was pulled through the water.
35. Frank got back to the dock.
36. Frank let go of the line.
37. Frank walked home.
38. Frank would never go hunting again.

APPENDIX B: STORY GRAMMAR ANALYSES FOR FRANK THE CRAB

Setting:

___Character: crab named Frank (*if no mention of name, still give credit*)

___Frank loved to find stuff

___Frank's house was full of junk

Initiating event:

___Stork told Frank about a can

Internal response:

___Frank wanted the can

Attempt:

___Frank was hunting for the can

Consequence:

___Boy found him

Attempt:

___Frank tried to hide in the hole

Consequence:

___Boy (+/– dog) found him (*if uses pronoun, still give credit*)

Initiating event:

___Boy threw Frank in the water

Attempt:

___Frank tried to swim to the top

Consequence:

___But he couldn't

Internal response:

___Frank was scared

___He wanted to go back home

Setting:

___Frank was tired

Initiating event

___He saw a box/got inside

Initiating event:

___A shark came

Internal response:

____Frank was afraid of the shark

Attempt:

___Shark put his nose in the trunk and shook it

Internal response:

___Frank thought he would never get home

Initiating event:

___Frank saw a worm on a hook

Internal response:

____He thought someone must be fishing on the dock

Internal plan/attempt

___He decided to hold on to the fishing line

___He held onto the fishing line

Consequence:

___He was pulled through the water/back on dock

Result:

___let go/went home

Resolution:

___He knew he would never leave his home again.

REFERENCES

Adams, A., Bourke, L., & Willis, C. (1999). Working memory and spoken language comprehension in young children. *International Journal of Psychology, 34,* 364–373.

Aram, D. M., Morris, R., & Hall, N. E. (1993). Clinical and research congruence in identifying children with specific language impairment. *Journal of Speech and Hearing Research, 36,* 580–591.

Baddelely, A. D., & Hitch, G. (1974). Working memory. In G. Bower (Ed.), *The psychology of learning and motivation* (Vol. 8, pp. 47–90). New York: Academic Press.

Bishop, D. V. M. (1994). Grammatical errors in specific language impairment: Competence or performance limitations? *Applied Psycholinguistics, 15,* 507–550.

Bishop, D. V. M., & Adams, C. (1992). Comprehension problems in children with specific language impairment: Literal and inferential Meaning. *Journal of Speech and Hearing Research, 35,* 119–129.

Bishop, D. V. M., & Edmundson, A. (1987). Language-impaired 4-year-olds: Distinguishing transient from persistent narrative impairment. *Journal of Speech and Hearing Disorders, 52,* 156–173.

Boudreau, D. M., & Hedberg, N. L. (1999). A comparison of early literacy skills in children with specific language impairment and typically developing peers. *American Journal of Speech Language Pathology, 8,* 248–263.

Bruner, J. (1986). *Actual minds, possible worlds.* Cambridge, MA: Harvard University Press.

Caspari, I., & Parkinson, S. R. (2000). Effects of memory impairment on discourse. *Journal of Neurolinguistics, 13,* 15–36.

Chapman, R. S., Streim, N. W., Crais, E. R., Salmon, D., Strand, E. A., & Negri, N. A. (1992). Child Talk: Assumptions of a developmental process model for early language learning. In R. S. Chapman (Ed.), *Processes in language acquisition and disorders* (pp. 3–19). Chicago: Mosby Year Book.

Clahsen, H. (1989). The grammatical characterization of developmental dysphasia. *Linguistics, 27,* 897–920.

Clahsen, H. (1999). Linguistic perspectives on specific language impairment. In W. C. Ritchie & T. K. Bhatia (Eds.), *Handbook of child language acquisition* (pp. 675–704). San Diego, CA: Academic Press.

Clifford, J. M. (1995). *Narratives from children with language impairment: An exploration of language and cognition.* Unpublished master's thesis, San Diego State University, San Diego, CA.

Crais, E. R., & Chapman, R. S. (1987). Story recall and inferencing skills in language/learning disabled and nondisabled children. *Journal of Speech and Hearing Disorders, 52,* 50–55.

Crosson, B. (2000). Systems that support language processes: Verbal working memory. In S. E. Nadeau, L. J. G. Rothi, & B. Crosson (Eds.), *Aphasia and language: Theory to practice* (pp. 399–418). New York: Guilford.

Duchan, J. F. (2004). The foundational role of schemas in children's language and literacy learning. In C. A. Stone, E. R. Silliman, B. J. Ehren, & K. Apel (Eds.), *Handbook of language and literacy* (pp. 380–397). New York: Guilford.

Eisenberg, A. R. (1985). Learning to describe past experiences in conversation. *Discourse Processes, 8,* 177–204.

Ellis Weismer, S. (1985). Constructive comprehension abilities exhibited by language-disordered children. *Journal of Speech and Hearing Research, 28,* 175–184

Ellis Weismer, S., Evans, J., & Hesketh, L. J. (1999). An examination of verbal working memory capacity in children with specific language impairment. *Journal of Speech and Hearing Research, 42,* 1249–1260.

Ellis Weismer, S., & Hesketh, L. J. (1993). The influence of prosodic and gestural cues on novel word acquisition by children with specific language impairment. *Journal of Speech and Hearing Research, 36,* 1013–1025.

Ellis Weismer, S., & Hesketh, L. J. (1996). Lexical learning by children with specific language impairment: Effects of linguistic input presented at varying speaking rates. *Journal of Speech and Hearing Research, 39,* 177–190.

Evans, J. L. (1996). SLI subgroups: Interaction between discourse constraints and morphosyntactic deficits. *Journal of Speech and Hearing Research, 39,* 655–660.

Evans, M. A., & Schmidt, F. (1991). Repeated maternal book reading with two children: Language-normal and language impaired. *First Language, 11,* 269–287.

Gardill, M. C., & Jitendra, A. K. (1999). Advanced story map instruction: Effects on the reading comprehension of students with learning disabilities. *Journal of Special Education, 33,* 2–18.

Gathercole, S. E., & Baddeley, A. D. (1990a). The role of phonological memory in vocabulary acquisition: A study of young children learning new names. *British Journal of Psychology, 81,* 439–454.

Gathercole, S. E., & Baddelely, A. D. (1990b). Phonological memory deficits in language disordered children: Is there a causal connection? *Journal of Memory and Language, 29,* 336–360.

Gathercole, S. E., & Baddelely, A. D. (1993). *Working memory and language.* Hillsdale, NJ: Lawrence Erlbaum Associates.

Gathercole, S. E., Willis, C., Emslie, H., & Baddeley, A. D. (1992). Phonological memory and vocabulary development during the early school years: A longitudinal study. *Developmental Psychology, 28,* 887–898.

Gaulin, C. A., & Campbell, T. F. (1994). Procedure for assessing verbal working memory in normal school-aged children: Some preliminary data. *Perceptual and Motor Skills, 79,* 55–64.

Goldman, S. R., & Rakestraw, J. A. (2000). Structural aspects of constructing meaning from text. In M. L. Kamil, P. B. Mosenthal, P. D. Pearson, & R. Barr (Eds.), *Handbook of reading research* (Vol. 3, pp. 311–336). Mahwah, NJ: Lawrence Erlbaum Associates.

Gopnick M., & Crago, M. (1991). Familial aggregation of a developmental language disorder. *Cognition, 39,* 1–50.

Graesser, A. C. (1997). Discourse comprehension. *Annual Review of Psychology, 48,* 163–189.

Graessser, A. C., Singer, M., & Trabasso, T. (1994). Constructing inferences during narrative text comprehension. *Psychological Review, 101,* 371–395.

Graybeal, C. M. (1981). Memory for stories in language-impaired children. *Applied Psycholinguistics, 2,* 269–283.

Gurney, G., Gersten, R., Dimino, J., & Carnine, D. (1990). Story grammar: Effective literature instruction for high school students with learning disabilities. *Journal of Learning Disabilities, 23*(6), 335–348.

Haden, C. A., Haine, R. A., & Fivush, R. (1997). Developing narrative structure in parent-child reminiscing across preschool years. *Developmental Psychology, 33,* 295–307.

Hayward, D., & Schneider, P. (2000). Effectiveness of teaching story grammar knowledge to pre-school children with language impairment: An exploratory study. *Child Language Teaching and Therapy, 16,* 255–284.

Heath, S. B. (1982). What no bedtime story means: Narrative skills at home and school. *Language in Society, 11,* 49–76.

Heath, S. B. (1986). Taking a cross-cultural look at narratives. *Topics in Language Disorders, 7*(1), 84–94.

Hemphill, L., Uccelli, P., Winner, K., & Chang, C. (2002). Narrative discourse in young children with histories of early corrective heart surgery. *Journal of Speech, Language, and Hearing Research, 45,* 318–331.

Hudson, J. A., & Shapiro, L. R. (1991). From knowing to telling: The development of scripts, stories, and personal narratives. In A. McCabe & C. Peterson (Eds.), *Developing narrative structure* (pp. 89–136). Hillsdale, NJ: Lawrence Erlbaum Associates.

Hughes, D., McGillivray, L., & Schmidek, M. (1997). *Guide to narrative language.* Eau Claire, WI: Thinking Publications.

Johnson-Laird, P. N. (1983). *Mental models: Towards a cognitive science of language, inference, and consciousness.* Cambridge, MA: Harvard University Press.

Just, M., & Carpenter, P. (1992). A capacity theory of comprehension: Individual differences in working memory. *Psychological Review, 99,* 122–149.

Klecan-Aker, J. (1993). An intervention programme for improving story-telling ability: a case study. *Child Language Teaching and Therapy, 9,* 105–115.

Lahey, M., & Bloom, L. (1994). Variability and language learning disabilities. In G. P. Wallach & K. G. Butler (Eds.), *Language learning disabilities in school-age children and adolescents* (pp. 354–372). New York: Macmillan.

Leonard, L. B. (1998). *Children with specific language impairment.* Cambridge, MA: MIT Press.

Liles, B. Z. (1985). Narrative ability in normal and language disordered children. *Journal of Speech and Hearing Research, 28,* 123–133.

Liles, B. Z. (1987). Episode organization and cohesive conjunctives in narratives of children with and without language disorders. *Journal of Speech and hearing Research, 30,* 185–196.

Liles, B. Z. (1993). Narrative discourse in children with language disorders and children with normal language: A critical review of the literature. *Journal of Speech and Hearing Research, 36,* 868–882.

Liles, B. Z., Duffy, R. J., Merritt, D. D., Purcell, S. L. (1995). Measurement of narrative discourse ability in children with language disorders. *Journal of Speech and Hearing Research, 38,* 415–425.

Liles, B. Z., & Purcell, S. (1987). Departures in the spoken narratives of normal and language-disordered children. *Applied Psycholinguistics, 8,* 185–202.

Mandler, J. M. (1978). A code in the node: The use of story schema in retrieval. *Discourse Processes, 1,* 14–35.

Mar, R. A. (2004). The neuropsychological of narrative: Story comprehension, story production and their interrelation. *Neuropsychological, 42,* 1414–1434.

Mayer, M. (1969). *Frog, Where Are You?* New York: Dial Press.

Mayer, M. (1973). *One Frog Too Many.* New York: Dial Press.

McCabe, A., & Bliss, L. S. (2003). *Patterns of narrative discourse.* New York: Allyn & Bacon.

McCabe, A., & Peterson, C. (1991). Getting the story: Longitudinal study of parental styles in eliciting narratives and developing narrative skill. In A. McCabe, & C. Peterson (Eds.), *Developing narrative structure* (pp. 217–253). Hillsdale, NJ: Lawrence Erlbaum Associates.

Merritt, D. D., & Liles, B. Z. (1987). Story grammar ability in children with and without language disorder: Story generation, story retelling, and story comprehension. *Journal of Speech and Hearing Research, 3,* 539–552.

Miller, P. J., & Sperry, L. L. (1988). Early talk about the past: The origins of conversational stories of personal experience. *Journal of Child Language, 15,* 293–315.

Miolo, G., & Chapman, R. S. (1999, June). *Predicting sentence comprehension in children: A comparison of three measures of working memory capacity.* Poster presented at the 20th annual symposium on Child Language Disorders, Madison, WI.

Montgomery, J. W. (1995). Sentence comprehension children with specific language impairment: The role of phonological working memory. *Journal of Speech and Hearing Research, 38,* 187–199.

Montgomery, J. W. (2000). Verbal working memory and sentence comprehension in children with specific language impairment. *Journal of Speech, Language, and Hearing Research, 43*(2), 293–308.

Montgomery, J. W. (2001). Relation of working memory to off-line and real-time sentence processing in children with specific language impairment. *Applied Psycholinguistics, 21,* 117–148.

Morrow, L. M., & Brittain, R. (2003). The nature of storybook reading in the elementary school: Current practice. In A. van Kleek & S. A. Stahl (Eds.), *On reading books to children* (pp. 140–158). Mahwah, NJ: Lawrence Erlbaum Associates.

Moser, R. M., & Johnston, J. R. (2004, June). *Beyond storage: Working memory and specific language impairment.* Poster presented at the Society for Research in Child Language Disorders, Madison, WI.

Nelson, K. (1986). *Event knowledge: Structure and function in development.* Hillsdale, NJ: Lawrence Erlbaum Associates.

Newcomer, P., & Hammill, D. (1997a). *Test of Language Development–3 Primary.* Austin, TX: Pro-Ed.

Newcomer, P., & Hammill, D. (1997b). *Test of Language Development–3 Intermediate.* Austin, TX: Pro-Ed.

O'Brien, E. J., & Albrecht, J. E. (1992). Comprehension strategies in the development of a mental model. *Journal of Experimental Psychology, 18,* 777–784.

Paul, R. (1996). Clinical implications of the natural history of slow expressive language development. *American Journal of Speech Language Pathology, 5*(2), 5–21.

Paul, R., & Smith, R. L. (1993). Narrative skills in 4-year-old with normal, impairment and late-developing language. *Journal of Speech and Hearing Research, 36,* 592–598.

Pearce, W. M., McCormack, P. F., & James, D. G. H. (2003). Exploring the boundaries of SLI: Findings from morphosyntactic and story grammar analyses. *Clinical Linguistics & Phonetics, 17,* 325–334.

Peet, B. (1964). *Ella the elephant.* Boston: Houghton Mifflin.

Peet, B. (1965a). *Chester the worldly pig.* Boston: Houghton Mifflin.

Peet, B. (1965b). *Kermit the hermit.* Boston: Houghton Mifflin.

Peet, B. (1975). *Cyrus the unsinkable sea serpent.* Boston: Houghton Mifflin.

Peterson, C. (1990). The who, when, and where of early narratives. *Journal of Child Language, 17,* 433–455.

Peterson, C., Jesso, B., & McCabe, A. (1999). Encouraging narratives in preschoolers: An intervention study. *Journal of Child Language, 26,* 49–67.

Peterson, C., & McCabe, A. (1992). Parental styles of narrative elicitation: Effect on children's narrative structure and content. *First Language, 12,* 299–321.

Preece, A. (1987). The range of narrative forms conversationally produced by young children. *Journal of Child Language, 14*, 353–373.

Pritchard, R. (1990). The effects of cultural schemata on reading processing strategies. *Reading Research Quarterly, 25*(4), 273–295.

Purcell, S., & Liles, B. Z. (1992). Cohesion repairs in narratives of normal language and language disordered school-aged children. *Journal of Speech and Hearing Research, 35*, 354–362.

Reilly, J., Losh, M., Bellugi, U., & Wulfeck, B. (2004). "Frog, where are you?" Narratives in children with specific language impairment, early focal brain injury, and Williams syndrome. *Brain and Language, 88*, 229–247.

Rice, M., Sell, M., & Hadley, P. (1991). Social interactions of speech- and language-impaired children. *Journal of Speech and Hearing Research, 34*, 1299–1307.

Ripich, D. N., & Griffith, P. L. (1988). Narrative abilities of children with learning disabilities and nondisabled children: Story structure, cohesion and propositions. *Journal of Learning Disabilities, 21*, 165–173.

Roth, F. P., Speece, D. L., Cooper, D. H., & De La Paz, S. (1996). Unresolved mysteries: How do metalinguistic and narrative skills connect with early reading. *Journal of Special Education, 30*, 257–27.

Rumelhart, D. E. (1975). Notes on schema for stories. In D. G. Bobrow & A. Collins (Eds.), *Representation and understanding* (pp. 2–34). New York: Academic Press.

Snow, C. E., & Dickinson, D. K. (1990). Social sources of narrative skills at home and at school. *First Language, 10*, 87–103.

Stein, N., & Glenn, C. (1979). An analysis of story comprehension in elementary school children. In R. O. Freedle (Ed.), *New directions in discourse processing* (pp. 53–120). Norwood, NJ: Ablex.

Stine, E. A., & Wingfield, A. (1990). How much do working memory deficits contribute to age differences in discourse memory? *European Journal of Cognitive Psychology, 2*, 289–304.

Strong, C. J., & Shaver, J. P. (1991). Stability of cohesion in the spoken narratives of language impaired and normally developing school-aged children. *Journal of Speech and Hearing Research, 34*, 95–111.

Sulzby, E., & Kadaravek, J. (1996). Parent–child language during storybook reading and toy play contexts: Case studies of normally developing and specific language impaired (SLI) children. *National Reading Conference Yearbook, 45*, 257–269.

Tabors, P. O., Snow, C. E., & Dickinson, D. K. (2001). Homes and schools together: Supporting language and literacy development. In K. K. Dickinson & P. O. Tabors (Eds.), *Beginning literacy with language: Young children learning at home and at* school (pp. 313–334). Baltimore: Paul H. Brookes.

Tager-Flusberg, H., & Cooper, J. (1999). Present and future possibilities for defining a phenotype for specific language impairment. *Journal of Speech, Language, and Hearing Research, 42*(5), 1275–1278.

Teale, W. H. (2003). Reading aloud to young children as a classroom instructional activity: insights from research to practice. In A. van Kleek & S. A. Stahl (Eds.), *On reading books to children* (pp. 114–139). Mahwah, NJ: Lawrence Erlbaum Associates.

Tomblin, J. B., Records, N. L., Buckwalter, P., Zhang, X., Smith, E., & O'Brien, M. (1997). Prevalence of specific language impairment in kindergarten children. *Journal of Speech Language and hearing Research, 40,* 1245–1260.

Towe, J. N., Hitch, G. J., & Hutton, U. (1998). A reevaluation of working memory capacity in children. *Journal of Memory and Language, 39,* 195–217.

Van Kleek, A., & Vander Woude, J. (2003). Book sharing with preschoolers with language delay. In A. van Kleek, S. A. Stahl, & E. B. Bauer (Eds.), *On reading books to children* (pp. 58–92). Mahwah, NJ: Lawrence Erlbaum Associates.

Watkins, R. V. (1997). The linguistic profile of SLI. In L. B. Adamson & M. A. Romski (Eds.), *Communication and language acquisition* (pp. 161–185). Baltimore: Paul H. Brookes.

Weschler, D. (1991). *Weschler Intelligence Scale for Children–III.* San Antonio, TX: Psychological Corporation.

Westby, C. E. (1991). Learning to talk—Differences. In C. Simon (Ed.), *Communication skills and classroom success: Therapy methodologies for language learning disabled students* (pp. 181–218). San Diego, CA: College-Hill Press.

14

Developmental Considerations in Addressing the AAC Needs of Children With Severe Disabilities

Stephen N. Calculator
University of New Hampshire

The field of augmentative and alternative communication (AAC) continues to evolve in terms of both technological developments and applications of this technology in addressing the functional communication needs of children for whom speech is insufficient to meet these needs, either temporarily or permanently. As the field has evolved, so too have beliefs about the role of developmental considerations in establishing AAC systems for particular individuals. In this chapter, this question focuses on one population in particular: children with the most severe disabilities, those functioning at prelinguistic or emerging linguistic levels of communication. Children with the most severe disabilities exhibit intellectual function in the severe to profoundly impaired range, accompanied by significant difficulties in adaptive behavior. Many of these children have accompanying sensory, motor, physical, and perceptual disabilities. A large proportion of these children are either not speaking at all or unable to convey more than a few basic wants and needs through speech. They are thus often considered candidates for AAC systems.

AAC AND DEVELOPMENTAL CONSIDERATIONS

Early in the development of thinking about AAC practice, some investigators (e.g., Chapman & Miller, 1980; Owens & House, 1984; Shane & Bashir, 1980) proposed that criteria for determining who was eligible for AAC support be based on notions drawn from the typical sequence of communicative development. For example, because typically developing children generally began talking after attaining cognitive skills such as symbolic play, object permanence, and means–ends ability, typically associated with Piaget's sensorimotor stage V, this level of symbolic behavior was thought to be a necessary prerequisite for considering children for AAC systems. Later investigators (e.g., Kangas & Lloyd, 1988; Reichle & Karlan, 1985) questioned the empirical bases for using these criteria. Specifically, they questioned the use of these criteria to exclude children who failed to demonstrate a particular level of cognitive functioning or to demonstrate a significant gap between their cognitive and language skills. Rowland and Schweigert (2003), in attempting to answer this question, reviewed research examining the relationship between language development and children's performance on various Piagetian tasks in the areas of object permanence, means–ends, symbolic play, and imitation. They concluded that although correlational relationships are seen in children without disabilities, causal relationships have not been demonstrated. Moreover, discrepancy formulas (e.g., language in relation to cognition) for determining eligibility for communication services, program dismissal, prognosis, and determining severity of a communication disorder have also come into question.

Current thinking sees the relationship between the cognitive and linguistic domains as complex. For example, some children have been found to demonstrate language abilities that exceed their mental age (Miller, Chapman, & Bedrosian, 1977). In addition, children who show no gap between language and cognitive skills have been shown to derive as much benefit from language instruction as those children with significantly higher cognitive than language scores (Cole, Dale, & Mills, 1990).

Current practice in AAC, as a consequence, operates on a basis of zero exclusion. All nonspeaking individuals, irrespective of their demonstrated levels of impairment, disability, and handicap, are seen as potential beneficiaries of AAC intervention. Despite the fact that developmental considerations are not incorporated into the decision to provide AAC services, the content of these services needs to be matched to the language, cognitive, motor, sensory, perceptual, and related capabilities of the individual, based on developmental level. Thus, a broad spectrum of activities that include not only symbolic but, when the situation calls for it, presymbolic forms of communication needs to be individually matched to potential AAC users. Yet few guidelines are available to allow the clinician to make these matches efficiently. For example, we cannot point to a score on a psychological test or subtest or cite a particular cutoff score and state with confidence that a child should be able to understand the concept of, for example, Minspeak, a semantic compaction system used to accelerate rates of message transmission in devices manufactured by the Prentke Romich Company, a leading manufacturer in the field. Nor can we identify cognitive predictors associated with the successful use of different symbol systems that might be used to represent vocabulary on other AAC devices.

There are now numerous devices on the market, and manufacturers are introducing new systems regularly. Still, there is an absence of data that allow a prediction to be made about which device will work best for each client at each developmental level. Certainly we must look beyond the devices per se to cognitive and motor demands each makes on the user and design instruction that both precedes and follows their introduction. AAC interventions often begin with a "try and see" or dynamic assessment approach (Weitz, Dexter, & Moore, 1997), which includes trial therapy approaches derived from baseline assessment information and frequent reevaluations of progress to verify the appropriateness of an AAC program. In applying this model, the clinician might also periodically probe for collateral changes in cognitive status as communication skills improve.

Calculator (2000) noted that information derived not only from direct observation but from careful interviewing of parents and teachers regarding children's rate of learning, trajectory of learning, retention of information, and feedback about how long it typically takes them to grasp new skills can help in making these initial decisions. Initial response to the introduction of an AAC system, through dynamic assessment methods, can also provide useful information. The readiness and efficiency with which a child grasps and retains operational characteristics of an aid are unequivocal predictors of the suitability of that particular aid, as well as related systems. Circumstances that help and hinder students' learning are also cited as important considerations. These may include variations in sensory and perceptual input, response mode, environmental modifications, arrangement of symbols, and symbol type among many factors.

Rowland and Schweigart (2003) proposed an alternative set of cognitive factors to consider, not in determining candidacy, but in matching AAC systems to users. These include:

- *Awareness* refers to understanding the distinction between oneself and the rest of the world. It includes learning about contingencies, including social contingencies, of one's actions. Awareness also incorporates "theory of the mind," the ability to understand and consider the thoughts, goals, desires, and intentions of someone else who may perceive a situation differently than you do.

- *Communicative intent* implies there is a purposeful communicative act. The idea here is the child is not dependent on the listener's interpreting and ascribing meaning and intent to the utterance but instead does so him or herself. The issue of intentionality in AAC has been discussed elsewhere (Iacono, Carter, & Hook, 1998). Maternal responsiveness has been cited as an important factor in fostering intentional communication, which, in turn, has been associated with subsequent language acquisition (Yoder & Warren, 1999).
- *World knowledge* refers to general experience and provides a foundation for understanding relationships between objects, oneself and others. Rowland and Schweigert link world knowledge to children's motivation to communicate in different situations, based on their previous experiences.
- *Memory* relates to the ability to store information and build on past experiences. It includes sensory, short term, or, working and long term memory.
- *Symbolic representation* refers to the ability to represent meaning through some type of code or representation. With increasing communication skills, the distance between the symbol and the referent may increase and the symbol may become increasingly abstract.
- *Metacognitive skills* allow children to talk about their own cognitive processes, including how they learn. These are especially important for individuals who use more sophisticated AAC systems where symbol organization and rate acceleration techniques may come into play.

Still, efficiency could be improved if there were some guidelines available for narrowing choices among systems and devices based on child characteristics and developmental level. In the remainder of this chapter, we discuss how information from a variety of sources can be used to inform this kind of decision making.

Let us start with the basic question of how cognition and language assessment baseline data might best be applied to AAC decision making in children with the most severe disabilities. We then proceed to other developmental considerations. If a child's communication skills were poorer than expected, given his or her measured level of cognitive ability, we would expect this child to benefit immediately from AAC programming. We would also expect this child to be able to benefit from symbolically more complex forms of AAC than the child with lesser cognitive skills. AAC would be conceptualized as a means toward more effective communication, but not necessarily an endpoint. Ultimately, we would strive not only to bring the child's communication skills on a par with current cognitive level, but to use language concepts learned through AAC to advance cognitive level as well, as they do in typical development.

For instance, Calculator (1997a) discussed ways of targeting means–end behavior in a communicative context. Conversational partners might present additional opportunities and reasons for children to communicate, and, if called on, might be seen by children as vehicles for having their wants and needs met. One example would be an activity in which the child needed to use an adult to obtain an object. The adult could place attractive objects in sight but out of reach and allow the child to receive them only when a targeted communicative signal (at first just a glance toward the object, later a gesture or vocalization combined with the glance, later still a point or indication of a symbolic representation of the desired end). Similarly, object permanence could be addressed within a communicative context by turning the activity into a "peek-a-boo" game in which the child was required to communicate in a targeted way to the adult that he or she wants to see the hidden object.

APPLYING DEVELOPMENTAL MODELS

The applicability of a normal language developmental model for clinical intervention with children using AAC systems was the subject of a paper by Gerber and Kraat (1992). The investigators listed several difficulties in applying a normal model of development to a population of children who rely on AAC systems:

- How applicable are data on a relatively small, homogeneous sample of children to the diverse children we see?
- Are these children truly comparable to normal developing children, given that, unlike children with typical development, they often demonstrate uneven patterns of development among areas such as cognition, language and social interaction, and within the various aspects of language development (semantics, syntax phonology, pragmatics)?
- What about the role of experience and chronological age? Would we expect a nonspeaking 6-year-old with a developmental level of 18 months to talk about the same things as a normal developing child at the same developmental level?
- How applicable is a model based on expressive production measures (e.g., MLU) for children with no speech?

Gerber and Kraat (1992) argue that interventions for these children might target functional communication needs of these children, even if that means violating typical sequences of acquisition. Still forms, content, and uses of language addressed in intervention would be based largely on these children's developmental capacities.

Despite these difficulties, there are several constructs from normal language development that are useful in thinking about helping children through the progression from absent to competent communication. These include classifications of preverbal communication, theories of the development of word meaning, and the transition to multisymbol utterances. For example, in the area of preverbal communication, children with severe disabilities who rely on AAC have been reported to progress from *perlocutionary* communication (i.e., in response to internal states without clear intentionality) to *illocutionary* communication (intentional, nonverbal behaviors executed through gaze, gestures and preverbal vocalizations) and then to locutionary or symbolic communication (Bates, 1976; Cress, 2002; Siegel & Cress, 2002). We discuss how each of these constructs from typical language acquisition can be applied to work with severely impaired AAC users.

Speech Act Development

Perlocutionary Stage. Perlocutionary acts are assumed to be lacking communicative intent and are not felt to be goal directed. As such, they are dependent on others ascribing meaning to them in order for them to function as communicative acts. Thus the first stage of development is characterized by partner-perceived communication. Cress (2002) asserted, "AAC, and every other form of communication, starts at birth with social interaction and the earliest behaviors of children. There are no prerequisites to AAC, and no children or adults who are not ready for AAC" (p. 220). Thus, we may see AAC programs for some children with the most severe disabilities (i.e., those exhibiting language skills commensurate with the perlocutionary stage) that include as a first step teaching partners to interpret and respond to children's preintentional behaviors (Calculator, 1984). During this stage, communication is dependent on the partner's ability and willingness to ascribe meaning to the child's behaviors, which are not intended to be interactive with the partner. Perlocutionary behaviors include spontaneous behaviors such as responses to internal states (e.g., hunger and pain) and environmental events (a highly preferred item or greatly disliked item is presented and the child reacts). They also include intentional behaviors such as actions on objects (e.g., operating a toy, pushing away unwanted food) or environmental events that are not intended for a particular partner.

Effective communicators at the perlocutionary stage are able to use different cues, including intonational contours, facial expressions, gestures, and proxemics, to contribute meaning to their behaviors. When these "data" are lacking, the task for partners attempting to engage them in interaction becomes more complex. To address this, either the interpretive skills of the partner must be improved or the nonverbal repertoire of the child augmented.

Although the child's behaviors are unintentional, the reaction of the partner provides contingency and a foundation for the child's learning the effect of these behaviors on others. This provides a bridge to an understanding of causality and later uses of illocutionary and subsequent symbolic communication.

The perlocutionary stage is also important with respect to the development of gaze patterns. In particular, deictic gaze, where the caregiver follows the infant's gaze and perhaps then engages the infant with, or labels, the corresponding object, reinforces a communicative function. Mutual gaze in which the child and partner look at each other is also viewed as an important contributor to social interactions as well as the development of attachment behaviors in this stage.

Efforts might also be directed at altering partners' perceptions of children as communication partners. Children with severe disabilities may provide little feedback in response to partners' early attempts to engage them in social interactions. Over time, partners may perceive children as nonresponsive and/or noncommunicative and perhaps sense that their efforts to communicate with their children are futile.

At the same time, intervention might target children's behaviors, fostering the replacement of unintentional behaviors with voluntary communicative behaviors. Such behaviors might, in turn, engage partners in social interaction and provide sources of verbal input to further stimulate continued growth in language skills.

AAC interventions for children in the perlocutionary stage may include increasing responsiveness to partners as well as objects and events in the environment. Other efforts might foster intentionality and means–end behavior by promoting active engagement with the environment. Investigators have demonstrated positive changes in children's uses of intentional communication associated with teaching their parents to recognize and respond to their intentional behaviors (Yoder & Warren, 1998).

Children in the later phases of the perlocutionary stage emit behaviors intended to initiate and sustain interactions with their partners. They communicate with the expectation their partner will respond.

Also late in this stage, children demonstrate their understanding of the functional uses of objects, acting on objects in predictable and often appropriate ways. This can have clear implications for AAC interventions, for example, with respect to instruction with natural and enhanced natural gestures (Calculator, 2002). In the latter case, the child might be taught to produce a gesture associated with an object when the object is proximal but not in direct contact, in order to make a request. A child who has a repertoire of diversified, object-specific actions can be more readily taught to use these same gestures communicatively than the child whose actions on objects are undifferentiated or stereotypical.

Beukelman and Mirenda (1998) refer to children with the most severe disabilities as beginning communicators who rely primarily on non-symbolic modes of communication and do not typically demonstrate intentional communicative behaviors. These children are learning to use aided or unaided symbols to represent basic messages for communicative functions such as requesting, rejecting, sharing information, and engaging in conversations. Some of them may be using electronic devices with limited speech output capabilities for participation and communication.

These children need direct instruction to grasp the concept that they can use symbols to influence people and events in their surrounding environments. One way to accomplish this is to embed symbol instruction within systematic daily routines in which symbols and corresponding events co-occur regularly with routine antecedents. Scripting provides one potentially effective means of accomplishing this. The partner inventories messages that are typically produced during a given activity, the partner's own as well as the child's. Beukelman and Mirenda (1998) provide several illustrations of this technique and its various components, which include a touch cue (e.g., unzip coat), verbal cue (e.g., "It's time to take off your coat"), pause (wait 10 s and look for a response), verbal feedback ("I see you moved your arm here. Let's take off your coat"), and action (remove coat).

Illocutionary Stage. Illocutionary acts are intentional communicative acts that are conveyed primarily through gestures and vocalizations. Here, the child actively attempts to engage others in various ways, whether it is soliciting their attention (protodeclaratives) or requesting objects and actions (protoimperatives). In this stage the child's behaviors are directed purposefully at a conversational partner. We now see reciprocal social exchanges between the child and partner.

Partners can foster the acquisition of language and communication skills in the illocutionary stage by being taught and/or encouraged to establish joint reference with children and to engage children in joint action (McLaughlin, 1998). In joint reference, the adult and child are attending to the same object or event. In joint action, the adult engages the child in routines, scripted activities, and other action sequences with predictable antecedents and consequences that fully engage the child's attention and participation.

A communication signal inventory, or communication dictionary, is often useful for children at this stage. All of the child's communicative behaviors are listed along with their corresponding meanings and the consequence the child should receive from the partner in response to the particular behavior.

Implications for Teaching Illocutionary Functions. Three broad functions of communication have been identified in children as they make the transition from preintentional to intentional communication: (a) regulating others' behaviors by requesting or protesting objects or actions; (b) engaging others in social interaction by requesting a social routine or comfort, for example; greeting or calling, or, showing off; and (c) establishing joint attention by directing their partner's attention to an object, event, or topic and commenting or requesting information (Snell, 2002; Wetherby & Prizant, 1989).

Cress and Marvin (2003) pointed out that children using AAC are often at risk for having restricted communicative functions. Although they may express wants and needs, these children may be unable to convey other functions such as joint attention (commenting) or continuing social routines. Other communicative functions that appear early in development often include greetings, protests, requests for attention or objects, and termination of an activity (Reichle, Halle, & Johnson, 1993). It is important to note these functions are often first conveyed spontaneously via natural gestures and other preexisting methods of communication and not through AAC.

Locutionary Stage. In the locutionary stage we see the onset of symbolic communication. Initially, children may use a combination of gestures and vocalizations, first used in the illocutionary stage, to convey a variety of primitive speech acts (Dore, 1974). In this stage we see a transition to symbols and conventional language behaviors for expressing communicative intentions.

It is certainly appropriate to stress conventional methods of communication for children exhibiting skills at this stage of development. Idiosyncratic gestures, for example, might be replaced by a conventional system of gestures or signs that are more easily recognized. Gestures or any other form of communication, including of course graphic representations, should also target a variety of communicative functions. Owens (2004) noted the importance of ensuring that symbol training in this stage is functional and fulfills a broad range of communicative intentions. He pointed out a common pattern of training programs that deteriorate to the child's responding to cues such as "What's this?" with the mistaken hope that the symbol will be used spontaneously at a future time.

Rowland and Schweigert (2000) pointed out that presymbolic gestures and vocalizations form a foundation for subsequent symbolic communication. However, children who communicate with vocalizations and gestures may not necessarily go on to learn symbolic forms of communication such as manual signs or spoken words. Rowland and Schweigert attribute this to children's difficulties understanding the one-to-one correspondence between a spoken sound or gesture and its referent, deficits in representational skills, and gross and fine motor limitations. In their investigation, children were able to bridge from the use of gestures to progressively more abstract forms of tangible symbols. Interestingly, the investigators reported collateral improvements in the speech of several of their children following the introduction of tangible symbols. Although no causal relationship can be stated, the investigators propose that addressing one symbol system appeared to generalize effects to another.

There is evidence of children in this stage who are unable to generalize symbol usage from one communicative function (labeling) to another (requesting) (Glennen & Calculator, 1985). To combat this, it is recommended that language intervention programs provide ample opportunities for children to gain experience using symbols functionally across settings and partners, conveying a full range of communicative intents. It is not enough to build a lexicon based on 50 pictures, where the only evidence is the child's ability to label each stimulus in a confrontational naming task. Owens (2004) recommended initially selecting a single communicative function for each new lexical item. However, additional functions should be taught if the child is to be expected to employ his or her communication display most efficiently.

Also significant in the locutionary stage is the need to capitalize on children's nonverbal behaviors. Pointing to graphic symbols should be augmented by vocalizations, facial expressions, gestures, pointing, and other sources of supplementary information for message clarity. Too often we see augmented communicators relying on aided systems of communication exclusively, providing no supplementary cues to their listeners via alternate channels. For example, different intonation contours and eye gaze could clarify when a question was being asked and to what the question referred.

As children progress deeper into the locutionary stage, Halliday's (1975) taxonomy of communicative functions may be useful in classifying as well as targeting intents of one- and two-word (symbol) messages. Conversational skills might also be worked on in this stage, particularly aspects such as topic initiation and turn taking.

Children using AAC frequently adopt a relatively passive style of interaction in which they function primarily in the respondent role. They answer questions posed of them, provide information requested, but rarely initiate new topics. Also, interactions involving augmented communicators are often of brief duration. Intervention goals might thus target both the content and breadth of children's interactions.

Symbol Iconicity. The visual relationship between a symbol and its referent is called *iconicity*. A symbol is deemed to be iconic when it "readily depicts a referent or some easily identifiable aspect of a referent" (Blischak, Lloyd, & Fuller, 1997, p. 40). The degree of iconicity needed to facilitate communication through a first AAC device is an important consideration during the transition from illocutionary to locutionary communication. Schlosser and Sigafoos (2002) found evidence that more iconic symbols were learned more readily than other symbols in this stage. Iconicity is certainly an important variable to consider when selecting an initial AAC symbol set to introduce initial vocabulary.

Fast Mapping. In order to account for the rapid growth of vocabulary demonstrated by preschool-aged children, investigators have proposed that children begin with incomplete maps or hypotheses of word meanings after only a few exposures, and then, with repeated exposure, these meanings become increasingly adult-like (Carey & Barlett, 1978; Rice, 1989). Cress and Marvin (2003) suggested that children who use AAC may understand and produce words differently than speaking children in that their words are more strongly tied to context and are organized differently.

Although speaking children may produce words not in their repertoire that they have learned through incidental exposure, the child using AAC may be constrained by the symbols made available to him or her. Implications of this are clear. Parents, teachers, clinicians, and others are encouraged to model and repeatedly expose children to novel symbols in a variety of contexts and not wait until a child demonstrates comprehension of a particular concept before providing the means and opportunity to use that concept in daily interactions.

We might look at this in terms of input and output modalities. Partners might accompany their speech with aided (e.g., graphic symbols) input, providing a language model for their child. They might also incorporate the child's AAC system in expanding messages produced by the child, as well as other discourse conventions (e.g., extensions, scaffolding, and recasts) that might foster their child's more effective use of the aid. Content of the child's device might thus be organized not only with the child's communication skills and needs in mind but also as a source of communication/language instruction via incidental teaching in daily interactions with teachers and others.

Types of Words. In examining the types of words or symbols used by children who rely on AAC, we may be able to take our cues from literature on typically developing children as well as children with developmental disabilities. In their review of multiple investigations, Wilkinson and McIlvane (2002) reported the basic category level is the most salient and earliest developing basis for categorization in children. Thus "dog" is preferable to the superordinate category label "pet" as well as the subordinate-level "Rover." The following discussion, related to semantic features, functional core, and prototype theory, presents implications with respect to how words and concepts might be best taught.

Applying Semantic Theories. Semantic theories help to explain how children develop mental concepts that are represented by words, and the ways in which the words and concepts relate. Three theorists continue to influence current thinking about semantic development in typical children. All three theories have significant implications for how we might design intervention programs for children relying on AAC systems in the locutionary stage of development.

Semantic Features. Clark's (1973) semantic feature hypothesis proposed that children organize vocabulary according to perceptual features such as shape, size, texture, and color. Over time, the features they use to define a particular word align more closely with that of the adult meaning as certain features are added and others drop out. This theory has some interesting implications for AAC. For one, given the motor, sensory, and perceptual disabilities experienced by many children using AAC, the relative salience they assign to particular features in defining a corresponding concept may differ from that of a typical child. There are also implications as to how symbols are depicted in terms of their relative ease of acquisition, retention, and generalizability. How do features such as size, color, and other perceptual attributes of the symbols themselves foster or impede acquisition of the corresponding concepts they represent?

Functional Core. Nelson's (1974) functional core hypothesis suggested children's meanings were based on their direct physical experience or actions on objects in their environment, and the movements that resulted. For children with multiple disabilities using AAC, once again such experiences might be limited and/or distorted, resulting in constrained or altered word meanings Where the child cannot engage the environment on his or her own, assistive technology might play an important compensatory role. Partners can also be supportive, for example, by arranging the environment such that it is optimally accessible to the child.

Prototypes. Bowerman's (1978) prototypic complex hypothesis proposes that children develop a model for what a concept depicts based on their corresponding experiences. Over time, the model or prototype changes. The prototype is often the referent that is most frequently used with the adult speech model and the one that was used first when the word was used. It appears the prototype is based on both perceptual and functional characteristics. This would underscore the value of providing valid, naturalistic experiences to children that offer a variety of stimulus contingencies. This is consistent with the concept of general case instruction (Chadsey-Rusch & Halle, 1992). In this technique, a skill is taught across a broad array of contexts, with multiple partners, with different variations, in order to promote generalization.

These three theories encourage us to envision children playing an active role in semantic development, formulating word meanings based on their personal experiences and changing conceptualizations. These are primarily self-selected from a bounty of verbal input to which they are exposed. To the contrary, for the child with a severe handicap who is using AAC, any symbols that are made accessible are selected and placed by someone else with minimal knowledge of the child's corresponding familiarity and experience with the concept. Rather than proceeding through a series of changing word meanings, as do typical children, the child using AAC may be expected to convey the adult meaning at the moment the symbol is affixed to his/her communication display.

Once again, we have no longitudinal data on the semantic development of children with the most severe disabilities who are using AAC systems. To what extent do these children display overextensions of word meanings and what are the bases of these behaviors? To what extent do they rely on perceptual characteristics, functional attributes, personal experiences, and imagined prototypes in assembling word meanings? Are there other factors operating with respect to their lexical development that are uncommon to typically developing children? Nonetheless, the developmental approach suggests several components of typical word learning that it would be advantageous to include in the initial symbol vocabularies of AAC users. These include:

- Providing direct sensory experience not only with objects themselves, but with their conventional use. Thus, play with a brush and pretending to brush hair may be necessary before using a picture to refer to a brush.
- Contrasting objects with different features and providing vocabulary for each member of the contrasting pair, so that features can be abstracted by the child. For example, *sock* might be taught in conjunction with *glove* or *mitten,* and the features of each contrasted verbally and through demonstration by the clinician.
- Using both prototypic and less prototypic exemplars of vocabulary concepts to help users grasp the conceptual range of the new symbol. For example, the term *shoe* might be taught with a child's shoe, a lady's high heeled shoe, and sneaker.

On to Two-Word (Symbol) Messages

Once again, information about typically developing children can greatly inform our practices with children using AAC systems at this stage of development. In particular, as children progress to multisymbol messages, it would be useful to track the variety and prevalence of semantic–syntactic rules (e.g., agent–action, action–object, demonstrative–entity, entity–locative, possessor–possession, and attribute–entity) they express. Furthermore, intervention for children at this stage might include modeling and prompting their use of symbols to express the full range of semantic-syntactic rules.

Cress and Marvin (2003) pointed out that children communicating at the single-word (symbol) level may express a limited range of semantic functions, conveying the single function of behavior regulation, consisting of requesting or rejecting objects or actions. They might be unable to use their lexicon for other functions such as agent, action, object, label, recurrence, attribute, and possession. Children need access to the symbols necessary to convey these semantic functions and knowledge of how to use them. Children can also be taught to combine symbol use with nonverbal behaviors, such as eye gaze and gestures, to convey a broader range of semantic functions.

This implies that when introducing a first lexicon to a child, we should consider introducing words that can serve a range of semantic functions. For example, although nouns may comprise the greatest proportion of items on a child's communication display, other kinds of symbols are necessary to allow word combinations to arise. Early symbol sets, like typical early vocabularies, should include not only nouns but verbs (*see, do, go*), adjectives (*pretty, dirty, big*), and social words (hi, bye-bye, night-night).

Grammar. Issues related to morphology and syntax have not been explored systematically in the AAC literature and have not been highlighted in AAC interventions (Sutton, Soto, & Blockberger, 2002). As Sutton et al. pointed out, children using AAC are constrained by the syntactic and morphological features of their systems. Unlike typical children, who have ample opportunities for production practice and feedback with different syntactic forms and morphological markers, children with severe speech disorders may rely on verbal input for the bulk of this learning if such structures are not accessible to them on their communication displays. Conversely, language comprehension may often present as a relative strength as it is not limited by characteristics of the AAC system.

Sutton et al. pointed out that graphic displays often contain a preponderance of nouns because verbs are difficult to display. This certainly impacts children's abilities to compose phrases and sentences. Children using AAC also rely on their listeners to interpret their messages and fill in missing information. This process of coconstruction is essential in avoiding and resolving conversational breakdowns. For example, the child may point to a single picture (e.g., "cup") and the adult glosses an entire phrase or sentence ("oh, you want some juice").

There is a vast input–output asymmetry experienced by children with severe disabilities who are using AAC systems in terms of syntactic and morphological information. In other words, the speech input they receive is far richer than the output they generate.

Typically developing children rely on word order to cue meaning in their auditory comprehension of language, and rarely exhibit word order problems in their spoken output. Similarly, children with cognitive impairments have not typically been found to encounter difficulties with word order. Conversely, examinations of AAC output reveal grammatical errors that include confusions of word order (see Smith & Grove, 2003, for review of this literature). This suggests that as AAC users begin to transition from single symbol to multisymbol output, attention to word order is essential. Students might be provided with color-coded templates that allow them to place symbols in correct order, for example.

Special Considerations in Teaching a First Language Through AAC

The young child who is learning to use AAC may be in the process of acquiring his or her native spoken language at the same time, and these two systems, spoken English and AAC, involve different methods of accessing, composing, and transmitting messages. Similarly, the discourse style associated with AAC may engender conversational rules that depart significantly from those associated with "normal" spoken discourse. We might thus expect to see both overlap as well as divergence in descriptions of the language acquisition process of children who use AAC in relation to those who rely on speech.

Understanding Language. Weitz et al. (1997) discussed ways in which AAC use can enhance English language comprehension. For example, they pointed to instances in which children's abilities to follow conversational exchanges, directions, or questions are aided by their partner's uses of visual representations (e.g., manual signs, gestures, and pictures) to augment their spoken messages. AAC systems may also help children acquire the structures of language. This has been evidenced by children whose output is significantly more complex structurally with their AAC system than when speaking.

Communicative Symmetry. A final issue concerns the degree to which communication between speakers and AAC users is symmetrical and reciprocal. For example, one might conjecture a child would be more likely to experience success with an AAC system in an environment in which his or her messages were responded to regularly than in an environment in which messages were ignored, redirected, and rejected. Sigafoos (1999) provides a helpful review of investigations designed to foster opportunities for individuals to communicate, creating needs to communicate, and providing functional consequences following communication attempts. This includes an explanation of several methods of engineering environments (e.g., missing item forms, interrupted behavior chain, incomplete presentation, delayed assistance, and wrong item format) to enhance probabilities of communicative exchanges occurring. Thus, children introduced to an AAC system that allows for successful communication may avoid the danger of having their communicative attempts "extinguished" by repeated failures to achieve their intentions through speech.

Iacono (2003) reviewed literature pertaining to adults' inabilities to interpret and respond contingently to the often ambiguous communicative signals of infants with severe disabilities. This can set in motion a cycle in which the child becomes progressively less motivated to act on the environment and assumes a passive role in interactions with the caregiver. This same pattern can persist as the child matures and continues to use communicative behaviors that are either idiosyncratic or highly ambiguous. Such children may find themselves engaged in interactions characterized by high rates of conversational breakdowns and asymmetry, in terms of their partners assuming primary responsibility for initiating, maintaining, and terminating most exchanges (Calculator & Dollaghan, 1982; Light, Collier, & Parnes, 1985).

Parents have been found to be able to perhaps foster the prelinguistic development of their children with disabilities by being responsive to their children's communicative attempts (Yoder & Warren, 1998). Instructional programs designed to enhance parents' input to their young language-learning children have been found to share several features in common. These programs tend to be child oriented, in that parents are taught to follow their child's lead and respond to their child's focus of attention. Second, emphasis is placed on promoting interaction. Parents are encouraged to allow sufficient time for their children to respond, decrease directiveness, and adopt more nurturant discourse styles. Third, parents are taught to model language by commenting on ongoing activities, using short, simple utterances, and expanding or extending their child's turns (Beukelman & Mirenda, 1998).

CONCLUSIONS

Decisions to provide AAC systems to prelinguistic children with severe impairments are no longer made exclusively on the basis of cognitive level, as current thinking favors making AAC systems available to any individual who needs to acquire a more effective form of communication, regardless of mental age. However, both research and practice rely heavily on understanding of the typical sequence of development in order to appropriately match devices and symbol systems to clients, to select speech acts and vocabulary to teach to the user, to guide the transition from single- to multisymbol communication, and to facilitate reciprocity between speakers and AAC users. Despite the important ways in which communication through AAC differs from speech communication, a developmental model remains relevant in many aspects of AAC practice, as it does in so many other aspects of communication disorders. This holds true with respect to the content as well as the sequence of instruction. At the same time, the individual who relies on AAC necessitates our augmenting developmental considerations with an eye to the functional consequences of our actions.

REFERENCES

Bates, E. (1976). *Language in context.* New York: Academic Press.

Beukelman, D., & Mirenda, P. (1998). AAC strategies for beginning communicators: Building opportunities and nonsymbolic communication. In D. Beukelman & P. Mirenda (Eds.), *Augmentative and alternative communication* (2nd ed., pp. 265–294). Baltimore: Paul H. Brookes.

Blischak, D., Lloyd, L., & Fuller, D. (1997). Terminology issues. In L. Lloyd, D. Fuller, & H. Arvidson (Eds.), *Augmentative and alternative communication* (pp. 38–42). Boston: Allyn & Bacon.

Bowerman, M. (1978). The acquisition of word meaning: An investigation in some current conflicts. In N. Waterson & C. Snow (Eds.), *The development of communication* (pp. 263–287). New York: John Wiley.

Calculator, S. (1984). Prelinguistic development. In W. Perkins (Ed.), *Language handicaps in children* (pp. 67–71). New York: Thieme-Stratton.

Calculator, S. (1997a). AAC and individuals with severe to profound disabilities. In S. Glennen & D. DeCoste (Eds.), *Handbook of augmentative and alternative communication* (pp. 445–471). San Diego: Singular.

Calculator, S. (2000). Augmentative and alternative communication. In E. Pritchard Dodge (Ed.), *The survival guide for school-based speech-language pathologists* (pp. 345–366) San Diego: Singular.

Calculator, S. (2002). Use of enhanced natural gestures to foster interactions between children with Angelman syndrome and their parents. *American Journal of Speech-Language Pathology, 11,* 340–355.

Calculator, S., & Dollaghan, C. (1982). The use of communication boards in a residential setting: An evaluation. *Journal of Speech and Hearing Disorders, 47,* 281–287.

Carey, S., & Bartlett, E. (1978). Acquiring a single new word. *Papers and Reports on Child Language Development, 15,* 17–29.

Chadsey-Rusch, J., & Halle, J. (1992). The application of general case instruction to the requesting repertoires of learners with severe disabilities. *Journal of the Association for Persons with Severe Handicaps, 17,* 121–132.

Chapman, R., & Miller, J. (1980). Analyzing language and communication in the child. In R. Schiefelbusch (Ed.), *Nonspeech language intervention strategies* (pp. 159–196). Baltimore: University Park Press.

Clark, E. (1973). What's in a word? On the child's acquisition of semantics in his first language. In T. E. Moore (Ed.), *Cognitive development and the acquisition of language* (pp. 65–110). New York: Academic Press.

Cole, K., Dale, P., & Mills, P. (1990). Defining language delay in young children by cognitive referencing: Are we saying more than we know? *Applied Psycholinguistics, 11,* 291–302.

Cress, C. (2002). Expanding children's early augmented behaviors to support symbolic development. In J. Reichle, D. Beukelman, & J. Light (Eds.), *Exemplary practices for beginning communicators* (pp. 219–272). Baltimore: Paul H. Brookes.

Cress, C., & Marvin, C. (2003). Common questions about AAC services in early intervention. *Augmentative and Alternative Communication, 19,* 254–272.

Dore, J. (1974). A pragmatic description of early pragmatic development. *Journal of Psycholinguistic Research, 3,* 343–350.

Gerber, S., & Kraat, A. (1992). Use of a developmental model of language acquisition: Applications to children using AAC systems. *Augmentative and Alternative Communication, 8,* 19–32.

Glennen, S., & Calculator, S. (1985). Training functional communication board use. A pragmatic approach. *Augmentative and Alternative Communication, 1,* 131–141.

Halliday, M. (1975). *Learning how to mean: Explorations in the development of language.* New York: Arnold.

Iacono, T. (2003). Pragmatic development in individuals with developmental disabilities who use AAC. In J. Light, D. Beukelman, & J. Riechle (Eds.), *Communicative competence for individuals who use AAC* (pp. 323–360). Baltimore: Paul H. Brookes.

Iacono, T., Carter, M., & Hook, J. (1998). Identification of intentional communication in students with severe and multiple disabilities. *Augmentative and Alternative Communication, 14,* 102–114.

Kangas, K., & Lloyd, L. (1988). Early cognitive skills as prerequisites to augmentative and alternative communication use: What are we waiting for? *Augmentative and Alternative Communication, 4,* 211–222.

Light, J., Collier, B., & Parnes, P. (1985). Communicative interactions between young nonspeaking physically disabled children and their primary caregivers: Part I. Discourse patterns. *Augmentative and Alternative Communication, 1,* 74– 83.

McLaughlin, S. (1998). *Introduction to language development*. San Diego: Singular.

Miller, J., Chapman, R., & Bedrosian, J. (1977, October). *Defining developmentally disabled subjects for research: The relationship between etiology, cognitive development, and language and communicative performance*. Paper presented at the second annual Boston University conference on language development, Boston.

Nelson, K. (1974). Concept, word, and sentence: Interrelations in acquisition and development. *Psychological Review, 81*, 11–56.

Owens, R. (2004). *Language disorders: A functional approach to assessment and intervention*. Boston: Pearson Education.

Owens, R., & House, L. (1984). Decision-making process in augmentative communication. *Journal of Speech and Hearing Disorders, 49*, 18–25.

Reichle, J., Halle, J., & Johnson, S. (1993). Developing an initial communicative repertoire: Applications and issues for persons with severe disabilities. In A. Kaiser & D. Gray (Eds.), *Enhancing children's communication: Research foundations for intervention* (pp. 105–138). Baltimore: Paul H. Brookes.

Reichle, J., & Karlan, G. (1985). Decision rules for the adoption of augmentative techniques. In R. Schielelbusch & L. Lloyd (Eds.), *Language perspectives II* (pp. 321–339). Austin, TX: Pro Ed.

Rice, M. (1989). Children's language acquisition. *American Psychologist, 44*, 149–156.

Rowland, C., & Schweigert, P. (2000). Tangible symbols, Tangible outcomes. *Augmentative and Alternative Communication, 16*, 61–78.

Rowland, C., & Schweigert, P. (2003). Cognitive skills and AAC. In J. Light, D. Beukelman, & J. Reichle (Eds.), *Communicative competence for individuals who use AAC* (pp. 241–275). Baltimore: Paul H. Brookes.

Schlosser, R., & Sigafoos, J. (2002). Selecting graphic symbols for an initial request lexicon: Integrative review. *Augmentative and Alternative Communication, 18*, 102–123.

Shane, H., & Bashir, A. (1980). Election criteria for the adoption of an augmentative communication system: Preliminary considerations. *Journal of Speech and Hearing Disorders, 45*, 408–414.

Siegel, E., & Cress, C. (2002). Overview of the emergence of early AAC behaviors. In J. Reichle, D. Beukelman, & J. Light (Eds.), *Exemplary practices for beginning communicators* (pp. 25–57). Baltimore: Paul H. Brookes.

Sigafoos, J. (1999). Creating opportunities for augmentative and alternative communication: Strategies for involving people with developmental disabilities. *Augmentative and Alternative Communication, 15*, 183–190.

Smith, M., & Grove, N. (2003). Asymmetry in input and output. In J. Light, D. Beukelman, & J. Reichle (Eds.), *Communicative competence for individuals who use AAC* (pp. 163–195). Baltimore: Paul H. Brookes.

Snell, M. (2002). Dynamic assessment. *Augmentative and Alternative Communication, 18*, 163–176.

Sutton, A., Soto, G., & Blockberger, S. (2002). Grammatical issues in graphic symbol communication. *Augmentative and Alternative Communication, 18*, 192–204.

Weitz, C., Dexter, M., & Moore, J. (1997). AAC and children with developmental disabilities. In S. Glennen & D. DeCoste (Eds.), *Handbook of augmentative and alternative communication* (pp. 395–431). San Diego: Singular.

Wetherby, A., & Prizant, B. (1989). The expression of communicative intent: Assessment issues. *Seminars in Speech and Language, 10,* 77–91.

Wilkinson, K., & McIlvane, W. (2002). Considerations in teaching graphic symbols to beginning communicators. In J. Riechle, D. Beukelman, & J. Light (Eds.), *Exemplary practices for beginning communicators* (pp. 273–321). Baltimore: Paul H. Brookes.

Yoder, P., & Warren, S. (1998). Maternal responsivity predicts the prelinguistic communication that facilitates generalized intentional communication. *Journal of Speech, Language, and Hearing Research, 41,* 1207–1219.

15

What Else About Comprehension? Examining Young Children's Discourse Comprehension Abilities

Linda M. Milosky
Syracuse University

Elizabeth Skarakis-Doyle
University of Western Ontario

Snow and Goldfield (1983) assert that from the very beginning of language acquisition, children are "bathed in an environment of extended discourse, whether it be conversation or narration." To "break into" their language community and become full participants, children must be able to navigate at the discourse level of comprehension. Many accounts of the development of comprehension in infancy and toddlerhood consider relatively small linguistic units—syllables, words, combinations of words, and then sentences—with the intent of demonstrating how children's comprehension skills are built in a relatively bottom-up fashion. Such accounts and the data that support them provide insight into aspects of this complex process. However, contemporary thought suggests that comprehension of language elements such as the word or sentence cannot account for the understanding of larger discourse units. Thus, this chapter seeks to consider the phenomenon of early discourse comprehension and to make a case for the importance of studying and assessing discourse level processing in young children.

In the early years of the Symposium on Child Language Disorders held in Madison, WI, as speakers described research that compared children with language impairments to typically developing children, the participating children typically would be matched on MLU, and the variables of interest typically involved aspects of language production. At the end of each talk, Robin Chapman would raise her hand and ask some variant of the question "What about comprehension?" Indeed, in 1981, she presented a paper with that title, and she went on to describe what was known about typical children's developing comprehension skills.

This chapter is the product of a decade-long dialogue between the authors, inspired by Chapman's intellectual heritage. When we had each been engaged in clinical practice in the 1970s, we had independently become convinced of the clinical importance of children's comprehension abilities during a time when focus was largely on analyzing the productive aspects of children's language. Assessment of "connected language" comprehension, particularly in young children, was not addressed in the literature or in clinical practice. Happily, the clinical predictive value of children's comprehension skills has since been empirically validated (cf. Johnson et al., 1999). However, during a time when much of the field was focusing on children's language production, Chapman's early and enduring interest in children's language comprehension reaffirmed our separate and mutual decisions to explore children's understanding of discourse. Her 1978 chapter in Kavanagh and Strange's volume made clear how children used comprehension strategies to make sense of the language directed at them in everyday interactions. We were brought together by our mutual interest in this sense-making, as we were convinced it reflected how children used their knowledge of the world in understanding language and competently engaged in communication. As researchers, her ideas supported us in our exploration of comprehension of discourse-level phenomena and committed us to shaping our questions and methodologies with greater ecological validity.

In our view, oral discourse comprehension is the understanding of a series of utterances in a specific context, in which the listener often must make numerous inferences about the events and the speaker, using linguistic, paralinguistic, extralinguistic, and metalinguistic information in order to fully appreciate the speaker's intent. As such, the study of discourse comprehension requires examination of how listeners use context in order to arrive at an interpretation that matches speaker intent. The studies discussed in the first half of the chapter therefore examine aspects of how the listener comprehends speaker intent, a key element of conversational comprehension. The second half of the chapter focuses on narrative comprehension and the evidence that young children are, in fact, processing narrative discourse. These foci reflect Chapman's exhortation to look at larger units of discourse in order to understand the child's language-learning experiences.

DETERMINING COMMUNICATIVE INTENT

Language used in the service of communication is rich with potential meaning. A single utterance may convey a multitude of meanings, depending on how, when, where, and by whom it is uttered and by whom it is heard. Speakers must convey their intent in ways that observe conventions and that achieve the desired effect in the listener's mind. Thus, speakers make contributions that are assumed by the listener to be relevant to the context and to be "making a point." Listeners, in turn, in order to discern the intent of an utterance, not only must connect it to prior utterances but may be required to consider a host of other knowledge sources that may influence interpretation of the utterances. The listener may need to consider the speaker's use of the physical environment as given or shared information. She may need to consider how gestures, emotional expression conveyed by prosody, facial expression, or other movement may change or at least shade the meaning of an utterance. She must bring to bear her prior history of events and people in order to consider how any one utterance is being used and hence is to be understood.

Thus, in developing comprehension of language in the service of communication, children must come to automatically process a host of verbal, nonverbal, and environmental cues, as well as activate their prior knowledge regarding these cues and the situations in which they have encountered them—they must call on their world knowledge in order to fully interpret utterances. As Chapman indicated in 1981, children as listeners must come to understand the speaker's intent by inferring what the speaker is assuming about the listener's knowledge state and desires, inferring the speaker's beliefs and goals, and assessing the degree to which they share various communicative conventions with the speaker. Although such sophisticated processing may seem to be only within the repertoire of older children and adults, it has become increasingly evident that preschool children use their knowledge of the world and of speakers in the course of communicative interaction to infer speaker intent and act accordingly. However, for children who cannot readily integrate the variety of situational and paralinguistic cues with a verbal message, noncomprehension may result and may be perceived as socially inappropriate or, in the case of behavioral directives, may be seen as noncompliance. Among those who study young children's language comprehension and difficulties with comprehension, focus has largely been on the challenges posed by relatively concrete interpretation of the linguistic elements of the message. The process of integrating linguistic and nonlinguistic sources of information in order to achieve comprehension of message intent is one that has received relatively little attention. However, as we advance theories of language impairment that are processing based and that postulate difficulties with cross-modality processing (Gillam, Cowan, & Marler, 1998) and higher cognitive integration, our models and our interventions will need to further consider the demands of integrating multiple cues in order to understand the subtleties of communicative intent.

The studies described in this section attempt to explore aspects of children's comprehension of another's communicative intent and the relation of these skills to language abilities. They examine: (a) the nature and frequency of early nonliteral intents directed at children, (b) the cues that are used to signal these nonliteral intents, (c) young children's ability to infer a speaker's desire, and (d) the emotion inferences that children might make in a given discourse situation that would allow them to infer a speaker's attitude, a critical element of determining intent. These studies are united by their focus on how children come to understand that communicative intent is determined situationally and in relation to the particular speaker, a key feature of comprehension in context. They reflect an enduring interest in the considerable, although generally effortless, amount of inferencing that occurs with each utterance in a conversation

COMMONALITY OF NONLITERAL INTENT

The degree to which a speaker's intent is evident in the linguistic elements of a message varies greatly, depending on the speaker, situation, and utterance itself. Investigations of comprehension of communicative intent quite naturally tend to focus on instances in which intent differs from literal meaning of the linguistic message or where ambiguity of intent exists. By nonliteral intent, we are referring to an utterance or series of utterances in which the speaker does not intend for the listener to attend to the conventional form/meaning of the words or actions. These intents may include, but are not limited to, idioms, irony, metaphors, hyperbole, rhetorical questions, and indirect requests.

Although indirect requests are probably the most frequent nonliteral form studied by researchers examining young children's comprehension, there is ample evidence that children frequently are exposed to nonliteral intents other than indirect requests during the preschool years. For example, Milosky and Goldberg (1993) found a rate of idiom use of 3.6 per minute in the dinner-time talk of the parents and siblings of preschool-aged children, with 37.1% of the idioms used occurring in utterances directed to the preschoolers. Sell, Kreuz, and Coppenrath (1997) found nonliteral uses to be as frequent as approximately 2 per minute in talk between parents and preschool children, with almost one-third (32%) of these utterances containing forms other than indirect requests (i.e., idioms, hyperbole, rhetorical questions, etc.) Thus, children are called on to comprehend many forms of nonliteral intent during the preschool years. If by mid to late preschool children are already being exposed to so many nonliteral forms, how are even younger children being introduced to the nature of nonliteral intent?

TEASING AS AN EARLY NONLITERAL INTENT

One early opportunity for nonliteral intent occurs during pleasurable playful teasing sequences between young children and their parents. Keltner, Capps, Kring, Young, and Heerey (2001) defined teasing as "an intentional provocation accompanied by playful off-record markers that together comment on something relevant to the target" (p. 234). Keltner et al. make clear that the purpose of a tease is to have an effect (often humorous) on another; their definition also makes clear that when language is used to convey the provocation, a child must engage multiple sources of information in service of the required nonliteral comprehension.

As Reddy (1991) has noted, very young children initiate and engage in early teasing in the form of offer–withdrawal sequences (offering of an object and then not giving it, while smiling or laughing). Reddy argues that the child's initiation of such teasing sequences may be related to the later understanding of deception and pretense and can reveal information about understanding of other's minds. Such so-called mind-reading skills clearly are essential for discerning the intent of a spoken utterance.

Parents also initiate linguistically based playful teasing. Young children are therefore provided with early, frequent practice in inferring nonliteral intent. To date, observations of such teases have consisted of very small-sample, ethnographic studies that have largely focused on parents' socialization goals in perpetrating these teasing episodes within White working-class (Miller, 1986), Kaluli (Schieffelin, 1986), and Mexicano (Eisenberg, 1986) communities. Based on these descriptions, therefore, we sought to conduct further analyses of how parents initiate and engage their children in playful teasing and how children indicate comprehension of an adult's teasing intention, particularly when the teasing involves language. We chose to focus on both the linguistic and nonlinguistic cues in these episodes in order to gain a better sense of early nonliteral exposure, and we have sought to examine these teasing episodes in light of children's language abilities, given the difficulties that older children with language impairments are reported to have with nonliteral language comprehension and with social interactions in general.

We began our investigation of this early form of nonliteral communication by seeking information about the frequency of playful teasing exchanges, then examined the reasons parents initiate such exchanges, explored the general structure of these exchanges, and finally probed the variation that may occur with children at different language levels. In order to accomplish these goals, we (Milosky & Stevens, 2000) questioned parents about their use of teasing and we examined parent-initiated playful teases gathered in a seminaturalistic manner from 15 parent–child dyads. In this study, 5 of the children, mean age 4-0 (4 years 0 months), had language impairments, 5 were same-aged typically developing peers, and 5, mean age 2-3, were younger, language-matched typically developing children.

Parental reports confirmed our belief that playful teasing was common, at least among parents of typically developing children. Seven out of 10 parents of typically developing preschool children reported that they engaged in playful teasing "often," or at least on a daily basis. Even with a small sample, parents of children with language impairment, though, were less likely to report frequent playful teasing; only one parent of five did so. Three of the remaining parents in the LI group indicated that they "sometimes" made attempts to tease their child, and the last parent indicated that she only "rarely" did so. Further exploration of the influence of children's language abilities on the frequency of parental teasing is therefore warranted. Having a preliminary idea of the general frequency and the potential impact of language level on that frequency, we went on to explore why parents engaged in these playful teases.

The goals or reasons offered for initiating playful teasing were largely affiliational or related to controlling behavior. Parents indicated that teasing was "another form of showing you love [the child] and like being around him," "making life more fun … [to] broaden his perspective sometimes," or to "have fun with interactions." Others parents reported that teasing had been used to help with difficult transitions, distract the child, cheer the grouchy child up, or simply to elicit certain behaviors (e.g., assistance with dressing).

Having a sense of the function of these exchanges at least from the parents' perspective, we then examined the structure of these teases. In the context of playful, teasing exchanges with young children, it has been reported (Eisenberg, 1986; Miller, 1986; Schieffelin, 1986) that parents often initiate such exchanges by making a patently false statement ("This is my blanket" while referring to the child's blanket) or by performing an action that deliberately violates norms (saying "It's time to go. Let's put on your shoes" and then placing a shoe on an ear, rather than a foot).

These deliberately false statements or actions constitute the "intentional provocation" of the Keltner et al. (2001) definition. The off-record markers in such parent–child exchanges, which signal the nonliteral intent, are likely to include nonverbal markers such as smiles, raised eyebrows, or prosodic distinctions.

In order to analyze the structure, we gathered examples of teasing episodes in a seminaturalistic manner. Parents were instructed to play with their children, and in the course of play to initiate tease interactions of the type they might typically use at home, with no particular structure specified. They were also asked to initiate some teases that we had structured for them (e.g., deliberately mislabeling an object) in an attempt to determine if we could elicit children's responses to teases that would be similar across dyads. We videotaped and coded parents' and children's movements, facial expressions, and paralinguistic cues. When asked to initiate typical teases (without any cues/structure provided by experimenters), the most common provocations that parents used were mislabeling of objects, withholding of desired objects, and claims that violated the child's knowledge of routines. Analysis of the tapes revealed a multiplicity of cues that parents used as off-record markers in order to signal teasing intent. These included very frequent smiles, prolonged mutual gaze, glaring, eye-widening, object-related movements (e.g., offers, withdrawals), parental body movements (leaning forward, tilting the head to the side), and touching or tickling the child. Paralinguistic cues included exaggerated prosody, laughter, and audible intakes of breath. Although it might be suggested that children are responding only to these nonlinguistic off-record markers, the fact that not all teases were successful argues against such an interpretation.

In order for a tease to be successful, a child must recognize the violation and also must recognize that it was the intent of the speaker to be playful or to have fun. The child is, in essence, distinguishing between the literal content of the utterance or action and the nonliteral intended meaning as signaled by the off-record markers (Keltner et al., 2001). Teases were deemed successful when children smiled or laughed at the provocative remark or responded with exaggerated (i.e., playful) prosody within 5 s of the parents' remark. In the unstructured, free-play situation, in total 93 tease interactions were observed, with roughly equal numbers across the 3 groups. Success rates varied among the groups: 46% of the teases directed at children with language impairments were successful, 71% of teases directed at their age-matched peers were successful, and 21% of the teases directed at the younger, language-matched peers were successful. In the structured interactions, success rate appeared markedly different among the groups, with 73% of the teases involving typically developing children being successful, and 27% of those with children with language impairments and

20% of those with younger, typically developing children being successful. These data suggest that typically developing 4-years-olds are generally able to read their parents' off-record markers and generate responses that are indicative of comprehending these teases, even when the nature of the teases was structured by the experimenter. However, the apparently lower success rates in the LI and LA groups in the teases that we attempted to structure suggest that teases may need to be highly routinized or familiar in order to be successful in children with lower levels of language abilities and/or general world knowledge. Replication with a larger cohort will illuminate the issue further.

In a subsequent larger scale study, we have therefore sought to conduct detailed examination of parent-initiated scripted exchanges. In particular, we wished to examine how parents of much younger children used verbal and nonverbal cues to signal nonliteral intent, the sequencing of these cues, the consistency of these cues, and the children's responses. Therefore, we (Burnett, Milosky, Hayes, & Neuman) are currently examining teasing sequences in 30 parent–child dyads, with children ranging in age from 18 to 32 months. In this study, we have interviewed parents about the frequency, types, and styles of playful teasing they employ with their children and their children's responses. We have videotaped the parents playing with their children, and we have encouraged them to include the types of playful teases that they would typically engage in, as reported in their interviews. We also have obtained measures of the children's language abilities (MacArthur Communicative Development Inventory; Fenson et al., 1993) and their general development (Ages and Stages Questionnaire; Bricker & Squires, 1999).

Our analyses to date have revealed four main types of teases reported by and demonstrated by mothers: mislabeling of objects or pictures, misuse or misplacement of objects, false claims of possession ("This is mine"), and mock physical challenge routines ("I've got your nose"). We have chosen first to examine the verbal components of mislabeling teases, as deliberate mislabeling may be considered (and therefore may resemble) language teaching routines. Analysis of the verbal interactions in object mislabeling teases demonstrated by 23 out of 30 mothers revealed that almost 70% of these teases were initiated with a question (e.g., "Is this a pig?" while pointing to a cow). Thus, even when deliberately or insincerely making an "error" and hoping to be caught, mothers were more likely to signal this intent by asking a question rather than making a statement ("That's a pig"). If the child did not correct the mother or otherwise indicate recognition of a mislabel, in about half the interactions, the mother revised the tease, stating it in a different way or providing a different mislabeling of the same object to perpetuate the tease. We currently are analyzing the nonverbal elements of the teases and the relation of parent and child behaviors to language abilities. We wish to further delineate the nonverbal cues parents are using to communicate affect/attitude when engaging in the teases. We believe that this reading of affect or the speaker's attitude toward the utterance is a critical element not only for playful teasing but also for comprehension of later developing, subtler communicative intents.

DETERMINING A SPEAKER'S DESIRE

Frequently, to make an inference about intent, a listener engaged in a communicative interaction formulates hypotheses about what a speaker's point is or what the speaker ultimately wants. Naturally, many of the experimental techniques for investigating children's knowledge about a speaker's or a character's desires or state of mind have involved considerable verbal skill. However, recent studies in the areas of new word learning and children's early desire psychology (Akhtar & Tomasello, 1996; Astington & Gopnik, 1991; Baldwin & Tomasello, 1998; Meltzoff, Gopnik, & Repacholi, 1999; Tomasello, 2001; Tomasello & Barton, 1994) have afforded a means of observing aspects of young children's knowledge about others' state of mind with tasks that require little or no verbal comprehension or production. Evidence of children's early awareness of others' desires (particularly when those desires differ from the child's) is critical to building an understanding of comprehension of intent, and we sought to examine whether such a skill might be related to language development. We therefore adapted a task previously used by Repacholi and Gopnick (1997) to examine the relation between children's ability to infer another's desires (a basis for comprehension of indirect requests as well as other indirect forms) and their language abilities. Repacholi and Gopnick had used the task to determine what very young children implicitly know about other people's desire, particularly when those desires may be different from their own. They assessed 14-month-old and 18-month-old children's ability to understand that an adult's food preference was different from their own. While presenting two different foods (crackers and broccoli), the experimenter expressed a food preference vocally (making sounds reflecting either pleasure or displeasure), by facial expression and by nodding or shaking her head. Half the time the adult indicated that she preferred the same food the child preferred (matched) and half the time the adult's preference was different from the child's (mismatched). The examiner then requested (both gesturally and verbally) that the child give her some food. The authors found that some 18-month-olds were able to recognize another's desire and act on it, offering, for example, broccoli instead of crackers; surprisingly, they found no relation between performance on the food preference task and a vocabulary report measure that assessed the children's production of mental state words. However, given the relatively limited vocabulary of many 14-month-olds, the language measure may not have exhibited sufficient variability to detect relationships, with means on this measure suggesting floor effects.

Therefore, to further determine how performance on such a desire task might be related to age and certain language abilities, we (Voleti & Milosky, 2003) administered the food preference task to children between the ages of 14 months and 30 months. Using a within-subjects design in which children received the matched and mismatched condition in counterbalanced fashion, we also administered three measures of language: informal language comprehension tasks, the MacArthur Communicative Development Inventory, and the same internal state language questionnaire employed by Repacholi and Gopnick (1997). Like Repacholi and Gopnick, we too did not find a relationship between internal state words in the child's expressive vocabulary and task performance, despite having a much greater range of scores on internal state words than they did. However, we did find that children who performed the task correctly (offered the adult the food the adult preferred but the child did not) had significantly higher MCDI vocabulary scores than did children who offered the adult the food they themselves preferred. This relationship was exhibited on both raw scores and percentile scores; consistent with these findings, we found no difference in mean chronological ages between children who did and did not perform correctly. We did not find a relationship between language comprehension and correct performance, but did find that task compliance was related to language comprehension abilities. Thus, knowing and acting on what someone else may want, even at early ages on a largely nonverbal task, may be linked to language development. This finding is consistent with Tomasello's (2001) conclusion that perceiving another's nonverbally communicated intention may be an important element in the process of learning new words.

INFERRING EMOTIONAL RESPONSES IN SOCIAL SITUATIONS

In addition to considering speaker desires, the emotion a speaker is likely to experience in a given situation also often must be inferred by the listener in order to comprehend that speaker's intent. For example, if I know you are angry in a given situation, I am much more likely to interpret "That's really great!" as a nonliteral, ironic statement rather than as a literal statement of delight. Therefore, investigation of children's inferences about a character's likely emotional response in a situation may yield further information about the nature of social conversational discourse comprehension and the sources of social difficulties for children with language impairments. Ford and Milosky (2003) investigated the ability of children with and without language impairments to infer how a story character might feel in a given situation. Stories were presented in three modalities—visual (pictures), auditory (orally presented sentences), and combined (pictures and orally presented sentences)—in order to determine how responses might change when language demands were minimized. We asked children to select a line drawing of the face that portrayed how the main character might feel after each three-element story. (Sample story: "Twinky wanted a teddy bear for his/her birthday. S/he opened a present with a big fluffy teddy bear. Twinky was ___." Line drawings depicted happy, sad, mad, or surprised.) Children had been tested to ensure their ability to both label and identify these line drawings of facial expressions, and all were able to do so. Despite this basic level of knowledge regarding the targeted emotions, we found that children with language impairments did not infer emotions in the stories as well as children without language impairments did. Furthermore, when errors were made, the children with language impairments were more likely than their typical peers to infer an emotion of the opposite valence (e.g., selecting happy instead of sad). If such a pattern of performance were carried over into actual social situations, the consequences could be quite negative. When we examined how the children's general language and cognitive abilities may have influenced task performance in the visual-only condition (perhaps minimizing language processing), we found that language skills, as measured by the comprehension subtests of the Clinical Evaluation of Language Fundamentals–Preschool (CELF–P; Wiig, Secord, & Semel, 1992) accounted for 46% of the variance in performance, with nonverbal cognition, as measured by the Kaufman Assessment Battery for Children (K-ABC; Kaufman & Kaufman, 1983), not accounting for any additional variance. Thus, children's general language comprehension abilities appear to be closely linked with their ability to make the inferences necessary for successful social interaction, even when the information was not conveyed through verbal channels, a finding consistent with Gernsbacher's (1990) concept of a "general comprehension skill." It is also consistent with arguments that many nonverbal tasks may be verbally mediated by children; thus it is plausible to consider whether language deficits may impede the meaningful interpretation of nonlinguistic elements of social situations and/or the integration of linguistic and nonlinguistic cues in those situations.

CONSTRUCTING DISCOURSE REPRESENTATIONS

As indicated earlier, inferring a character's emotional response should occur as part of the process of forming a mental representation of a situation, and indeed, the active, constructive comprehender seems to anticipate such emotional responses when processing discourse (Gernsbacher, Goldsmith, &

Robertson, 1992). However, there has been little research on young children's online processing of discourse and the nature of the difficulties children with language impairments may experience in anticipating characters' internal responses to events. Therefore, Ford, in her dissertation study, examined whether young children with and without language impairments developed discourse-based expectations about a character's emotional response to common situations, employing an online response time comprehension measure based on Gernsbacher's methodology. Findings (Ford & Milosky, 2005) suggest that, as a group, children with language impairments may not be developing a mental representation of the discourse whole when presented with a story about an emotionally evocative situation, even when that story is presented simultaneously visually (animated pictures on a computer screen) and verbally (orally presented sentences). Thus, these children seem to have difficulty integrating information across pictures and/or utterances in order to make an inference about an internal state, although their chronological peers did do so. Language ability alone did not best account for children's performance; instead, a combination of language ability and vocal response time (as measured by a minimally linguistically demanding task) provided the best fitting model. In addition, language ability as measured of CELF–P did not predict children's score on a social competence scale, but response time on the inferencing task and drawing of facial expressions did. These findings further affirm that in order to unravel the complex relationship between language and social competence, we need to use various tasks that tap knowledge of and ability to read the linguistic and nonlinguistic cues that are likely to arise in a social discourse situation.

THE CHALLENGES OF EXPLORING CONVERSATIONAL COMPREHENSION

Conversational discourse is one primary context for socialization and for language learning. As the studies already described highlight, understanding a speaker's intentions, beliefs, desires, and affect is critical for the development of discourse comprehension and social competence. The further elucidation of the social difficulties demonstrated by many children with LI must include examination of comprehension and production in ways that fully capture the complexity of conversational discourse. As children mature, their conversational contributions must increasingly take account of the previous speaker's utterances, and the mental representations that are developed are ones that incorporate both parties' utterances. The child therefore must rapidly switch between comprehension and production skills. The representation formed during conversation also must allow for flexibility or shifting, with considerable need for rapid inferencing skill, as topics evolve or change, and as expectations about what the other person will say are violated. We have much to learn about the nature of children's comprehension of conversation, particularly at the level of the discourse whole, rather than viewing conversation as a series of utterances. However, emerging work on the nature of young children's narrative discourse representations has begun to provide evidence, using creative methodologies, that preschool-aged children do form language-based representations beyond the sentence level.

EMERGING NARRATIVE REPRESENTATIONS

Young children are regularly exposed to narratives during the language learning years, with story listening being perhaps the most common experience with narrative discourse, at least in Western societies (Dickinson & Snow, 1987; Nelson, 1996). Although this is a common activity of early childhood, young children are generally presumed to have very limited understanding of stories. Even mothers seem to expect very little in the way of understanding a story line. Early studies of mother–child storybook reading exchanges revealed (Snow & Goldfield, 1983) that storybook discourse centers around picture description rather than a thematically organized event. Although prevailing wisdom suggests reading stories is of great benefit to the young child, and, indeed, reading experts such as Paris and Paris (2003) claim that narrative competence is a fundamental cognitive skill influencing early reading development, little is known about the what, when, and how of story comprehension development. Nelson (1996) has suggested that children may employ both gestalt and analytic processes in beginning to understand stories, just as in language development generally. Indeed, she suggests that story understanding may begin in terms of "bits and pieces" but notes that "much more systematic analysis of this topic over the years from 2 to 6 is needed" (p. 210). What follows is one research group's efforts in this endeavor.

The journey began with creating methodological procedures from which valid inferences could be made. As with all of comprehension, evidence that it has occurred must be inferred from responses to input such as requests to act or speak. Hence, it is often the case with young children that compliance rather than comprehension is measured. Engaging yet "devious" measures (Hirsh-Pasek & Golinkoff, 1991) are needed to uncover a young child's understanding of discourse in general and story in particular. Memory demands, expressive language skill, and task compliance, as noted earlier, confound efforts to measure young children's discourse understanding (McCabe, 1996). Ideally, a measure of young children's discourse comprehension would limit memory demands, would require a nonverbal or brief verbal response, and would employ a task that was engaging to young children.

Heeding Chapman and Kohn's (1978) advice to look to the world of the child when attempting to uncover what a child understands, Skarakis-Doyle and colleagues turned to the routine of storybook reading to develop two innovative procedures to address the challenge of assessing young children's discourse comprehension and comprehension monitoring (i.e., the ability to know when you have not understood).

Young children have a great fondness for hearing a favorite storybook over and over again, often to the dismay of the story reader. As the routine for story events is established over the multiple readings, a caregiver will often engage the child in the storytelling by pausing and allowing the child to say what comes next. Further, should the unwitting caregiver make an error in reading the familiar story, even the child as young as 30 months will admonish, correct, or at least look quizzically at the adult. The implication from both these observations is that in order to participate in such interactions, even a very young child has laid down some representation for the story discourse. We reasoned, then, that such interactions might provide a window into the very young child's understanding of story type discourse. From them, the Joint Story Retell (JSR) (Dempsey & Skarakis-Doyle, 2001; Skarakis-Doyle & Wootton, 1995) and the Expectancy Violation Detection Task (EVDT) (Skarakis-Doyle, 2002) were created to measure the oral story comprehension of children 2½ to 4 years of age. The JSR and EVDT simulate the naturalistic activity of story reading observed in parents and their young children that were described earlier. These procedures require little expressive language ability. Memory demands are controlled in several ways. First, comprehension is measured while the child hears the story, rather than after the story is completed as is done when comprehension questions are administered. By doing this, the entire story representation does not have to be held in working memory. Second, memory demands are eased by utilizing story content that is familiar to the child, that is, routine events.

Over the course of a decade of development, both commercially available children's books and one specifically written for our work have been utilized with these procedures. The fundamental feature across the story stimuli used was that they were script-like in nature. Nelson (1996) has proposed that event knowledge in the form of a script is crucial for the young child entering a linguistic world. Scripts provide the context in which language is learned, used and understood. Key script concepts of actors, actions, and props (i.e., objects) are also those semantic categories prevalent in early language development. Such script structure, although not identical, is recognized as highly similar to that of story. Information must be structured in order for discourse comprehension and comprehension monitoring to proceed successfully. Hence, it may be that cognitive-linguistic abilities, comprehension, and comprehension monitoring emerge in the context of the child's event knowledge, just as Nelson and colleagues have shown for other linguistic developments. Motivated by Nelson's model, the content and the structure of the stories chosen were routine childhood events such as bath time, toileting, and bedtime.

The stories utilized contained core elements for the routine event. For example, in the bath-time story such elements as soap, water, and undressing for a bath were included. Additionally, optional acts and slot fillers that support these core elements were also present; for example, in the bath-time story the child tested the bath water. All stories were composed of five episodes organized around a central goal, that is, taking a bath, going to bed, or using the toilet. Each episode, in turn, was comprised of a sequence of goal directed activities. All stories had approximately 400 words and 30 sentences. All were patterned storybooks; thus, vocabulary words, sentence patterns, and episodes were repeated and a distinct rhythmic or song-like refrain was incorporated into the text at similar intervals. Each page of text was accompanied by a color illustration, and analyses were conducted to ensure that the presence of illustrations did not provide additional cues that would confound an interpretation of the child's understanding (Dempsey & Skarakis-Doyle, 2001; Skarakis-Doyle, 2002). An example from a story is provided in Table 15.1.

JOINT STORY RETELL

The JSR is essentially a cloze procedure adapted for oral presentation. It is grounded in the assumption that a listener can utilize redundancy in spoken text to retrieve a word or phrase and hence demonstrate comprehension of a surrounding passage, just as is done when implemented in assessment of reading text (Dietrich, Freeman, & Griffin, 1979). The child retells an edited version of the story along with the examiner, using the fill-in-the-blank or "cloze" procedure. Key story elements are omitted, and comprehension ability is demonstrated by the child's accuracy in providing those elements when the examiner pauses. Studies of interrater and test–retest reliability as well as, internal consistency (Dempsey, Skarakis-Doyle, & Lockwood, 2000) have demonstrated that the JSR meets the criteria for reliability set out by McCauley and Swisher (1984). In addition, Dempsey and Skarakis-Doyle (2001) demonstrated its validity as a measure of story comprehension. Notably, in this study and subsequent work (Skarakis-Doyle, Dempsey, & Lee, 2002, 2004), the JSR consistently shows a strong and significant relationship to comprehension questions, the traditional measure of story comprehension. Dempsey and Skarakis-Doyle (2001) also demonstrated that although expressive language abilities

TABLE 15.1
Examples of Measures of Oral Story Comprehension

Story Stimulus

One day a little girl named Sarah made very messy mud-pies in the backyard. Sarah's mom took one look at her and said, "Splish, splash, Sarah needs a bath. Mommy says you're dirty and she can't have that." (From "Splish Splash," Skarakis-Doyle & Wooton, 1995).

Joint Story Retell

One day a little ___ (girl) named Sarah made very messy ___ (mud-pies) in the backyard. Sarah's mom took one look at her and said, "Splish, splash, Sarah needs a bath. Mommy says you're dirty and she can't have that."

Event Violation Detection Task

One day a little named Sarah made very messy mud-pies in the **bathroom** (backyard). Sarah's mom took one look at her and said, "Splish, splash, Sarah needs a bath. Mommy says you're dirty and she can't have that."

played a significant role in predicting performance on comprehension questions, it did not for the JSR, suggesting it could be a viable alternative for measuring language comprehension in children with limited expressive language (i.e., children who were very young or with expressive language impairment). Having confidently established that JSR is measuring what it was intended to and was useful with very young children, the authors then employed it in a series of investigations seeking to better understand the nature of emerging oral story comprehension.

VOCABULARY AND DISCOURSE COMPREHENSION

Rice and Watkins (1996) suggest that receptive vocabulary is a powerful index of language ability and may thus be predictive of narrative comprehension. Conventional wisdom suggests that although knowing the meaning of individual words is important to the understanding of a narrative, it is just one of a complex of abilities that are integrated into the service of understanding discourse. Dempsey, Lee, and Skarakis-Doyle (2004) examined the relationship between vocabulary knowledge and narrative comprehension in normally developing children between 30 and 70 months old. Both a measure of general receptive vocabulary (Peabody Picture Vocabulary Test–III, PPVT–III; Dunn & Dunn, 1997) and vocabulary specific to the story were investigated, as was verbal memory, given its important relationship to vocabulary. Story-specific vocabulary had only a moderately weak relationship with story comprehension, consistent with what conventional wisdom would suggest. Interestingly, general receptive vocabulary had a moderately strong relationship to story comprehension, but when working memory was controlled statistically, no further significant relationship was found. Rationally and empirically, vocabulary knowledge was demonstrated as a necessary contributor to story comprehension but was not found to be as pivotal to the process as some have suggested. These findings led to further examination of the constructs contributing to a young child's story comprehension.

CONSTRUCTS UNDERLYING DISCOURSE COMPREHENSION

For the past 30 years, researchers interested in language acquisition have been guided by theories of language based on adult competence, yet have recognized that the developing system should be studied in its own right and have done so. Often theories based on the assumptions of a fully developed or fully competent system were too powerful to provide a parsimonious explanation of a developing system. Chapman (2000) reminds us of the fundamental insight that new forms and meanings emerge out of "old" or existing forms of behavior. Given the unstable and incomplete state of a young child's linguistic and cognitive systems, the constructs that could underlie emerging narrative comprehension might be found within the child's existing repertoire. Building on their previous work, Skarakis-Doyle, Dempsey, and Lee (2002) investigated variables that both were widely noted in the literature as fundamental constructs in narrative comprehension and were recognizable components of a young child's cognitive-linguistic system. Once again the JSR was employed as the measure of story comprehension. They found for children developing normally who were between 30 and 70 months of age that although verbal working memory accounted for the great majority of variance when predicting story comprehension performance, general language ability (measured both by receptive vocabulary and a general index of expressive development) and inferencing ability also made unique contributions to predicting story comprehension performance. Although these results suggest that story comprehension strongly depends on working memory even for young children, it does not fully account for the emerging discourse comprehension system as some have suggested (Daneman & Blennerhassett, 1984).

GIST COMPREHENSION AND EMERGING DISCOURSE COMPREHENSION

Given that a role for inferencing in story comprehension was empirically established in the previous study, Dempsey, Skarakis-Doyle, and Lee (2002) continued to investigate the emergence of gist understanding in children who were normally developing between the ages of 30 and 70 months of age. Comprehending the "gist" of a story is held as the hallmark of narrative comprehension because it requires both the understanding of ordered events and the human response to them. Participants in the study were presented traditional factual and gist questions with the latter varying in the transparency of the main character's intention. The most sophisticated gist question, which was asked first, queried the main character's social intention, "Why did Sarah keep asking her mom for things?"; the next level queried motivation for her physical actions, "Why did Sarah keep starting to leave the room?"; and finally, the most basic gist question simply queried the main character's basic desire, "Did Sarah want to take a bath?" Analyses revealed that gist knowledge was differentially related to a child's level of factual understanding, that is, comprehension of physical act motivation and basic desire were both moderately and significantly correlated with accuracy on the content questions. Children who had a better grasp of the facts also had better understanding of the main character's desire and motive for her action. But as would be expected, developmental differences were also revealed. While the most transparent inference about the character's desire emerged among the youngest children, understanding of motivation for physical action of leaving the bathroom emerged among the older children, and the understanding the social intention of the character was not even grasped by children at age 5 yrs consistent with theory of mind research.

THE EXPECTANCY VIOLATION DETECTION TASK

The EVDT is based on the assumption that by deliberately violating a child's expectations about a story, we gather evidence of what expectations have been developed and provide opportunities for young children to indicate their understanding (Markman, 1981). The EVDT is an altered version of the story in which key script components are changed or "violated." Over the course of developing this procedure a number of different types of violations have been utilized, including:

- Within component, actor, action object substitutions—In this type of violation the substitution was within the semantic class but was implausible or inappropriate to the story. We infer that to recognize these violations the child minimally invoked world knowledge of the relationships of actors and actions or objects and actions that were "probable event" and whether those events "fit" the routine event described in the story (Skarakis-Doyle, 2002).
- Within story, actor, action violations—In this type of violation, one story character was substituted for another or an action was replaced with one occurring from another place in the story (Skarakis-Doyle &

Milosky, 1999). We infer that to recognize these violations the child presumably had a representation for specific information of precisely who did what and when for the stimuli story and could not respond using only general knowledge about entities and actions.

- Goal violations—Actions were inserted in the story that were plausible and could fit the story context but that disrupted progress toward accomplishing a central goal of the story (Skarakis-Doyle & Milosky, 1999). We infer that to recognize these violations, presumably the child had developed a macrostructure of the story discourse (Hudson, 1988).
- Violations of content produced with unique prosody—the content of commands or rhythmic repetitive phrases were substituted with phrases not within the story (Skarakis-Doyle & Milosky, 1999). We infer that responses to these violations may indicate that children had a representation for information encoded in a highly salient prosodic envelope.

Children are read the original script-based story (the same as used in the JSR) and then introduced to the EVDT during a modeling/practice period. An example from the EVDT can be found in Table 15.1. The child is then reread the altered version of the story and instructed to catch silly or out-of-place elements in the story they had just heard. Verbal and nonverbal responses occurring within 5 s of the violation are coded for frequency and type. Comprehension monitoring (or the ability to know when you haven't understood) is demonstrated by the child's reaction to the altered story components (Skarakis-Doyle, 2002). As with the JSR, investigations into the psychometric rigor of the EVDT have been conducted (Dempsey et al., 2000; Skarakis-Doyle, 2002). The EVDT also meets the standards for reliability set forth by McCauley and Swisher (1984). The high interrater reliability achieved is particularly important given that subtle nonverbal responses may be considered indices of detection. In the early 1980s researchers identified the importance of recording nonverbal indexes of comprehension monitoring such as facial expressions of puzzlement, smiles, or shifts in eye gaze. Such responses are thought to be more sensitive to emerging comprehension monitoring abilities because they require little overt awareness of comprehension breakdown and because they are easier to produce. Indeed, they may in part or whole be involuntary. Skarakis-Doyle (2002) found these types of responses to be particularly robust with a false-positive rate of less than 1%.

Empirical evidence was also accrued to support the claim that the EVDT was measuring emerging comprehension monitoring. Several types of converging evidence were obtained. Evidence of expected performance differences over time is a particularly illuminating form of evidence for validity (Messick, 1995). Skarakis-Doyle (2002) found a correlation of .71 between age and the EVDT. Although children as young as 30 months demonstrated emerging ability to detect story violations, performance steadily improves with age, as expected. Several investigations of concurrent validity, correlating the EVDT with a traditional discourse comprehension measure (i.e., comprehension questions), have yielded a moderate and significant relationship (Dempsey, Jacques, Skarakis-Doyle, & Lee, 2002; Dempsey & Skarakis-Doyle, 2001; Skarakis-Doyle & Milosky, 1999). However, the moderate magnitude of this relationship indicates that although the EVDT, in part, measures primary comprehension, as do comprehension questions, it may be measuring additional ability as well. This is precisely what we would expect for a measure of comprehension monitoring that also entails additional cognitive processes.

To further understand what the EVDT was measuring and how it did so, Dempsey et al. (2002) investigated the role that the knowledge of truth conditions played in a child's ability to detect violations. Comprehension monitoring requires that one is aware of when the expectations that one has for discourse material are not realized, that is, that what one believed to be true about the material was not presented as such. This entails knowledge of the relationship between a phrase and its referent in the world, or the "truth conditions" of an assertion. Normally developing children between the ages of 30 and 61 months were examined for the comprehension monitoring of a script-based story utilizing the EVDT and additionally on an adaptation of Pea's (1982) sentence verification task. This task evaluated understanding of the following conditions in a picture pointing task: true affirmatives—the phrase (This is a ___) and pictured referent matched; false affirmatives—the phrase (This is a ___) did not refer to the picture referent; true negatives—the phrase (This is not a ___) and its negative did not describe the pictured referent; and false negative—the phrase (This is not a ___) and its negation accurately described the pictured referent. Facility with the verbal logic of truth conditions, particularly affirmative conditions, was found to contribute at least in the detection phase of comprehension monitoring. With increasing understanding of what the EVDT was measuring, it was also employed to investigate the nature of emerging discourse representation in young children.

DISCOURSE REPRESENTATION—HOW, WHAT, AND WHEN

As has already been noted, listening to a story being read aloud is likely to be a child's first exposure to narrative discourse, and if the story is one that the child is fond of, he or she is likely to hear it repeatedly. In a period of emerging language abilities, what would be the nature of a young child's early discourse representation for given narrative? Skarakis-Doyle and Milosky (1999) were challenged by this problem. They examined these questions: How much of a representation of the story do young children construct when they are exposed to a story for the first time? What elements do they comprehend and remember? How does this change with age between 36 and 59 months? The EVDT was employed to determine whether children would create a discourse representation that was sufficient to form expectations for the material based on one presentation of an engaging story (i.e., a global-level "fast map"). Use of the EVDT permitted investigation of the potential nature of the representation by examining responses to several different types of violations of the story material, each of which probed a different discourse element. Children did respond verbally and nonverbally in a robust manner to the violations in the EVDT. Responses times to each of the types of violations were similar; however, children in this age range were most sensitive to violations embedded in a unique prosodic envelope (i.e., content embedded in a song or rhyme), then to substitutions of actors and actions within the story, and finally to disruption to goal structure. Children responded to more violations of all types as they got older. These children had indeed formed expectations for the material, suggesting that a representation of sufficient completeness had been created after only one exposure to a story.

The previously described program of research demonstrated that the JSR and EVDT can measure story-type discourse comprehension and monitoring in children between the ages of 2½ and 4 years. These measures permit advances in our knowledge of a child's early attempts at understanding the types of discourse that they are exposed to early in life. We now have an emerging picture of what the young child's capabilities may be. Such developmental data can provide the foundation for early identification of language comprehension impairments. The imperative for such an application is clear when the severely disabling condition that results from such impairments is considered. Johnson et al. (1999) reported that the single most accurate predictor of long-term negative outcome was status of language comprehension. Thus, the ability of the JSR and EVDT to accurately detect language comprehension deficits in young children is being investigated. In a pilot study, Skarakis-Doyle and Wootton (1995) examined potential differences in performance on these two measures by children with language impairment (LI). Comparing eight children with LI to age-matched controls (language status was controlled statistically), they found that the children with LI performed significantly less accurately than did control children on both the JSR and EVDT. Further, they found that when children with LI did detect violations on the EVDT, the latency of initial nonverbal detection was significantly slower for the children with LI than for control children. However, as noted by Plante and Vance (1994), statistical significance speaks only to the fact that the variance associated with each group's performance on the experimental measures is above chance level. It does not address the question of a measure's ability to accurately predict group assignment (i.e., children with language comprehension impairments as impaired and children with normal developing language as such). In research funded by the Hospital for Sick Kids and the Ontario Ministry of Health and Long Term Care, Skarakis-Doyle et al. (2004) replicated the findings of the earlier pilot work with children with LI and conducted additional discriminative analyses on the JSR and EVDT. In a group of 44 children between the ages of 36–61 months, the two measures had overall classification accuracy of 81.6% and 94.7%, respectively. As measures of early discourse comprehension, the JSR and EVDT demonstrate excellent psychometric rigor on all accounts. In addition to examining these measures individually, we investigated the discriminative ability of a comprehensive battery of comprehension measures that included lexical (PPVT–III; Dunn & Dunn, 1997), grammatical (Grammatical Morphemes subtest of Test for Auditory Comprehension of Language, TACL–III; Carrow-Woolfolk, 1999), and these discourse-level measures. Outstanding overall identification accuracy was achieved (100%) with this battery of comprehension measures, as well as superb sensitivity and specificity in identification. Although this battery provides accurate identification, that is not its primary purpose, because the individual measures did so with acceptable adequacy using Plante and Vance's 1994 suggested standards. More importantly, it provides a rigorous and clinically efficient means for identifying language comprehension impairments at several different levels. It can be administered in approximately 30 min and would provide direction for establishing treatment goals at multiple levels of comprehension. Such multilevel assessment and treatment procedures are critically important to early intervention efforts.

CONCLUDING REMARKS

It has been our goal, in keeping with Chapman's heritage, to emphasize that the examination of discourse-level phenomena is critical to any account of language development or disorder. It is only at this level that one truly begins to examine language in the service of communication, an overriding concept that Chapman emphasized in her teachings and writing. Driven, in part, by the relative paucity of assessment tools for conversational and narrative discourse level phenomena, particularly during the preschool and early school-age years, we have reported on some of the questions that have motivated our research and some of the tasks we have used to assess comprehension of those phenomena.

The current focus on early literacy experiences has begun to advance the study of discourse comprehension in young children and further highlights the need to understand, in depth, how and when children begin developing expectations for discourse structure and content. In exploring emerging conversational and narrative comprehension, it is key that we understand the underpinnings of flexible language comprehension—being able to create a whole that is more than the sum of the parts. By using prior knowledge such as scripts, and making inferences about events, motivations, a speaker's attitude, or a character's affective responses, children become able to truly determine the full import of a series of utterances—the meaning of both what is said and what is not said.

We spoke, at the beginning of this chapter, of the need for children to break into their language community. Language is the primary means by which children become part of their social community. Because we have evidence of the continued social difficulties of some children with language impairments, with the increased likelihood of psychiatric diagnoses in adulthood (Beitchman et al., 2001), the role that reduced language comprehension plays in such difficulties must be fully explored. We must provide children with skills and strategies that allow them to do more than "nod and smile" (Blalock, 1982) in the face of rapid conversational exchanges or extended narratives. Chapman's enduring lesson for both researchers and clinicians is that we must look not only at what the child says but also at what the child understands, and her work reminds us of the need to appreciate the mental richness of the comprehension process. Perhaps it is fitting, given the recent release of the final *Stars Wars* movie, to close with a repetition of Chapman's 1981 use of Ben Kenobi's exhortation to Luke Skywalker: "Seeing is with the mind, Luke, not the eyes."

REFERENCES

Akhtar, N., & Tomasello, M. (1996). Two-year-olds learn words for absent objects and actions. *British Journal of Developmental Psychology, 14*(Pt. 1), 79–93.

Astington, J. W., & Gopnik, A. (1991). Developing understanding of desire and intention. In A. Whiten (Ed.), *Natural theories of mind: Evolution, development and simulation of everyday mindreading* (pp. 39–50). Cambridge, MA: Basil Blackwell.

Baldwin, D. A., & Tomasello, M. (1998). Word learning: A window on early pragmatic understanding. In E. V. Clark (Ed.), *The Proceedings of the Twenty-ninth Annual Child Language Research Forum* (pp. 3–23). Chicago: Center for the Study of Language and Information.

Beitchman, J. H., Wilson, B., Johnson, C. J., Atkinson, L., Young, A., Adlaf, E., et al. (2001). Fourteen-year follow-up of speech/language-impaired and control children: Psychiatric outcome. *Journal of the American Academy of Child & Adolescent Psychiatry, 40*(1), 75–82.

Blalock, J. W. (1982). Residual learning disabilities in young adults: Implications for rehabilitation. *Journal of Applied Rehabilitation Counseling, 13*(2), 9–13.

Bricker, D., & Squires, J. (1999). *Ages and Stages Questionnaires: A parent-completed child-monitoring system* (2nd ed.). Baltimore: Paul H. Brookes.

Carrow-Woolfolk, E. (1999). *Test for Auditory Comprehension of Language* (3rd ed.). Austin, TX: Pro-Ed.

Chapman, R. S. (1978). Comprehension strategies in children. In J. Kavanagh & W. Strange (Eds.), *Speech and language in the laboratory, school, and clinic* (pp. 308–327). Cambridge, MA: MIT Press.

Chapman, R. S. (1981, June). *What about comprehension?* Paper presented at the Symposium on Research in Child Language Disorders, Madison, WI.

Chapman, R. S. (2000). Children's language learning: An interactionist perspective. *Journal of Child Psychology & Psychiatry, 41*(1), 33–54.

Chapman, R. S., & Kohn, L. L. (1978). Comprehension strategies in two and three year olds: Animate agents or probable events? *Journal of Speech & Hearing Research, 21*(4), 746–761.

Daneman, M., & Blennerhassett, A. (1984). How to assess the listening comprehension skills of prereaders. *Journal of Educational Psychology, 76*(6), 1372–1381.

Dempsey, L., Jacques, J., Skarakis-Doyle, E., & Lee, C. (2002, November). *The relationship between preschoolers' comprehension monitoring ability and their knowledge of truth conditions.* Paper presented at the Annual Convention of the American Speech Language and Hearing Association, Atlanta, GA.

Dempsey, L., Lee, C., & Skarakis-Doyle, E. (2004, June). *Understanding the constructs underlying narrative comprehension in young children: The role of vocabulary.* Paper presented at the Symposium on Research in Child Language Disorders, Madison, WI.

Dempsey, L. F., & Skarakis-Doyle, E. (2001). The validity of the joint story retell as a measure of young children's comprehension of familiar stories. *Journal of Speech-Language Pathology & Audiology, 25*(4), 201–211.

Dempsey, L., Skarakis-Doyle, E., & Lee, C. (2002, July). *Emergence of narrative comprehension in preschoolers: Understanding the gist.* Paper presented at the Symposium on Research in Child Language Disorders, Madison, WI.

Dempsey, L., Skarakis-Doyle, E., & Lockwood, S. (2000, November). *Assessing preschooler's discourse comprehension: The reliability of the JSR.* Poster presented at the American Speech Language and Hearing Association Annual Convention, Washington, DC.

Dietrich, T., Freeman, C., & Griffin, P. (1979). Assessing comprehension in a school setting. In R. W. Shuy (Series Ed.) & P. Griffin (Vol. Ed.), *Papers in applied linguistics: Linguistics and reading series* (Vol. 3, pp. 1–16). Arlington TX: Center for Applied Linguistics.

Dickinson, D. K., & Snow, C. E. (1987). Interrelationships among prereading and oral language skills in kindergartners from two social classes. *Early Childhood Research Quarterly, 2*(1), 1–25.

Dunn, L., & Dunn, L. (1997). *Peabody Picture Vocabulary Test* (3rd ed.). Circle Pines, MN: AGS.

Eisenberg, A. R. (1986). Teasing: Verbal play in two Mexicano homes. In B. B. Schieffelin & E. Ochs (Eds.), *Language socialization across cultures* (pp. 182–198). New York: Cambridge University Press.

Fenson, L., Dale, P., Reznick, J., Thal, D., Bates, E., Hartung, J., Pethick, S., & Reilly, J. (1993). *MacArthur Communicative Development Inventories (CDI).* San Diego, CA: Singular.

Ford, J. A., & Milosky, L. M. (2003). Inferring emotional reactions in social situations: Differences in children with language impairment. *Journal of Speech, Language, & Hearing Research, 46*(1), 21–30.

Ford, J. A., & Milosky, L. M. (2005, June). *The time course of emotion inferencing: Differences in children with language impairment*. Poster presented at the Symposium on Research in Child Language Disorders, Madison, WI.

Gernsbacher, M. A. (1990). *Language comprehension as structure building*. Hillsdale, NJ: Lawrence Erlbaum Associates.

Gernsbacher, M. A., Goldsmith, H. H., & Robertson, R. R. (1992). Do readers mentally represent characters' emotional states? *Cognition & Emotion, 6*(2), 89–111.

Gillam, R. B., Cowan, N., & Marler, J. A. (1998). Information processing by school-age children with specific language impairment: Evidence from a modality effect paradigm. *Journal of Speech, Language, & Hearing Research, 41*(4), 913–926.

Hirsh-Pasek, K., & Golinkoff, R. M. (1991). Language comprehension: A new look at some old themes. In N. A. Krasnegor & D. M. Rumbaugh (Eds.), *Biological and behavioral determinants of language development* (pp. 301–320). Hillsdale, NJ: Lawrence Erlbaum Associates.

Hudson, J. A. (1988). Children's memory for atypical actions in script-based stories: Evidence for a disruption effect. *Journal of Experimental Child Psychology, 46*(2), 159–173.

Johnson, C. J., Beitchman, J. H., Young, A., Escobar, M., Atkinson, L., Wilson, B., et al. (1999). Fourteen-year follow-up of children with and without speech/language impairments: Speech/language stability and outcomes. *Journal of Speech, Language, & Hearing Research, 42*(3), 744–760.

Kaufman, A., & Kaufman, N. (1983). *Kaufman Assessment Battery for Children*. Circle Pines, MN: AGS.

Keltner, D., Capps, L., Kring, A. M., Young, R. C., & Heerey, E. A. (2001). Just teasing: A conceptual analysis and empirical review. *Psychological Bulletin, 127*(2), 229–248.

Markman, E. (1981). Comprehension monitoring. In W. P. Dickson (Ed.), *Children's oral communication skills* (pp. 61–94). New York: Academic.

McCabe, A. (1996). Evaluating narrative discourse skills. In K. N. Cole & P. S. Dale (Eds.), *Assessment of communication and language* (Vol. 6, pp. 121–141). Baltimore, MD: Paul H. Brookes.

McCauley, R. J., & Swisher, L. (1984). Use and misuse of norm-referenced tests in clinical assessment: A hypothetical case. *Journal of Speech & Hearing Disorders, 49*(4), 338–348.

Meltzoff, A. N., Gopnik, A., & Repacholi, B. M. (1999). Toddlers' understanding of intentions, desires and emotions: Explorations of the dark ages. In P. D. Zelazo & J. W. Astington (Eds.), *Developing theories of intention: Social understanding and self-control* (pp. 17–41). Mahwah, NJ: Lawrence Erlbaum Associates.

Messick, S. (1995). Validity of psychological assessment: Validation of inferences from persons' responses and performances as scientific inquiry into score meaning. *American Psychologist, 50*(9), 741–749.

Miller, P. (1986). Teasing as language socialization and verbal play in a white working-class community. In B. B. Schieffelin & E. Ochs (Eds.), *Language socialization across cultures* (pp. 199–212). New York: Cambridge University Press.

Milosky, L., & Goldberg, L. (1993, November). *Idiomatic input to preschool children.* Poster presented at the American Speech-Language-Hearing-Association Annual Convention, Anaheim, CA.

Milosky, L., & Stevens, A. (2000, June). *Playful teasing episodes in interactions between preschoolers and their parents.* Poster presented at Symposium for Research on Child Language Disorders, Madison, WI.

Nelson, K. (1996). *Language in cognitive development: Emergence of the mediated mind.* New York: Cambridge University Press.

Paris, A. H., & Paris, S. G. (2003). Assessing narrative comprehension in young children. *Reading Research Quarterly, 38*(1), 36–76.

Pea, R. D. (1982). Origins of verbal logic: Spontaneous denials by two- and three-year olds. *Journal of Child Language, 9*(3), 597–626.

Plante, E., & Vance, R. (1994). Selection of preschool language tests: A data-based approach. *Language, Speech, & Hearing Services in Schools, 25*(1), 15–24.

Reddy, V. (1991). Playing with others' expectations: Teasing and mucking about in the first year. In A. Whiten (Ed.), *Natural theories of mind: Evolution, development and simulation of everyday mindreading* (pp. 143–158). Cambridge, MA: Basil Blackwell.

Repacholi, B. M., & Gopnik, A. (1997). Early reasoning about desires: Evidence from 14- and 18-month-olds. *Developmental Psychology, 33*(1), 12–21.

Rice, M. L., & Watkins, R. V. (1996). "Show me x": New views of an old assessment technique. In K. N. Cole & P. S. Dale (Eds.), *Assessment of communication and language* (Vol. 6, pp. 183–206). Baltimore, MD: Paul H. Brookes.

Schieffelin, B. B. (1986). Teasing and shaming in Kaluli children's interactions. In B. B. Schieffelin & E. Ochs (Eds.), *Language socialization across cultures* (pp. 165–181). New York: Cambridge University Press.

Sell, M. A., Kreuz, R. J., & Coppenrath, L. (1997). Parents' use of nonliteral language with preschool children. *Discourse Processes, 23*(2), 99–118.

Skarakis-Doyle, E. (2002). Young children's detection of violations in familiar stories and emerging comprehension monitoring. *Discourse Processes, 33*(2), 175–197.

Skarakis-Doyle, E., Dempsey, L., & Lee, C. (2002, July). *The emergence of narrative story comprehension in young children: An examination of underlying constructs.* Poster presented at the Symposium on Research in Child Language Disorders. Madison, WI.

Skarakis-Doyle, E., Dempsey, L., & Lee, C. (2004, June). *Identification of discourse comprehension impairments.* Poster presented at the Symposium on Research in Child Language Disorders, Madison, WI.

Skarakis-Doyle, E., & Milosky, L. (1999, June). *Assessing discourse representations in preschool children: Elements of a global fast map.* Poster presented at the Symposium on Research in Child Language Disorders, Madison, WI.

Skarakis-Doyle, E., & Wootton, S. (1995). An investigation of the ability of children with developmental language impairment to use everyday knowledge in comprehension. In D. MacLaughlin & S. McEwen (Eds.), *BUCLD 19: Proceedings of the 19th Annual Boston University Conference on Language Development* (Vol. 2, pp. 599–610). Somerville, MA: Cascadilla Press.

Snow, C. E., & Goldfield, B. A. (1983). Turn the page please: Situation-specific language acquisition. *Journal of Child Language, 10*(3), 551–569.

Tomasello, M. (2001). Perceiving intentions and learning words in the second year of life. In M. Tomasello & E. Bates (Eds.), *Language development: The essential readings* (pp. 111–128). Malden, MA: Blackwell.

Tomasello, M., & Barton, M. E. (1994). Learning words in nonostensive contexts. *Developmental Psychology, 30*(5), 639–650.

Voleti, R., & Milosky, L. M. (2003, November). *Relation between young children's language abilities and their interpretation of adult intents.* Poster presented at the American Speech-Language-Hearing Association Convention, Chicago.

Wiig, E., Secord, W., & Semel, E. (1992). *The Clinical Evaluation of Language Fundamentals—Preschool.* San Antonio, TX: Psychological Corporation.

16

The Developmental, Interactionist Perspective: An Afterword

Robin S. Chapman
University of Wisconsin–Madison and Waisman Center

PROLOGUE

How do children learn to talk? That was the question I took to graduate school at Berkeley and later research at the University of Wisconsin–Madison. It has been my great joy to have learned much from the children I studied, and to have had extraordinary students and colleagues, the authors of these chapters among them, who have spelled out many of the answers to that question, and its companion, *What about comprehension?*, opening up many new and important arenas of study, particularly in the area of child language disorders.

My questions arose from the intense arguments at the beginning of the 1960s between Noam Chomsky and B. F. Skinner about how linguistic knowledge could be accounted for—triggered, special, idealized, universal linguistic competence versus learned, language-specific, stimulus-response chains of exclusively verbal performance. Neither account seemed satisfactory. My texts and teachers were the developmental psycholinguists: Roger Brown and the students of his original psycholinguistic seminar, including Dan Slobin, who argued for the roles of cognitive operating principles in children's processes of listening and speaking, and the importance of cross-linguistic study. The painstaking longitudinal studies of form, content, function, and context in young children's speech by Brown, Susan Ervin-Tripp, and Lois Bloom provided data on "rule" acquisition in action—and in context. The anthropologists Dell Hymes and John Gumperz made us think about speakers' reasons for talking and broadened our thinking to multiple languages and bilingual speakers. Researchers in child development—Piaget, Vygotsky—stretched our perspective to cognitive and social domains. The philosopher John Searle made us think about speech acts. And as my own generation developed, we profited from the late Liz Bates's leadership of research on communicative performance (Slobin & Tomasello, 2005), and her advocacy for the interactionist, emergent perspective on child language development that I share today and have summarized earlier in this book (Chapman, this volume).

Why don't children learn to talk? In these chapters, my colleagues offer evidence from a variety of developmentally disabled populations that language learning is dependent on social, cognitive, motor, and working memory skills of the learner—and world knowledge, experience, and the nature of the interactional input. They argue for the continuing ways that a developmental perspective is important to research on children's language disorders, and the limits and alternatives to that perspective in particular populations. They also underscore the extraordinary progress we have made in understanding the sources of individual differences in language learning; in broadening our evidential basis for identifying children at risk for language disorders; in tracing specific conditions to the transactional effects of environment, biology, and genetic origins; in extending our studies to a variety of specific populations; in developing tasks for assessing pragmatic development; and in developing new methodologies for analyzing language production and comprehension across many speakers, languages, and communication tasks, including narrative and incidental word learning.

This afterword briefly speaks to these themes of the preceding chapters, considers what might be the next steps in our 21st-century research agenda, and revisits the role of developmental and interactionist considerations in our theories of language acquisition and disorder.

THE ROLE OF INFORMATION PROCESSING IN DEVELOPMENT: INTEGRATING OVER TIME

Early textbooks in our field contrasted developmental approaches not only with linguistic, modular accounts, but with informational processing approaches, treating them as competing accounts of children's language acquisition and disorder. As the chapters in this book make clear, the dichotomy between developmental and information-processing approaches was a false one, arising from a failure to distinguish time scale. Developmental change *is* the accumulation of moment-to-moment change as it arises in perception, extends to the time-scale of learning, and, with extended use of varied action across days and months, becomes a new developmental achievement.

In Ellis Weismer's work on late talkers (this volume), we find research that relates information-processing outcomes, ranging from a millisecond time scale to longer term developmental progress. The fast mapping of novel words at 2½ years differentiates late talkers and the comparison group, and predicts developmental progress measured by mean length of utterance a year later. The addition of standardized measures of vocabulary production and comprehension at 2½ substantially increases the explained variance at 3½. This is one of the first studies to incorporate processing measures as predictors of subsequent development; Ellis Weismer's longitudinal account effectively unifies theory into a dynamic systems approach to SLI, rather than either a developmental or an informational-processing one alone.

In the work reported here by Abbeduto and McDuffie we find a similar careful analysis of the contribution of attention following (latency to redirect attention to the object signaled by the adult) in the joint activity paradigm to the child's success in fast mapping, and the significant correlation of both with developmentally later gains in receptive and expressive vocabulary, in individuals with autism and fragile X syndrome. Here, too, the information-processing and developmental accounts are linked, and evidence obtained for the mediating role of attention following in language learning.

THE LEARNING CYCLE: ONE NEW ASPECT AT A TIME

Learning is the link between the scales of information processing and developmental change. The generalization that "new forms first express old functions" and "new functions are first expressed by old forms" that Chapman (this volume) uses to characterize acquisition of new words and structures was first made by Werner and Kaplan and extended in elegant longitudinal detail by Bloom (1973). Bloom's own analyses of the single-word utterances of Allison's first three transcripts showed that single words did not stand for whole phrases or sentences but rather revealed the child's learning to speak "one word at a time" about events, with successive one-word utterances taking up different aspects of the event.

Crais (this volume) extends the principle again to children's use of gesture in routines and subsequent communicative uses, showing the importance of considering gestural roots of communicative competence and lexical development. Her work demonstrates the way in which gestures come to have communicative significance in interaction with others, and can then be extended to other meanings and uses.

The power of this developmental principle is that it offers a route into learning even when the child's system is atypical, as Calculator (this volume) describes for augmentative systems users: Whatever actions are currently in the repertoire can be used to express new meaning; whatever meaning the child currently communicates can be mapped to new forms that are understood by a wider circle of listeners.

The same principle offers a way into understanding and remapping echolalic communications of individuals with autism, or developing vocabulary in the context of the communicative uses they already control (see Paul, this volume)—although the acquisition pattern may be "atypical," the underlying developmental principle is the same. And its developmental use consists not in rejecting inappropriate form and content, but in modeling substitute forms for use: We do not insist on adult pronunciation, or all the syllables of a word, or expected content. We put communication first.

Children who are developing bilingually, as Kay-Raining Bird demonstrates for children with Down syndrome (this volume), also show this one-new-aspect-at a time; in early vocabulary acquisition, words tend to be used in one or the other language, although they are understood in both. Typically we accept such limitations in children's early word use and acquisition; we do not ask that the meaning of "light" or "ball" be confined to adult category instances, or pronounced in the way adults do, or used in all communicative functions at once. Importantly, Kay-Raining Bird's work confirms in a developmentally disabled population that early bilingual environments do not slow the usual pace of acquisition.

MULTIDIMENSIONAL LEARNING AND DEVELOPMENT

Kent and Vorperian (this volume) show us that speech development, as a precursor and intrinsic facet of language, must be considered simultaneously across multiple domains: auditory, motor, visual, and interaction. Further, they demonstrate that the course of sensorimotor mapping extends from infancy to late teenage years. The dynamic nature of that learning is underscored by children's need to accommodate differing growth trajectories for the larynx, face, and cranial structures subserving speech over that time period.

The interactive, contextual nature of that learning is underscored by infants' sensitivity to the statistical structure of spoken language input and its correlation with visible mouth movements of the speaker and (nonidentical) productions by the infant. The possibility of mirror neurons, or other auditory-motor mappings, that link auditory pattern to the child's own production patterns by age 8 months suggests the way in which "rehearsal" functions of auditory working memory may subserve subsequent nonword repetition and fast-mapping performance in production.

Kent and Vorperian's account of possible neurons mirroring speech sound recognition could, additionally, be extended to mirror neurons of other's actions, focus of attention, and communicative intents, providing a basis for the kind of early social knowledge that the Child Talk model (Chapman, this volume) has claimed to play a role in early mappings, and a potential target of early damage in autistic spectrum disorders.

MULTIPLE DIMENSIONS IN POPULATIONS WITH LANGUAGE LEARNING PROBLEMS

This volume includes studies of a variety of populations—children with SLI (Ellis Weismer; Boudreau; Dollaghan; Klee; Milosky & Skarakis-Doyle); children with cognitive impairment, including Down syndrome (Kay-Raining Bird), fragile X syndrome (Abbeduto & McDuffie, Johnson-Glenberg), and children on the autism spectrum of disorders (Paul et al.); children with neonatal and environmental risk factors (Johnson); children who are bilingual (Miller). The work mades clear that language learning can be delayed or accelerated with respect to other domains, and also fractionated, or dissociated, in differing ways in the different populations' courses of learning. These specific behavioral phenotypes are an active and exciting focus of much current research.

Context

Johnson-Glenberg (this volume) proposes, in her analysis of the skills of learners with fragile X, that the pattern of learning itself may be atypical in this population—that these individuals are more likely to learn the context associated with the learning task as well as the task, making later recall of irrelevant information better, but retrieval of the learned content in new contexts more difficult. This hypothesis offers a behavioral translation of the biochemical and neurophysiological differences thought to characterize the syndrome at a synaptic level. In typically developing children, in contrast, initial mapping of context with learning (e.g., remembering where an object was hidden, in the fast-mapping task) is quickly overridden by subsequent learning opportunities, unless context continues to serve a communicative function.

Working Memory

The role of working memory, particularly verbal working memory, in language disorders is demonstrated here in a number of studies, but its effect appears primarily when the task challenges limited resources. For example, Boudreau (this volume) offers a resource capacity account of narrative skill in children with SLI, who reach a stage where they do fairly well in retelling simple stories, but when confronted with complex plots show significant problems not only in retaining plot elements, but in the lexicon and syntax used to convey what they do remember. And it is in this form of the task that working memory predicts performance.

Ellis Weismer (this volume) demonstrates that MLU increases in a microgenetic study of repeated storytelling over a period of weeks occurs for both typically developing and late-talker groups in the low script condition, but only for the comparison sample, not the late talkers, in a high script condition with multiple production demands. Thus, processing demands interact with capacity in determining what is learned.

Communicative Uses

The children on the autism spectrum are a particularly interesting group for a theory of acquisition, in that the difficulties they encounter can persist in the pragmatic domain, and the semantic aspects of emotional and mental state language, even when language learning takes place. One might argue that the formal aspects of language learning are spared—but this view appears refuted by Paul's (this volume) longitudinal data on very young children (16–37 months) suspected of an ASD diagnosis at study entry. Almost 40% of this group are reported to be without speech at 18 months, and those who do speak show an anomalous pattern of poorer language comprehension than word and speech production.

As Paul points out, the tasks associated with comprehension assessment are more removed—decontextualized—from the likely early learning contexts than those associated with production, and the dissociation disappears as the children develop. The measures of language use continue to show regulatory, but not interactional, uses, and comprehension learning takes place for items of interest to the child, but not for items in the joint interaction space to which the adult attempts to shift the child's interest. Nor is child-directed speech likely to elicit heightened attention.

These findings, atypical for most language learners, carry the strong implication that our usual language interventions, based on heightening the naturalistic, communicative parent–child interactions in play, will radically fail for children on the autistic spectrum. As Paul points out, language interventions based on joint attention, social (as opposed to means–ends) communicative goals, and child-directed speech will be significantly less effective for this population.

A developmental framework allows for the discovery of departures from the typical pattern, but these limitations of attention and use require a rethinking of effective interventions. What aspects of the environment does the child attend to and find interesting? Language input can be responsive to the child's focus of attention. What are the uses of language of interest to the child? Contexts in which language use can obtain access to objects or activities—or actually manipulate the nonsocial environment directly, as in voice-controlled computer programs—may prove more effective than play contexts where joint attention is shared, for this population.

THE DEVELOPMENTAL COURSE: NOT A STRAIGHT LINE

A consequence of the nonlinear underpinnings of development, in tasks of shorter time scale, is that development itself shows nonlinearities. If this were not the case, our interventions could not succeed—small differences in amount and focus of clinical intervention could not yield the success they do.

Ellis Weismer's finding that late talkers identified at age 2 are, for the most part, "caught up" by age 5, in the sense of performing within normal test range, reflects the fact that developmental trajectories can be nonlinear—that, as Paul (1996) and Rescorla (2002) have also demonstrated, late talkers can "catch up" to test norms. Comparison to the controls matched for socioeconomic status and nonverbal cognition showed continued, substantial delay, however, as Paul and Rescorla also found. Thus, our norm-reference definitions of SLI may miss children whose skills are not referenced to their cognitive achievements (more on this issue later).

The failure to identify frank specific language impairment (SLI) at age 5 through age 2½ indicators is disappointing, on the one hand, and encouraging for child outcomes, on the other. One-third of Ellis Weismer's sample had speech, or speech and language, therapy in the period between 2 and 5, and parental interactional patterns in this relatively high socioeconomic sample may have been supportive of progress in the late talker group as well. If these same children had entered environments with multiple risk factors, or accelerated education demands, the outcomes might not have been so successful, as Johnson (this volume) reminds us.

Identification of effective clinical markers for SLI is also the subject of the work Klee, Gavin, and Stokes (this volume) report for American English, British English, and Cantonese speaking children. Klee and his colleagues show that age, utterance length, and lexical diversity, in combination, are sensitive and specific discriminators of SLI at ages 4 and 3—but not at age 2—in the children they've studied, underscoring once more the age-restricted range of effective predictors. Both utterance length and lexical diversity contribute unique variance to the prediction of SLI, demonstrating across language, culture, and dialect that simple measures obtainable from computer analyses of children's talk can identify children accurately.

Paul (2000) has pointed out the cost, to the child, family, and society, of incorrectly predicting that late-talking children will later show SLI. Identification of SLI is typically made without reference to other cognitive domains, unless frank cognitive impairment is present. However, Ellis Weismer's evidence suggests that expressive language, nonword repetition, and verbal working memory measures will continue to be domains of relative weakness in 5-year-old children who were late talkers, despite performance on nonverbal cognition and narrative comprehension and retell tasks similar to the comparison sample.

Here a dynamic systems approach to development can be helpful (Abbeduto, Evans, & Dolan, 2001). Markers of language learning impairment are not constant across life span—for example, the difficulties in past-tense marking exhibited by 5-year-olds are not present earlier; nor can verbal working memory measures or expressive language pick out the child at 8 months who will have later problems. But measures reflecting the success of the immediate past new learning—for example, canonical babbling at 8 months, productive vocabulary at 2 years, or fast-mapping skills at 2½, grammatical morphology of nouns during early word combinations and of verbs later—all have a chance of indicating, sensitively, current difficulties in mastering the next set of developments in language learning.

Dynamic assessment varying task difficulty and amount of contextual support, and microgenetic tasks tracing change in performance with practice over short time spans can be helpful if we know the developmental "next step" confronting children; the information-processing and learning time-scales can inform the developmental scale.

THE COURSE OF DEVELOPMENT: WHAT'S LEARNED?

The classical account of language acquisition described children as learning linguistic rules. The interactionist account views the emergence of "rule-governed" behavior as cumulating from a developmental, incremental process of learning from input and interaction. Dollaghan (this volume) offers an innovative connectionist analysis of verb use by children of high and low MLU, asking whether verbs can be viewed as "hubs" in a network of lexical connections, meaning that they afford links to multiple other lexical nodes in the process of sentence construction. Indeed, she finds evidence that verbs that are high frequency (top 20%) for children account for a far greater proportion of multiword utterances in the high MLU group than the low MLU group. We might expect to find this pattern replicated at a later developmental time for the low MLU group—when MLU had increased to the high MLU groups' level.

A challenge facing emergent, interactionist accounts of language development is the further construction of connectionist models that can yield predictions of the differing trajectories and phenotypes of language use and comprehension. These models will have to incorporate multidimensional aspects of learning—the early sensorimotor mappings that Kent and Vorperian (this volume) discuss; the social, object, action, spatial, and causal domains of knowledge that children develop (Chapman, this volume); and the differing degrees of connectivity among these domains in differing populations.

MEASURING LANGUAGE DEVELOPMENT: MLU AND NUMBER OF DIFFERENT WORDS

The ability to predict outcomes for children, given observations at an earlier time, is a key concern in the field of child language disorders. For prediction to succeed, observations must be both valid and reliable. Our focus on analysis of language samples—the real outcomes of interest—rather than proxy test scores arises from the desire to have valid measures. Miller (this volume) details the considerable work that has gone into creating computer support for language transcript analysis in English, and its extension to Spanish, in the SALT program.

Notable in this history was the decision to let the user define additional codes, rather than to require extensive coding of predetermined categories as the CHILDES system requires, and the inclusion of conversational context, allowing discourse analyses to be made. Miller and Leadholm (1995) developed reference databases of conversational and narrative language samples for children 3 to 13 years of age that have served as critical developmental reference data bases for the field. The power of computer support for analysis has greatly enhanced our ability to carry out longitudinal and large-*n* work, and its power remains to be exploited for large-*n* studies of pragmatic aspects of language use.

Miller's most recent work extends the promise of computer-assisted analysis to Spanish and a controlled narrative sampling context. He and his colleagues have worked on gathering and analyzing 5,000 narratives a year, obtained from bilingual, Spanish–English-speaking children, over 3 years. This undertaking would have been impossible without SALT—and indeed, hardly possible with it. The creation of new utilities to manage such a large database, a Spanish look-up dictionary to identify root word forms automatically in this highly inflected language, and utilities to facilitate mass insertion of codes and make a reality of our vision of 20 years ago: Together, these yield the ability to create reference databases locally, for populations of particular interest.

The narrative retellings that Miller reports are particularly interesting for the light they shed on lexical access. The stories are presented both verbally and as a wordless picture book, and retellings from kindergartners through third graders use surprisingly few of the words from the script—5 to 12 words of the possible 87. When the children's vocabulary use is analyzed, however, synonyms and near synonyms are supplied for almost 40 of the 87 script categories by third grade. With pictured content, story formulation appears driven more by picture–semantic word links from long-term store than by connections from short-term memory "fast mapping" of script words to referents.

One might expect that Miller's participants would reveal fast-mapped comprehension for a much larger fraction of the script vocabulary—illustrating, again, the need to assess comprehension to evaluate beginning learning. But the production data underscore the multiple systems that feed information to online language production—making the timing of lexical access a potentially important component of utterance production and the complexity of those utterances. (I note that these data also disconfirm the claim of our Child Talk model that memory for talk produced and encountered will play a continuing important role in utterance formulation.)

WHAT ABOUT COMPREHENSION?

The need to ask this question is dramatically illustrated in Kent and Vorperian's chapter here, as they show the necessity for infant speakers to map speech production onto speech perception as a way of anchoring their changing productive means to effective perceptual outcomes.

The continuing importance of considering comprehension skill is highlighted in a number of the chapters. Thal, Tobias, and Morrison (1991) showed that late talkers with comprehension problems are more at risk for subsequently identified specific language impairment than those without. Ellis Weismer, in her population-based study of SLI in Iowa kindergartners, has demonstrated that expressive language impairment co-occurs with comprehension skill impairment to a greater or lesser degree; the pattern fits a continuum model rather than a binary typology of expressive-only or receptive–expressive child language disorder.

And—perhaps most compelling of all—Calculator (this volume) discusses the group of children and adults without effective communicative means, for whom an adequate assessment of comprehension and motor control is the prerequisite to the design of augmentative communicative systems.

WHAT ABOUT PRAGMATICS?

Our understanding of pragmatic development, particularly comprehension, in typically developing and language-impaired children has required creativity in inventing naturalistic tasks that reveal children's inferences about speaker affect, intent, situation, the protagonist's goals and feelings, and the expectations of listeners. The work by Milosky and Skarakis-Doyle (this volume) is extraordinary for its innovative focus on the origins of nonliteral language understanding and the early stages of story comprehension and comprehension monitoring in toddlers and preschoolers.

Their analyses indicate the importance of both verbal working memory and speed of nonverbal, inferential reasoning in social and cognitive domains to the outcomes of discourse comprehension tasks. Additionally, Milosky and her colleagues have analyzed parent–child interaction patterns to show the substantial frequencies with which children are required to recognize nonliteral language uses—teasing, irony, metaphor—in everyday interaction. When these inventive methodologies and assessment instruments are extended to children with problems in social inferencing, such as those on the autistic spectrum, we may get a far more subtle understanding of the problems that arise in discourse comprehension than is currently available.

WHAT ABOUT INTERVENTION?

Johnson (this volume) urgently reminds us that vulnerable children offer challenges to parenting, and encounter challenges in chaotic environments, that can sabotage development of social attachment, language and cognitive skills, and effective communication strategies. Her transactional account of J, a child born to a mother on methadone maintenance, makes abundantly clear the importance of the emotional support offered by the communicative environment. No developmental model in our new century can ignore the environmental contributions along the developmental path—nature and nurture are inextricably intertwined, as transactional interactionist perspectives recognize.

What Johnson challenges us to do is to think beyond our traditional acquisition measures, with their narrow focus on size of word inventory, length of sentence, mastery of grammatical morphemes, number of story propositions recalled, comprehension of second-order theory of mind tasks—all useful measures of progress—to the affective and communicative roots of the child's experience of the social world. What measures can reflect the quality of children's lives, the quality of parenting they receive, the quality of life in the family, the quality of support for children's development in the community? What societal norms and expectations, what intervention programs offering family education and support, what individual acts can each of us undertake to nurture each child? How do we really leave no child behind?

Who Should Receive Intervention?

Ellis Weismer raises the question of where the estimated 7% of kindergartners come from with SLI, if not from late talkers. Perhaps if we were to combine known risk factors for development—including poverty, socioeconomic status (SES), and more direct measures of the quality of language input, with exposure to intrauterine and environmental toxins, we might more effectively identify, at an early age, children's whose need for intervention remained high at age 5. The new National Institutes of Health (NIH)-sponsored national longitudinal study of children offers an important opportunity to investigate predictors of language delay in a very large-n sample.

Ellis Weismer has shown that the practice of cognitive referencing—that is, asking if language achievements are consistently lower than nonverbal cognitive skills—is not defensible on the basis of obtained patterns for language impaired children. Indeed, failure to find a gap between nonverbal cognition and language was never a defensible reason for denying services; it simply suggested that a different set of causes for delay might be at work.

If language developmental rate can be variable, and reflect resilience in learning, it is also sensitive to multiple risk factors that cumulate in poorer outcomes. Johnson (this volume) suggests that, from the viewpoint of social policy, intervention for language learning is important whenever children's skills are at risk of not meeting school and community expectations, whether or not the lag qualifies as specific language impairment. Further, the intervention practices offered by speech-language clinicians have been drawn from practices accelerating language learning in typically developing children within the same cultures.

To do this is to argue, as Bruce Tomblin has, that specific language impairment is a category we impose, rather than one intrinsic to the child, and to broaden our diagnostic efforts to those children who will have the most need of intervention. I want to underscore the importance of separating the research question of who has a language impairment (e.g., ruling out environmental and cognitive contributions to the language delay/difference)—and the subsequent search for genetic markers or causes—from the clinical practice question of who should receive services from speech-language clinicians, where mismatch to the expectations of the educational, vocational, or community environments for performance in the native language needs to be the factor determining eligibility and likelihood of benefit.

Individuals who are learning the local language as a second language need support from bilingual—ESL (English as a second language), in the case of English—professionals; but they may also need support from speech-language clinicians if learning is a problem in the first language as well. I've been concerned and surprised, over the years, to see our careful research on identifying SLI as a clinical category used as a desideratum of who should receive services, particularly in populations with developmental disability, where every child needs services. My own view is that speech-language clinicians should be working with all children with language delay or developmental disabilities, in all the ways (classroom or family consultation, small group, one-on-one) that are fruitful, whether or not their language delay is commensurate with other cognitive delay.

Reconceptualizing Intervention as Curriculum and Community Activities

One implication of this view is that the home, classroom, and community are important sources of learning at all ages, and should be conceptualized as sources of skill acquisition for individuals with a wide range of communicative, language, and cognitive skill. The interactionist perspective leads one to look for language uses that have meaning in context—that give children powerful ways of expressing themselves. Examples can be found in writing programs that encourage children to tell their stories (Dyson, cited in Johnson's chapter), or summer programs performing Shakespearean plays, or student-run stores and newspapers, or student participation in creating digital videos, or the critical discourse and documentation of science labs, or the discussion and enactment of skills for making friends, assertive requesting, negotiating conflict, and making peace.

The vast number of language learning encounters in children's lives come not from clinicians, but from parents, caregivers, teachers, and the media. Interventions that support parents, improve day care settings, create communicative opportunities in the classroom, and recognize the power of the stories we offer our children will have great leverage.

FUTURE RESEARCH

What issues should future research address? Longitudinal learning in specific populations, neuroimaging of language processing, genetic routes of specific patterns of language disability, the efficacy of intervention methodologies, the role of environmental interventions, an expansion of theory-of-mind studies to the development of pragmatic competence broadly conceived—these are all topics that the researchers here are already tackling, and they are also the cutting-edge issues in the field. What awaits is the joining of these findings to the biological streams of research that are identifying mechanisms at levels from neurotransmitters to synaptic plasticity, amygdala and hippocampal function, and cortical and cerebellar structure and function, on the one hand, and on the other the investigation of the environmental factors at societal levels that contribute to improved or impaired quality of life.

ACKNOWLEDGMENTS

The writing of the chapter was supported by NIH grant R01-HD-23353 to the author and the core NIH grant to the Waisman Center.

REFERENCES

Abbeduto, L., Evans, J., & Dolan, T. (2001). Theoretical perspectives on language and communication problems in mental retardation and developmental disabilities. *Mental Retardation and Developmental Disabilities Research Reviews, 7,* 45–55.

Bloom, L. (1973). *One word at a time: The use of single word utterances before syntax*. The Hague: Mouton.

Miller, J. F., & Leadholm, B. J. (1995). *Language sample analysis: The Wisconsin guide.* Madison: Wisconsin Department of Public Instruction.

Paul, R. (1996). Clinical implications of the natural history of slow expressive language development. *American Journal of Speech-Language Pathology, 5,* 5–21.

Paul, R. (2000). Predicting outcomes of early expressive language delay: Ethical implications. In D. Bishop & L. Leonard (Eds.), *Speech and language impairments in children* (pp. 195–209). Hove, England: Psychology Press.

Rescorla, L. (2002). Language and reading outcomes to age 9 in late-talking toddlers. *Journal of Speech, Language, and Hearing Research, 45,* 360–371.

Slobin, D. I., & Tomasello, M. (2005). Thirty years of research on language, cognition, and development: The legacy of Elizabeth Bates. *Language Learning and Development, 1,* 129–149.

Thal, D., Tobias, S., & Morrison, D. (1991). Language and gesture in late talkers: A 1-year follow-up. *Journal of Speech and Hearing Research, 34,* 604–612.

Author Index

Note: f indicates figure; *n* indicates footnote; *t* indicates table.

A

C

F

H

L

M

N

O

P

R

S

U

V

W

Subject Index

Note: f indicates figure; *n* indicates footnote; *t* indicates table.

D

R